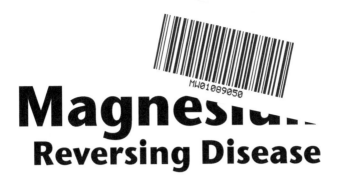

Magnesium
Reversing Disease

Magnesium
Reversing Disease

Thomas E. Levy, MD, JD

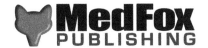

Disclaimer

This book is intended to be an information resource only. There is no intent that this book be used for any diagnostic or treatment purposes. A specific physician/patient or dentist/patient relationship is necessary before any medical or dental therapies are initiated. In no manner should this book, or any of the information in this book, be used as a substitute for diagnosis and treatment by a qualified medical and/or dental health-care professional.

To order additional copies of this book, contact:
MedFox Publishing, LLC
1-866-359-5589
www.MedFoxPub.com
Orders@MedFoxPub.com
2505 Anthem Village Drive, Suite E-582,
Henderson, NV 89052-5529

Dedicated to all health care
practitioners who truly make the
health and welfare of their patients
their top priority.

Acknowledgments

To Les and Cindy Nachman, whose friendship and support remain invaluable in my efforts to spread my medical messages around the world.

To David Nicol, a good friend and incredible editor.

To my wife Lis, and my daughter Daniela.

To my good friends and colleagues, Ron Hunninghake and Keith Skinner, who always give me valuable insights on whatever we might discuss.

Table of Contents

SECTION ONE:
The Evidence of Magnesium's Unparalleled Curative Power

— Chapter 1 —

— Chapter 2 —

SECTION TWO:
Applying Magnesium's Unparalleled Curative Power

— Chapter 16 —

Vitamin C Supplementation 251
An Essential Guide

— Chapter 17 —

Companion Supplements 305
Importance and Considerations

Magnesium Supplementation   319
An Essential Guide

Foreword

"A Touch of Genius"

I was shocked...and amazed!

Looking up from the latter pages of Dr. Tom Levy's 12th book, *Magnesium: Reversing Disease,* I realized that in my entire 43-year medical career, I had never before heard these two words, *magnesium & mitochondria,* being used together in the same sentence!

Here it is:

> **"...95% of the magnesium in the cell is in the mitochondria."**

Of course, I knew about both of these words. I knew they were related. I just didn't realize how INCREDIBLY RELATED they were!

When I graduated from medical school in 1976, we weren't much concerned about mitochondria, the powerhouse of almost every cell in the human body. Mitochondria were briefly alluded to in our basic microbiology course, along with the infamous Krebs Cycle. We learned enough to pass the written tests.

However, once we were in the hospital, we were doing the "real" work of medicine: seeing patients, doing physical exams, ordering tests, and prescribing treatments such as medication and surgery. For sure, _mitochondria_ didn't seem to have anything to do with it!

At that time, however, the word _magnesium_ was more meaningful to me. Why? During my third year of medical school my father developed chest pain in the small town where I grew up. Because he was a moderate smoker, his family doctor (my cousin) presumed it was angina and worried he might have a serious blockage in his coronaries. Dad was sent to a tertiary care hospital for a heart catheterization.

Interestingly, he was also having multiple premature ventricular contractions (PVCs) when he arrived at the hospital. PVCs are heartbeats that trigger too early and occur too frequently. Although they are generally benign, PVCs can spell trouble when they happen during a heart attack.

Fortunately, in addition to a whole battery of blood tests, Dad's assigned cardiologist correctly ordered a serum magnesium level to check out the PVCs. (I doubt that the cardiologist even gave a second thought about this being related to my Dad's mitochondrial health.) Dad's serum magnesium level was very low. Dad always had had an upset stomach and was an avid Tums user. For sure, all that calcium had been effective in neutralizing his stomach acid, but it had also prevented the proper absorption of magnesium from his diet. This explained the low serum magnesium and the PVCs.

I was in the cath lab when the cardiologist squirted Dad's coronaries. They were all clear! The nurses and I actually started cheering and clapping! Dad was awake and smiling broadly too. The only one not cele-brating was the cardiologist, as he appeared to be deep in thought. His fortunate discovery of low serum levels of magnesium and the proper response to it resulted in decisive actions that made a huge difference in my father's health, who was 53 at that time.

The cardiologist ordered an upper GI barium swallow and diagnosed an acid reflux problem that was causing the lower esophageal spasms that mimicked angina chest pain. These spasms were a direct conse-quence of Dad's low magnesium level.

The cardiologist told Dad to take SlowMag (an OTC form of magnesium) for the rest of his life. He did... and he lived until the ripe old age of 90.

He looked my father in the eye, right there on the cath table, and said, "Elmer, this would be a perfect time for you to quit smoking!" My Dad, being in a very teachable moment, never touched another cigarette. Hip Hip... Hurray!

That profound experience was my introduc-tion to the word *magnesium*...something I'll never forget. Now, the word *mitochondria*...essentially, that word meant nothing to me for the first 10 years of my medical practice as a family doctor. During that initial decade of my medical career, I never thought about any patient's mitochondria, nor did I ever measure serum magnesium levels like the cardiologist did. So, of course, I never saw the vital relationship between the two. I was your typical conventional doctor who listened to symptoms, did a few tests, made mental diagnoses, and then treated my patients with symp-tom-controlling medications.

Fortunately, in 1989, I ran into Dr. Hugh Riordan, the founder of *The Center for the Improvement of*

Human Functioning (now known as *The Riordan Clinic* since his passing in 2005.) Hugh was interested in disturbed cellular functioning as the root cause of all human disease. Spending untold time in The BioCenter Laboratory, he measured and analyzed nutrients and hormones...intra- and extracellular molecules that were necessary for the healthy functioning of cells.

When I joined Hugh Riordan that year, something amazing happened: I actually started to use the knowledge I had gained during the first two years of medical school. I started thinking about mitochondria, cellular membranes, the nucleus, ribosomes, lysosomes, and a whole new vocabulary of microbiologic thought that had somehow escaped my attention and the attention of most busy physicians.

That's when I first began reading the works of said Dr. Thomas Levy. (Little did I know that we would be traveling the world together, awakening health practitioners to that *Wonderful World Within You* – the title of Dr. Roger Williams delightful book about intracellular biology and nutrition that he wrote in hopes of inspiring his grandchildren to recognize the supreme importance of nutritional biochemistry.)

Now, Dr. Levy has done it, again. I mean, REALLY DONE IT! In this, his 12th, and what I believe is his <u>consummate work</u>, he has used two of the most powerful words in the biochemical vernacular...in the same sentence! Once again:

> **"...95% of the magnesium in the cell is in the mitochondria."**

Mitochondria make up 10% of the total weight of the human body. Without the mitochondria, our cells could only generate $1/19^{th}$ of the energy we now use to maintain health. One of the great emerging medical insights of our time is that the vast majority of the chronic illnesses have their origin in MITOCHONDRIAL DYSFUNCTION, which then leads to global cellular dysfunction, the hallmark of chronic illness.

This book contains over a thousand references to back up what I would call THE ULTIMATE CONCLUSION: chronic illness = cellular dysfunction = hidden magnesium deficiency.

Take a look at the chronic illnesses afflicting our globe today: Cancer – Heart Disease – Alzheimer's – Autoimmune "-itis disorders" – Digestive Disorders – COPD – Obesity – Diabetes –the innumerable viral and bacterial infectious diseases – Osteoarthritis and Musculoskeletal Disorders – many more. These are all covered in detail in this book! Their link to magnesium deficiency is beyond dispute. Modern medicine has managed to overlook its own scientific foundation in favor of the myopic view that drugs are the only way. (Although sometimes they are!)

These chronic illnesses are not only stealing quality of life from the majority of our fellow planetary inhabitants, they are also stealing health care resources in a dramatic way.

In 1960, the average annual cost of health care in the U.S. was $146.

By 2017, as reported by the centers for Medicare and Medicaid Services report, "National Health Expenditures Summary Including Share of GDP, CY 1960-2017", it had risen to an incredible $10,739!

My conclusion, and the conclusion of this book, is simple: we have allowed our medical care system to focus predominantly on symptoms, not causes. This treatment paradigm ignores biology and tout's pharmacology. Result: an unsustainable healthcare system. Allow me to quote Albert Einstein:

> "Any intelligent fool can make things bigger and more complex...it takes a touch of genius, and a lot of courage to move in the opposite direction."

This book is a clear road map to a better, simpler, and more rational way to reverse the great disease epidemics of our times.

Ron Hunninghake, MD
Chief Medical Officer
Riordan Clinic
Wichita, Kansas

Preface

It's been nearly five years since *Death by Calcium* was published. For several years prior to writing that book, the need to expose the real and imminent dangers of excessive calcium ingestion often surfaced as I ran across more and more peer-reviewed research demonstrating its incredibly negative health effects. What was worse, the dairy industry, supplement manufacturers, pharmaceutical companies, and physicians all over the country and throughout the rest of the world were (and still are) aggressively promoting this dangerous calcium over-consumption in the name of good health.

It is true that the body needs a limited regular dietary intake of calcium. What is not true is that an adult needs more than is found in a healthy diet in an individual with a normal vitamin D status that omits all but occasional dairy. In fact, over-consumption of calcium has been linked to increased all-cause mortality, heart disease, cancer, arthritis, and even dementia. And, contrary to the advertising promises, calcium does **not** prevent or even reduce the incidence of factures related to osteoporosis. The scientific proof of these facts is abundant and much of it is decades old, "hiding in plain sight" in the world-wide scientific literature. This means that the majority of healthcare practitioners in this country are either ignorant of or choose to ignore the research published in their own medical journals. My publisher and I thought it necessary to take this important warning to the health-conscious public, and so, *Death by Calcium* was born.

At that time, my suggested remediation of calcium toxicity was to avoid calcium supplementation, restrict its dietary intake, and to improve antioxidant and nutrient status with some specific dietary and supplement regimens, along with the proper adjustment of certain critical hormones – advice still important to follow.

Recently, however, MedFox suggested that I write a book on magnesium.

I must admit, my first reaction was rather tepid. A quick look online revealed a plethora of books on magnesium. Frankly, I initially felt that another magnesium book would just be a reproduction of what was already too available in bookstores and on the internet and would not be especially significant or noteworthy. But because I highly respect the advice of the folks at MedFox, I started to delve into recent magnesium research. What I found was astounding!

Not only did my research further confirm the information published in *Death by Calcium*, it also demonstrated beyond a shadow of a doubt that magnesium is actually the natural antidote for calcium toxicity *and* the intracellular damage it causes. This is a huge finding that still remains unappreciated. Excess intracellular calcium is present in all diseased cells, as well as in all cells affected by any poisoning or toxin exposures. This elevated intracellular calcium, along with the increased intracellular oxidative stress that it directly causes, must be remedied in order to resolve or improve any medical condition or toxin exposure. As it turns out, increasing the intracellular levels of magnesium is the natural antidote to this elevated intracellular calcium characteristic of all disease processes. The greater the magnesium uptake into these cells, the more that calcium is displaced and pushed out. Additional measures are available to help normalize intracellular calcium levels, but magnesium is the most important. Furthermore, the intracellular calcium levels will never normalize by any other measures if significant deficiencies of magnesium in the body remain unaddressed.

Many different agents will promote good health. However, magnesium, along with vitamin C, are head and shoulders above all other supplements. Certainly, there are many different vitamins, minerals, and nutrient agents that strongly support good health and are wonderful supplements to take on a regular basis. However, all treatment and/or supplement protocols will never result in optimal health if magnesium and vitamin C are not adequately supplemented on a regular basis as well.

I'm convinced, with the few rare situations involving magnesium excess or toxicity mentioned later in the book, that everyone will benefit from learning and applying the information presented herein. Prepare to be amazed and to find healing for much of what ails you as you explore and employ the wealth of information you now hold in your hands. You will quickly see that this is not just another magnesium book.

Thomas E. Levy, MD, JD

Introduction

Our incredible bodies are comprised of trillions of cells. At the foundational level, cells are built from of an enormous number of biomolecules of many different kinds such as lipids, proteins, enzymes, DNA, amino acids, etc. A simplified overview can be diagrammed like this:

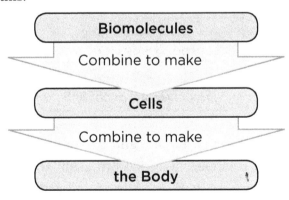

When biomolecules lose electrons through oxidation, they also lose all or most of their normal chemical reactivity, or biological function. A cell is deemed to be diseased when the quantity of oxidized biomolecules within the cell walls begins to disrupt normal cellular function. When the number of dysfunctional cells is sufficient to impair normal tissue or organ function, a diagnosis can usually be made, depending upon where, how, the extent, and the type of cells that are damaged. That can be represented like this:

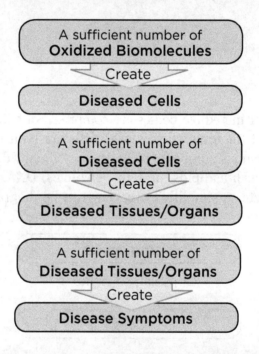

All pathogens, toxins, and poisons, directly or indirectly, promote increased intracellular oxidative stress (increased IOS) in the affected cells as more and more biomolecules are oxidized. One of the chief mechanisms for elevating IOS involves increased extracellular calcium entry into the cell via the calcium channels in the cell's membrane.

The Problem with Traditional Healing Paradigms

Traditional medicine has definitely produced many astounding and helpful breakthroughs. It is not the intent of the author to cast aspersions on all traditional health paradigms out of hand. There is certainly a proper place for some traditional methods and interventions. The important point is that many of the approaches employed by traditional health care practitioners have serious limitations because they fail to treat the underlying causes of disease pathologies. Rather, they are largely focused on symptom suppression/elimination. Symptoms, of course, are a manifestation of the disease, but they are not the disease, and blocking them in no way addresses the cellular pathology inside the diseased cells.

Maintenance drugs, surgery, chemotherapy, and radiation are the primary tools of the traditional healthcare practitioner. With the exception of a certain class of prescription drugs known as calcium channel blockers, these treatment modalities do not address the root problem. When these traditional treatment approaches are combined with good nutrition, focused supplementation, and proper care of the body, some restoration of health and wellness at the biomolecular level can result. However, such improvements occur in spite of the medical treatment rather than because of it.

Maintenance Drugs

As just noted, with few exceptions, maintenance drugs take aim at disease symptoms. Not only do most drugs fail to address the underlying problem of oxidized biomolecules, but directly or indirectly they *often generate more* oxidized biomolecules. That's not to say there isn't a place for medications, but most often they can only provide temporary symptom relief and may themselves cause other health problems. However, even when they do not generate the oxidation of more biomolecules, they still are "permitting" the underlying disease process to continue to evolve and worsen.

Surgery

Many surgical interventions are helpful and some are necessary. But, surgery never remediates pathologies due to oxidized biomolecules. As long as the conditions that are producing increased IOS are not addressed, surgery will only be a temporary fix.

Chemotherapy and Radiation

The main purpose of chemotherapy and radiation is to create enough oxidative stress in diseased cells to kill them. The major problem here is that the increased IOS induced by these chemicals is not and cannot be limited to diseased cells. Rather, it affects healthy cells as well, further expanding the population of diseased cells in the body.

The Functional Approach

Fundamentally, lasting health and wellness starts at the molecular level. Unless the underlying cause of any pathology is remediated, a patient can never achieve optimal health. It is the contention of the author that increased IOS is the cause of all disease and in fact, that it *is* the disease.

If that is true, and evidence for that position is abundant, the healthcare practitioner must employ whatever means are available to limit the causes of increased IOS and to heal (chemically reduce with electron donation) oxidized biomolecules through the use of antioxidants, hormones and other interventions. Much documentation showing that the major cause of increased IOS is an excess of intracellular calcium as has been thoroughly presented elsewhere (see *Death by Calcium* by the same author). This current work lays out the case for magnesium as the natural antidote for that calcium excess.

Section One reveals copious evidence for magnesium's unparalleled restorative and often curative power. Here the reader will be presented with the documented mechanisms by which magnesium works its "magic," not only at the cellular level but also throughout various tissues and organ systems in the body.

Section Two provides a strategy for applying magnesium's therapeutic powers in tandem with other interventions to achieve optimum health through prevention of further damage along with repair/reversal of existing damage.

We stand at the threshold of a new frontier in the practice of medicine that can lead to true health and wellness. Restoring oxidized biomolecules to the functional (reduced) state in combination with the prevention of chronically increased IOS provides real hope for reversing and even curing disease.

SECTION ONE:

The Evidence of Magnesium's Unparalleled Curative Power

Ignorance Has Consequences

Why isn't serum magnesium tested as a part of the routine laboratory profiles drawn by the vast majority health practitioners? Published research from the past few decades much more than justifies such tests, but most doctors are woefully unaware about the role this essential mineral nutrient plays in health and longevity. And now, the more recent research that is presented throughout this book indicates that regular monitoring of serum and intracellular magnesium levels is exponentially more important than ever imagined.

Essential Mineral Nutrient

Magnesium is the second most abundant cation (positively-charged ion) inside the cells of the body after potassium, and it is the fourth most abundant cation throughout the body. It is present in high concentrations in every metabolically active cell of the body, and, not surprisingly, it is essential for life as well as just good health.

Magnesium is an essential cofactor for hundreds of critical enzymes in the body, and it is known to be involved in **roughly 80%** of all the known metabolic functions in the body.[1,2] When essential enzyme cofactors such as magnesium are significantly diminished in concentration and availability, the overall enzyme activity in an area of diminished cofactor concentration is significantly diminished as well.

Magnesium has been found to be critical for the metabolism of ATP (a critical molecule involved in the delivery and dissemination of energy in all the cells of the body). It is also required for protein, DNA, and RNA synthesis, as well as for the synthesis of fatty acids and for the conversion of vitamin D into its active hormone form in the body.[3] Magnesium also plays a critical role in the production of glutathione, the most important and most concentrated antioxidant inside the cells of the body.[4-7] Inside the cell, magnesium works to keep sodium and calcium levels lower

*Magnesium is an essential cofactor for hundreds of critical enzymes in the body, and it is known to be involved in **roughly 80%** of all the known metabolic functions in the body.*

and potassium levels higher.[8] Arguably, there is no single molecule more critical for sustaining life and promoting health than magnesium. For example, few molecules are as critical as vitamin C. However, high doses of other antioxidants can **partially** compensate for an advanced deficiency of vitamin C. However, there are NO such even partially compensatory substi-

*...this unaddressed state of magnesium deficiency is not only the origin of many diseases, it reliably promotes and further aggravates **all** known diseases.*

tutes when magnesium is deficient. Only magnesium can alleviate the impact of a magnesium deficiency.

Ironically, as essential as magnesium is, it is often referred to as the "forgotten electrolyte," as clinicians continue to fail to realize its vital role in supporting optimal health in every tissue type and organ system of the body.[9] When a serum magnesium level is clearly low, the clinician **might** start magnesium supplementation even though it should **always** be initiated in that situation. Since magnesium does most of its work inside the body's cells, substantial body-wide deficiencies of magnesium are **common** even in the face of a normal serum magnesium level. And, much more often than not, this "hidden" deficiency remains unaddressed for the lifetime of the patient. As will be demonstrated in subsequent chapters, this unaddressed state of magnesium deficiency is not only the origin of many diseases, it reliably promotes and further aggravates **all** known diseases.

Body-Wide Impact

As will be discussed in much greater detail throughout the book, magnesium deficiencies have been associated with virtually all of the disease states that have been specifically studied for this relationship. Furthermore, many of the associated disease states substantially improve and sometimes even disappear upon a sufficient enough restoration of the depleted magnesium stores in the body. Some of the more significant conditions caused and/or worsened by magnesium deficiency include the following:

- ✓ Cardiovascular diseases (coronary and peripheral atherosclerosis, cardiac arrhythmias and QTc prolongation, hypertension, congestive heart failure; stroke)
- ✓ Metabolic syndrome
- ✓ Diabetes
- ✓ Chronic fatigue and fibromyalgia
- ✓ Kidney disease
- ✓ Osteoporosis and osteoarthritis
- ✓ COPD and asthma
- ✓ Calcium-containing stone formation anywhere in the body
- ✓ Preeclampsia and eclampsia
- ✓ Migraines and seizure disorders
- ✓ Depression and anxiety
- ✓ Dementias, neurodegenerative diseases, and seizure disorders
- ✓ Hearing loss

The Healing Mineral

Since magnesium is an important mineral in the structure of normal bone, most of the scientific literature that examines the relationship of magnesium to the support and promotion of good healing in

Just like insulin, which strongly promotes the transfer of magnesium from the extracellular to the intracellular space, magnesium supplementation by itself is a clear-cut healing agent.

general focuses on its ability to help heal bone fractures and promote bone growth.[10-13] However, when the effects of magnesium on healing not related to the bone are examined, the effects are still consistently very positive. Just like insulin, which strongly promotes the transfer of magnesium from the extracellular to the intracellular space, magnesium supplementation by itself is a clear-cut healing agent.

Magnesium serves as the most important calcium channel blocker in the body. It also appears to be a more general calcium antagonist and regulator of calcium metabolism.[14-19] And since excess calcium in the body, particularly inside the cell, lies at the root of all pathophysiology, magnesium is and remains the perfect antidote to mitigate all diseases.

In a randomized, double-blind, placebo-controlled trial on diabetic patients with foot ulcers, daily oral supplementation with only 250 mg of magnesium oxide nevertheless showed substantial benefits in terms of ulcer size, glucose metabolism, plasma total antioxidant capacity, and C-reactive protein level.[20] Another similarly conducted trial that involved the same dose

Not surprisingly, there appears to be a consistent linkage/relationship between intracellular magnesium levels, glucose metabolism, and glutathione, which are all factors that positively impact increased intracellular oxidative stress (increased IOS).

of magnesium oxide along with vitamin E produced much the same results on ulcer improvement, antioxidant capacity, lipid levels, C-reactive protein, and glucose control.[21] In another randomized, double-blind, placebo-controlled clinical trial, short infusions of magnesium directly before and during outpatient mastectomies both improved Quality of Recovery questionnaire scores and significantly reduced oral opioid doses post-procedure for pain control after discharge.[22] Acute ischemic stroke patients recovered more quickly when given a 24-hour infusion of magnesium sulfate.[23] Intravenous magnesium in rabbits with burns was shown to decrease burn area, wound depth, healing time, and size of healed scar.[24] Animal and cell studies have also demonstrated this ability of magnesium to support good wound healing.[25,26] Another animal study suggests that the early elevation of magnesium in wound fluid (along with a reduction in calcium level) is an activator of the important cell migratory response needed to initiate and sustain healthy healing.[27] Collectively, all of these studies logically indicate that any form of magnesium that eventually is able to raise intracellular magnesium levels and thereby lower intracellular oxidative stress will have a positive healing impact clinically.

Not surprisingly, there appears to be a consistent linkage/relationship between intracellular magnesium levels, glucose metabolism, and glutathione, which are all factors that positively impact increased intracellular oxidative stress (increased IOS). Insulin increases intracellular glutathione levels, decreasing intracellular oxidative stress.[28] Glutathione administrations increase intracellular glutathione levels, and they also improve intracellular magnesium levels. *In vivo* infusions increased magnesium levels inside red blood cells, and *in vitro* glutathione addition substantially elevated intracellular magnesium levels.[29] All of these positive effects also appear to be directly supported by the ability of another important antioxidant, vitamin E, to improve the action of insulin.[30] Another study concluded that a lowered glutathione intracellular status (increased IOS) reduced insulin effect (sensitivity) but that improving the intracellular glutathione levels via intravenous infusion significantly increased insulin effect and total glucose uptake.[31] Generally, a state of increased IOS inside the cells serves to worsen itself in a downhill positive feedback manner, until and if a direct intervention can "break the cycle" or at least slow it down (vitamin C, vitamin E, glutathione, magnesium administrations, etc.) by lessening that oxidative stress.

Diabetes and hypertension have long been observed to be diseases that frequently occur together, with substantial similarities in body type, inflammation and oxidative stress levels, and insulin resistance.[32] It has also been established that many diabetics have very low intracellular magnesium levels.[33] Intracellular magnesium levels are significantly depleted in hypertensive patients, and higher blood pressures are related to even lower intracellular magnesium levels.[34] Furthermore, in hypertensive patients the lower the intracellular magnesium level is, the less it will be elevated following insulin administration.[35] In other words, the intracellular magnesium needs some support independent of the amount of insulin present in order for the insulin to function optimally. The ionic status of the cytoplasm must be normalized as much as possible for insulin to have its full physiological impact in the first place. Although an argument can be made that one condition can help to "cause" the other, restoring magnesium levels would appear to be much more effective in resolving or stabilizing the underlying diseases and improving both the blood pressure and blood sugar than just giving more insulin to deal with the decreased insulin sensitivity (increased insulin resistance) characteristic of these diseases. In other words, it is more important to treat insulin resistance, at least initially, with magnesium and not just more insulin.

The Need for Magnesium Supplementation

While it might be technically possible for a limited number of individuals in good health to adequately support normal magnesium levels throughout the body with a perfect diet that is perfectly digested, such a situation is so rare that it should be effectively regarded as nonexistent. Many individuals, especially older ones, have multiple diseases or medical conditions that increase the magnesium demands of the body. Furthermore, many medications, especially

And for most individuals, these RDAs will be substantially below the amount of daily magnesium that should be absorbed/assimilated to maintain an optimal magnesium status.

diuretics and proton pump inhibitors (e.g., Prilosec or Nexium), can cause a chronic wasting of magnesium that is extraordinarily difficult to negate or overcome with magnesium supplementation. Other prominent magnesium-lowering agents include aminoglycoside antibiotics, some antiviral and antifungal agents, chemotherapy, and immunosuppressants.

For individuals who cannot afford or are otherwise not inclined to eat an organically-sourced diet on a regular basis, the amount of magnesium being consumed in a "regular" non-organic diet is nowhere close to even the dietary reference intakes (RDA) that are recommended at this time.[36] And for most individuals, these RDAs will be substantially below the amount of daily magnesium that should be absorbed/ assimilated to maintain an optimal magnesium status. RDAs for the daily requirements of vitamin C, for example, should be increased roughly 100-fold or more to optimize the intake of this nutrient for many people. The increased use of non-organic fertilizers and different forms of food processing simply prevents most food and food sources from having a reasonable content of magnesium in the first place. Some authorities assert that modern food processing depletes the magnesium content by 80 to 90%. Furthermore, it has been estimated that over the last 60 years the magnesium content in non-organically raised fruits and vegetables has decreased by 20 to 30%.[37] Even overeating such foods will not come close to sustaining a normal magnesium status in the body.

The magnesium content of drinking water can have a substantial impact on magnesium status and general health. Although it should not completely substitute for magnesium supplementation, it does appear that the magnesium content of drinking water can significantly support magnesium levels with significant positive health impact in the body.[38,39] In a sizeable meta-analysis of 10 different studies, it was concluded that the risk of death from coronary heart disease was significantly lower when drinking water with higher magnesium levels was consumed.[40] Higher magnesium drinking water levels also have been associated with a lower risk of ovarian cancer death and a lower risk of death from hypertension.[41,42] There is no good reason to believe that any similarly constructed studies on the impact of higher magnesium levels in the drinking water of a population would not favorably impact whatever other disease or condition is being examined.

All that said, most individuals, with just a few exceptions, should be supplementing with magnesium (see Chapter 18 for more detail).

Calcium Antagonist

*Magnesium's Primary
Function and Benefit*

The Toxicity of Excessive Calcium Ingestion

The medical literature is incredibly clear: Calcium is very toxic when chronically ingested in excessive amounts! Unfortunately, there is a profound ignorance about what peer-reviewed journals report, even among health care professionals regarded as experts in human physiology and clinical medicine. The untold sickness and death that results from not being aware of calcium toxicity is further magnified by the fact that many health care providers vigorously promote regular dairy consumption and even advocate calcium supplementation as beneficial for general health.

Since many health-conscious people wrongly regard significant ingestion of dietary calcium as an integral part of an optimally healthy lifestyle, the nearly universal promotion of calcium supplementation – especially by health professionals – makes total calcium intake an even greater public health concern.

It is best to regard calcium as a "toxic nutrient." That means it is absolutely essential for good health at a lower range of intake, but it becomes progressively more toxic the more it is ingested beyond this lower

Most Americans already consume too much calcium in the diet, so supplementation is actually dangerous for most people.

range. Although many nutrient supplements can be taken with no significant concern for reaching a toxic level of ingestion, this is definitely not the case with calcium. Most Americans already consume too much calcium in the diet, so supplementation is actually dangerous for most people.

The medical and scientific literature supporting the toxicity of excess calcium is substantial. Even calcium supplementation as minimal as 500 mg daily puts the supplementing individual at a greater risk of heart attack and stroke.[1-3] Furthermore, a much larger and prospective study that followed over 61,000 women over a very extended period of time (median of 19 years) examined mortality relative to overall daily calcium ingestion. This study not only demonstrated a significantly increased chance of premature death from heart disease among the women taking in the most calcium from dietary and supplemental sources, it also showed that high calcium intake was associated with an increased all-cause mortality.[4] A more recent study with men showed the increase in all-cause mortality from high calcium intake among men was even more dramatic than in women.[5] These increases in the chance of death from any and all diseases indicate that excess calcium equally harms all the cells of the body.

The above studies are further supported by research examining increased death risk with a very predictive medical test that is used to determine heart attack risk (coronary artery calcium tomography). The calcium score from this test is a direct and objective indicator of how much calcium has deposited in the coronary artery. Initially, a greater chance of death from coronary artery disease (heart attack) was found to correlate with increased calcium scores. However, since the increasing calcium deposition in the coronary arteries is really just the most visible display of excess calcium throughout the body, including inside of all the cells, it turns out that this test is also a good measure of the chance of death from any condition (all-cause mortality). Multiple studies now show that the higher the coronary calcium score, the greater the chance of dying from anything.[6-11]

Even calcium supplementation as minimal as 500 mg daily puts the supplementing individual at a greater risk of heart attack and stroke.

The Adverse Effects of Magnesium Deficiencies

Magnesium deficiencies have been found to be associated with just about every medical condition that has been examined in a scientifically sound manner. Research suggests that this is true because magnesium serves as a natural calcium channel blocker and as a general antagonist to calcium.[12,13] This is significant because these calcium channels literally pene-

Magnesium deficiencies have been found to be associated with just about every medical condition that has been examined in a scientifically sound manner.

trate and traverse the full width of the cell membranes throughout the body. As such, they are the primary determinants of how much calcium gets inside the cell. When calcium ingestion is high, more calcium eventually finds its way inside the cells, largely through these channels. When you have increased amounts of magnesium coming into the body, many of these channels are blocked, or otherwise inhibited from facilitating calcium entry into the cytoplasm.

The Health-Promoting Impact of Magnesium Administration

With all the health-promoting properties discussed elsewhere, and especially with its powerful effects on normalizing increased intracellular oxidative stress (IOS), magnesium is an ideal agent to add to any protocol to simply promote good healing. For all of the studies that have been done on magnesium, it is quite amazing that so few have investigated the direct effects of magnesium on the healing process. Many studies, on the other hand, demonstrate the positive effects of insulin on healing which provide a glimpse at magnesium's healing properties as well. That's because, in addition to its glucose-related metabolism function, insulin greatly facilitates the transfer/uptake of magnesium from the extracellular space into the intracellular space. Also, the numerous studies that have been done on magnesium and different diseases uniformly show that injuries, such as stroke due a loss of blood flow (ischemia), are reliably lessened by magnesium administration. Such studies are really only viewing cellular repair and healing from a different point of view.

The relatively few healing-property studies found on magnesium unrelated to bone repair, show that magnesium accelerates and improves the quality of healing (and/or lessens the extent of injury). In rats, adding a magnesium solution to a wound dressing substantially accelerated healing, including improved

...the numerous studies that have been done on magnesium and different diseases uniformly show that injuries, such as stroke due a loss of blood flow (ischemia), are reliably lessened by magnesium administration.

collagen deposition and new blood vessel formation.[14] In a randomized, double-blind, placebo-controlled trial, the postoperative quality of recovery, which in large part includes improved healing, was clearly enhanced by intravenous magnesium in patients undergoing outpatient mastectomy. [15]

Another randomized, double-blind, placebo-controlled trial with diabetic patients showed that the supplementation of magnesium and vitamin E signifi-

Since diabetics heal so poorly, magnesium's ability to promote healing in these patients logically suggests that it would support healing in the non-diabetic to an even greater degree.

cantly accelerated foot ulcer healing.[16] A similarly conducted trial also showed that magnesium **alone** resulted in largely the same improvements in diabetic foot ulcer healing.[17] Since diabetics heal so poorly, magnesium's ability to promote healing in these patients logically suggests that it would support healing in the non-diabetic to an even greater degree. And since magnesium can potentially normalize increased IOS in any cell in the body, there is every good reason to believe that magnesium would counter infections, neutralize toxic impact, and promote good healing everywhere in the body.

In an animal study, the local administration of magnesium promoted the healing of meniscal knee injuries. It was noted that the treated animals had enhanced tissue regeneration, less cartilage degeneration, and greater continued mechanical strength long after the repair. Additionally, it is extremely interesting that the magnesium appeared to enhance the recruitment and involvement of stem cells to the site of the lesion.[18] While not yet extensively studied, this could prove to be another major reason for the positive impact of magnesium in both enhancing tissue healing as well as in the prevention of tissue damage.

Calcium vs. Magnesium — The Antagonistic Relationship

As a practical point, then, it appears that calcium and magnesium have mutually antagonistic roles in the body and in cellular metabolism. A lot of one will limit and drive down the amount of the other in the body, and vice-versa. While there are practical obstacles to optimizing magnesium levels in the body, the literature indicates that lowering the excesses of intracellular calcium is only achieved naturally by the assimilation of sufficient amounts of magnesium.

Limitations on the degrees of excessive intracellular calcium concentration can also be achieved by the administration of prescription calcium channel blockers. In fact, the administration of such agents, especially in their long-acting forms, has also been shown to decrease all-cause mortality, a rare finding among prescription drugs. This clearly indicates again that the degree to which intracellular calcium elevations are increased is the single most critical factor currently known to determine how diseased a cell is.[19-23]

For this reason, it is usually desirable for anyone with elevated blood pressure (hypertension) that cannot be maintained within the normal range by magnesium and other nutrient supplementation to include one of the three major classes of long-acting calcium channel blockers as at least one of their prescription medicines for blood pressure. And if the blood pressure can be controlled by such a prescription calcium antagonist as a monotherapy, all the better.

However, a limited number of cell and animal

*Just as **increased** calcium intake has been shown to increase all-cause mortality, the **lower** magnesium levels that typically accompany or result from a state of calcium excess have also been shown to be associated with that increase.*

studies indicate that the prescription calcium channel blockers can negatively impact sex hormone and thyroid status.[24-26] While these hormones should always be monitored carefully and repeatedly over time to determine the need for addressing deficiencies, it would appear warranted to be even a bit more vigilant in following the hormone status on patients taking prescription calcium channel antagonists. And remember that magnesium as a calcium channel blocker is actually supportive of a normal thyroid and sex hormone status, further indicating that magnesium levels should first be optimized before relying completely on prescription calcium channel blockers to control blood pressure and other medical conditions.

Just as ***increased*** calcium intake has been shown to increase all-cause mortality, the ***lower*** magnesium levels that typically accompany or result from a state of calcium excess have also been shown to be associated with that increase. Furthermore, the lower the serum magnesium level, the greater the increase in all-cause mortality.[27-29] It was noted that death from all causes jumped by 40% for those subjects with a serum magnesium concentration below 0.73 mmol/L. Such a concentration is found in about 25% of the population.

Earlier investigators have suggested a normal range of serum magnesium levels to be between 0.75 and 1.0 mmol/L.[30] However, since this range reflects magnesium levels for most of the population, this "reference range" includes significant deficiency states as well. A serum magnesium level of 0.85 mmol/L would be a better starting point for a range less likely to be statistically associated with an actual state of magnesium deficiency.[31]

These magnesium levels reflect exactly what would be expected in light of the magnesium-calcium reciprocal relationship discussed elsewhere. However, significant trials looking at magnesium supplementation directly on all-cause mortality remain to be performed. Even so, it is reasonable to believe that increasing magnesium levels via supplementation would decrease all-cause mortality to the same degree that lowered levels increase it.[32] Nevertheless, the more quality studies examining the relationship of calcium, magnesium, and all-cause mortality, the better.

Although achieved by the intravenous administration of magnesium rather than oral supplementation, two studies stand out in demonstrating the importance of increasing magnesium levels in the body and decreased all-cause mortality. One study, performed in a double-blind randomized fashion, showed that a 24-hour infusion of magnesium sulfate preceded

This protocol also reduced all-cause mortality, in follow-up periods ranging between 1.0 to 5.5 years.

by a loading-dose injection in 2,316 suspected acute myocardial patients reduced cardiac mortality.[33] This protocol also reduced all-cause mortality, in follow-up periods ranging between *1.0 to 5.5 years*. A similarly impressive effect of decreasing all-cause mortality was seen in 194 consecutive acute myocardial infarction patients receiving a 48-hour infusion of magnesium sulfate. Again, the protective effect of the **one-time** magnesium infusion in decreasing the chances of dying from anything was seen after a mean follow-up period of 4.8 years.[34] These two studies by themselves should have changed the standard of care for acute myocardial infarction patients for the past two decades, but it has not changed.

The Slow Advancement of Clinical Medicine

Clinical medicine inches forward at an incredibly slow rate, when it advances at all. In the 34th edition (2014) of The Washington Manual of Medical Therapeutics, a guide very trusted and used by post-graduate medicine residents in training programs throughout the country, no mention at all is made of using magnesium in any capacity with patients presenting with chest pain and/or heart attack. Intravenous magnesium sulfate is only acknowledged in the manual as being of use as a "Second Line" therapy for asthma.

Whenever you hear of a new and exciting medical advance in the news, don't assume for a moment that it will be adopted promptly, or at all, in the routine treatment protocols. This is true even in our most reputable and famous hospitals and medical institutes throughout the country. Nevertheless, an important additional takeaway message from the two studies just cited is that one should never miss the opportunity to have magnesium added to an intravenous infusion, whatever the reason for the infusion. This would apply even in patients with kidney disease, although greater care to give the most appropriate dose would be necessary in that patient subset, since toxicity is a concern with the combination of intravenous application and decreased elimination in the urine.

The critical relationship between magnesium and calcium in the body is further highlighted by the effect of magnesium on areas in the body that have already developed hardened calcium deposits.

Lower serum magnesium levels, in conjunction with higher phosphorus and calcium levels, are associated with increased aortic valve calcification.

Magnesium administration, typically oral, reliably appears to dissolve pre-existing calcium deposits while preventing new deposits from developing.[35-37] Lower serum magnesium levels, in conjunction with higher phosphorus and calcium levels, are associated with increased aortic valve calcification.[38] Another study showed a significant association between calcium plaque buildup in the arteries and veins in the extremities (peripheral vascular calcification) and lower serum magnesium levels.[39] Furthermore, this finding was observed independent of serum calcium and phosphate levels.

As the research already presented demonstrates, there is an inverse relationship between serum magnesium and serum calcium levels: as one increases, the other decreases and vice versa. Additionally, as serum magnesium decreases, a propensity toward increased calcification occurs. Consistent with this inverse calcium/magnesium relationship, a very recent study has demonstrated that a higher calcium/magnesium ratio was a significantly more accurate indicator of increased all-cause mortality than low serum magnesium alone.[40]

This finding provides a new way to help track propensities for calcification. Monitoring the calcium/ magnesium ratio has the potential to make it much easier to determine calcification propensity and response to therapeutic interventions in the future. The opposite ratio (serum magnesium/calcium quotient) also appears to be a better indicator of magnesium status than the serum magnesium level alone. Emerging evidence suggests that a ratio of 0.4 is optimal, and 0.36 to 0.28 too low.[41]

Calcifications nearly always occur in the extracellular space. They do not generally occur inside the cell, since even an elevated intracellular level of calcium is much too low to allow for gross, large intracellular calcifications to occur. This is because extracellular calcium levels are as much as 10,000-fold more concentrated than intracellular calcium levels.[42]

Conversely, roughly 99% of the magnesium in the body is found inside the cells, consistent with their roles as natural antagonists that these important minerals play.[43] Even so, electron microscopic findings in animal studies have indicated some calcium deposition can occur inside the mitochondria and other intracellular organelles.[44-47] Consequently, it appears that increasing magnesium concentrations in both the extracellular and intracellular spaces are needed to optimize the ability of magnesium to inhibit the calcification process.[48,49] Much scientific literature, including animal and cell studies, has demonstrated that magnesium is an effective inhibitor of calcification throughout the body.[50-53]

Because of this, it appears that getting magnesium well-absorbed into the blood as well as inside the cells of the body should be an optimal goal of magnesium supplementation. Quite possibly, this is achievable with

Research shows that control/regulation of intracellular calcium metabolism also facilitates the ability of the body to neutralize significant toxic challenges.

a quality liposome-encapsulated form of magnesium taken orally, with or without other forms of magnesium. The impressive clinical effects of intravenous magnesium are probably due to the ability to get the blood and extra-cellular concentrations substantially higher than can be achieved with any of the regular oral supplementation forms of magnesium, which could then act to more effectively increase intracellular magnesium concentrations. Also, traditional oral forms of magnesium supplements tend to cause diarrhea well before the body/cell content of magnesium is optimal.

Research shows that control/regulation of intracellular calcium metabolism also facilitates the ability of the body to neutralize significant toxic challenges. All toxins exert their toxic effects by oxidizing biomolecules, or by causing them to be oxidized. Increased intracellular calcium concentrations are a primary mechanism by which toxins exert their toxic impact. It follows that lessening the intracellular calcium would be an effective strategy for lessening or blocking increased IOS completely.

Consistent with this model, it has been shown that toxic methylmercury exposure results in the loss of intracellular calcium homeostasis (equilibrium), resulting in elevated intracellular calcium levels and increased IOS.[54] Another potent toxin, formaldehyde, has been shown to increase intracellular calcium concentrations in exposed neurons.[55]

When an intracellular deficiency of it can be corrected, magnesium will wield a powerful antidote effect against toxins because of its antagonist effects against the high calcium concentrations seen in all toxin-induced cellular damage. For example, magnesium has been shown to have neuroprotective effects against the toxicity inflicted by lipopolysaccharide (a potent toxin often released by gram-negative bacteria as they die off) and its release of inflammatory mediators.[56] Even dose-related toxins such as glucose share the condition of increased IOS from excess calcium. Prolonged excess

When an intracellular deficiency of it can be corrected, magnesium will wield a powerful antidote effect against toxins because of its antagonist effects against the high calcium concentrations seen in all toxin-induced cellular damage.

glucose levels (hyperglycemia) initiate the degeneration in the tiny blood vessels of the retina seen in diabetic retinopathy by increasing free calcium levels in the cytosol (the inner aqueous component) of the afflicted cells.[57]

The oxidative status of the affected cells in Alzheimer's disease, Parkinson's disease, and amyotrophic lateral sclerosis (ALS) have been examined, and they all demonstrate a dysregulation of calcium that results in high intracellular levels of calcium with the accompanying increased IOS.[58-61] Much literature has documented the ability of antioxidants, especially vitamin C, to neutralize toxic damage by donating electrons to oxidized biomolecules, thereby restoring them to normal.[62] Without being a direct antioxidant molecule, magnesium appears to minimize such oxidative damage by decreasing intracellular calcium levels in toxin-exposed cells.[63]

Since magnesium lowers intracellular calcium levels and decreases increased IOS, a clear anti-toxin effect can generally be anticipated clinically when enough magnesium can be taken up by the toxin-exposed cells and tissues. And because of the important role that increased intracellular calcium has in increasing IOS in the cytoplasm, it appears that combining magnesium with prescription calcium channel blockers amplifies this antitoxin effect. This combination has been reported to serve as an effective antidote for acute organophosphorus insecticide poisoning, a form of poisoning that has never responded well to traditional forms of treatment.[64]

Animal studies have also confirmed the positive protective/antidote effects of magnesium, alone or in combination with another agent, against toxin-induced oxidative stress and radiation-induced oxidative stress. Magnesium administration decreased the inflammation in a hydrochloric acid-induced acute lung injury in rats.[65] In rats inflicted with radiation-induced brain injury, magnesium sulfate administration not only appeared to clearly lessen the injury, postmortem analysis of the brain tissues indicated that there was a reduction in calcium overload that resulted from this treatment.[66] In another rat study, magnesium sulfate clearly lessened the morbidity and even the mortality rate in animals given

Additional studies have also demonstrated that toxin exposures not only increase intracellular calcium levels, they also rapidly deplete intracellular magnesium levels.

doxorubicin, a chemotherapeutic agent known to consistently have significant toxic side effects, especially against the heart.[67]

If substantial doses of vitamin C were also added to such a combination, even better clinical results should be anticipated. While vitamin C, by itself, has had an extraordinary track record in the effective clinical treatment of a wide variety of poisonings and intoxications, it would appear that an even more optimal approach to a patient critically ill from a toxin exposure would be an infusion of vitamin C, magnesium, and a calcium channel antagonist. The vitamin C will neutralize the toxin directly as well as reduce poisoned (oxidized) biomolecules. At the same time, the magnesium and the prescription calcium channel blocker can rapidly decrease the elevated intracellular calcium seen in all poisonings, reducing the attendant elevated IOS that ultimately leads to greater cell morbidity and ultimately cell death when left unchecked. The addition of regular insulin and hydrocortisone to the treatment cocktail would further increase the intracellular levels of vitamin C while simultaneously

increasing intracellular magnesium and decreasing intracellular calcium and elevated IOS. All or at least part of
this treatment protocol should be the approach of poison
control centers around the world.

Multiple studies have now shown that
magnesium supplementation reliably
decreases the circulating levels of C-reactive
protein (CRP), a substance that reflects the
state of oxidative stress, or inflammation,
present in the body at any point in time.

Additional studies have also demonstrated that
toxin exposures not only increase intracellular calcium
levels, they also rapidly deplete intracellular magnesium
levels.[68,69] The toxicity of acute cocaine administration *in
vitro* also is quickly reflected in rises of intracellular free
calcium levels in the cerebral vascular smooth muscle
cells studied.[70] As would be expected, magnesium administration is effective in bringing down elevated levels
of calcium in the affected cells, largely or completely
negating the impact of a given toxin on those cells.[71,72]
In an animal study, magnesium was able to decrease
toxic effects (oxidation) when taken at the same time as a
known toxin.[73]

Further confirmation of the critical role that magnesium plays in calcium metabolism comes from studies
examining its effects on parameters of inflammation.
Basically, inflammation only occurs where there is
increased oxidative stress, and increased oxidative stress
results in inflammation. Effectively, they are synonyms,

at least in terms of their negative clinical impact. Multiple studies have now shown that magnesium supplementation reliably decreases the circulating levels of C-reactive protein (CRP), a substance that reflects the state of oxidative stress, or inflammation, present in the body at any point in time. Lowering intracellular calcium levels is essential in order to reduce increased oxidative stress body-wide.[74-76] Magnesium sulfate infusions also consistently and significantly lowered serum levels of CRP and IL-6 (another inflammation marker) in post-operative patients.[77]

The importance of this magnesium-calcium relationship is further demonstrated by studies that look at the way intracellular levels of magnesium and of calcium respond to different positive and negative physiological factors. Magnesium deficiency, in both animal and *in vitro* studies, appears to cause inflammation through the mechanism of increasing intracellular calcium levels, which then initiates the inflammatory response.[78] The disordered physiological processes (pathophysiology) involved in hypertension and states of increased vasoconstriction (as is seen in hypertension) consistently involve elevated intracellular calcium levels along with decreased intracellular magnesium levels. Intracellular potassium levels tend to also decrease in conjunction with the lowered intracellular magnesium levels.[79,80] It has also been shown that the administration of agents that provoke vascular muscle constriction increase cytoplasmic calcium levels while decreasing cytoplasmic magnesium levels.[81,82]

Platelets, which do not have nuclei but do contain cytoplasm, have also had their magnesium and calcium levels studied. In patients with normal blood pressure versus patients with hypertension who were either treated or untreated, similar patterns of increased calcium and decreased magnesium were seen when blood pressure was not controlled. As it came under control, these patterns were less pronounced.[83] The same patterns were also found in red blood cells from patients with essential hypertension (a persistently high blood pressure without an evident cause).[84] In the lymphocytes of hypertensive and normotensive rats, similar levels of calcium and magnesium were seen, and the supplementation of magnesium not only lowered blood pressures, but brought calcium levels down while raising magnesium levels.[85,86]

RECAP

Magnesium properties that reduce, or cause to be reduced, increased IOS:

1. Serves as a calcium channel blocker, decreasing intracellular concentrations of calcium
2. Serves as a calcium antagonist and calcium regulator
3. Serves as an antitoxin by decreasing intracellular concentrations of calcium
4. Primarily reduces insulin resistance, allowing insulin to better reduce intracellular oxidative stress by the further promotion of more magnesium entry into the cells, along with improved vitamin C cellular uptake

Heart Health

Magnesium and Cardiovascular Diseases

Adequate magnesium intake is critical for maintaining normal vascular smooth muscle tone and blood pressure. It is also essential for preventing and mitigating the development of atherosclerosis leading to angina pectoris and myocardial infarction. Magnesium deficiency is an important factor in the origin or cause of many arrhythmias, as well as in the development of congestive heart failure.[1] It is now quite clear that serum magnesium is an unreliable indicator of intracellular magnesium levels, except when the serum magnesium has been very low for a long period of time. Even those with normal serum levels often have a significant overall magnesium deficiency. In fact, due to many exogenous factors, it has been suggested that the vast majority of people in the modern world run the risk of subclinical but substantial magnesium deficiency, warranting regular magnesium supplementation in nearly everyone at risk of heart disease and other chronic diseases.[2]

Coronary Artery Disease

A large number of studies have demonstrated that magnesium deficiency and low magnesium intake are consistently associated with an increased risk of coronary artery disease and atherosclerosis. It is also associated with the abnormal laboratory abnormalities seen in metabolic syndrome. Metabolic syndrome, which typically involves at least three of the following:

- ✓ abdominal obesity
- ✓ high blood pressure
- ✓ elevated triglycerides
- ✓ low HDL lipoproteins
- ✓ elevated fasting glucose levels

is very strongly associated with an increased risk of heart disease and diabetes, as well as increased all-cause mortality.[3] A large meta-analysis (a statistical analysis of multiple studies) concluded that low dietary intake of magnesium increased the incidence of metabolic syndrome, and that higher intakes lessened the incidence.[4] Randomized, double-blind clinical trials have shown that magnesium supplementation is effective in the treatment of metabolic syndrome.[5]

A chronically low serum magnesium level, which reliably indicates body-wide magnesium depletion, is associated with an increased risk of death due to coronary artery disease.[6,7] Higher dietary intake of magnesium was associated with a reduced cardiovascular mortality in a large Japanese study.[8] A similar result was seen in a study on Hawaiian adults over a 30-year follow-up period.[9]

Coronary artery calcification has long been established to correlate with an increased risk of heart attack. These calcification scores have also been correlated with all-cause mortality, or chance of death from any disease or medical condition. An elevated calcium-magnesium ratio in the hair has also been

A large number of studies have demonstrated that magnesium deficiency and low magnesium intake are consistently associated with an increased risk of coronary artery disease and atherosclerosis.

associated with coronary artery calcification in an adult group of patients.[10] All of this is consistent with the studies showing that increased calcium intake increases all-cause mortality, while increased magnesium intake would be expected to decrease all-cause mortality.

Myocardial infarction, the most significant manifestation of advanced coronary artery disease for many individuals, also appears to be associated with, or partially provoked by, depressed serum magnesium levels. One study found decidedly lower serum magnesium levels in myocardial infarction patients compared to normal controls.[11] Although there has been some debate over its benefits in myocardial infarction patients, two significant studies demonstrated that a prolonged infusion of magnesium sulfate in the coronary care unit provided both short-term and long-term benefit. In each case, the infusion was started immediately after diagnosis or coincident with the treatment to re-establish blood flow (reperfusion) to the areas deprived because of the heart attack. This therapy appears to substantially reduce all-cause mortality for up to five years following the treatment.[12,13] Other similar studies not demonstrating this positive outcome possibly did not infuse magnesium soon enough, or a conclusion of no benefit in mortality reduction was inappropriately concluded because the study period only extended for 30 days after treatment.[14-16]

Arrhythmias

Arrhythmias are heart conditions in which the heartbeat is irregular, too fast, or too slow. Combinations of these three characteristics also occur. Many of the most common arrhythmias are associated with low magnesium levels and a large percentage of arrhythmia patients even have documented intracellular magnesium deficiencies.[17] Not surprisingly, such individuals have been shown to have positive clinical responses to magnesium administration. The upper heart chamber arrhythmias are some of the most common of all, often starting as isolated early atrial beats (premature atrial contractions). When left unaddressed, many individuals with these irregular beats progress to intermittent and even sustained rapid heart rhythms (tachycardias). These rapid rates are either regular in nature (supraventricular or atrial tachycardia) or highly irregular and even chaotic in nature (atrial fibrillation). Many clinicians have been effectively preventing and treating these arrhythmias with magnesium for many years.[18] The incidence of premature contractions, of both ventricular and supraventricular origin, have been clearly lessened by the oral administration of magnesium over a 30-day period.[19]

Postoperative cardiac patients often have arrhythmias; preventing and/or controlling them is

Many clinicians have been effectively preventing and treating these arrhythmias with magnesium for many years.

an important therapeutic objective. In a meta-analysis of seventeen clinical trials with a total of 2,069 patients, magnesium administration pre-cardiac surgery resulted in a dramatic lessening of postoperative cardiac arrhythmias. Supraventricular arrhythmias were down 23%, atrial fibrillation in particular by 29%, and ventricular arrhythmias by 48%.[20]

Another meta-analysis of five trials with a total of 348 pediatric heart surgery patients compared the preventive capacity of magnesium supplementation with placebo administration on the incidence of postoperative arrhythmias. There was an overall 66% reduction of arrhythmia incidence in the magnesium group.[21] A larger meta-analysis of twenty-two studies compared patients taking magnesium with patients taking a placebo. It concluded that the magnesium takers had a significantly lower incidence of both supraventricular and ventricular arrhythmias after surgery to bypass obstructed coronary blood vessels (cardiac revascularization surgery).[22] An even larger meta-analysis of thirty-five studies found magnesium administration significantly reduced the incidence of atrial fibrillation following cardiac surgery.[23]

Another recent study also showed that a substantial oral dose of magnesium was as effective

*There was an overall 66%
reduction of arrhythmia incidence
in the magnesium group.*

as an intravenous administration of magnesium in preventing postoperative arrhythmias after coronary bypass surgery.[24]

Ventricular tachycardia is an especially worrisome arrhythmia putting the patient at a significant risk of sudden death. In one especially dangerous form of this arrhythmia known as torsades de pointes, the repolarization period of the myocardial cells (the QT interval), following heart contraction is prolonged (see Figure 3.1). When this occurs the ventricular tachycardia often degenerates into ventricular fibrillation, which rapidly proceeds to cardiac arrest and death. In a case report of a patient who took cocaine and methadone and presented with low potassium and magnesium levels and a critically unresponsive case of torsades de pointes, magnesium replacement played a major role in resolving the arrhythmia.[25] QT interval prolongation, sometimes leading to ventricular tachycardia, is recognized as one of the most dangerous cardiovascular toxic effects of a number of anticancer drugs, and the recommended treatment for it is the infusion of magne-

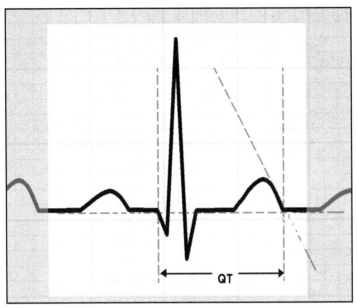

Figure 3.1: the QT Interval

sium. If not resolved promptly, electrical cardioversion is also indicated. The other common cardiovascular toxicities from chemotherapy also occur in the presence of lowered magnesium levels, most likely as the consequence of the magnesium deficiency itself. These toxicity-related outcomes include arrhythmias, coronary artery disease, stroke, hypertension, thrombosis, and heart failure.[26]

Complex ventricular arrhythmias are often seen in heart failure, typically occurring in the presence of low magnesium levels. In 68 patients who were able to complete the study protocol, magnesium supplementation was very effective in significantly alleviating and even abolishing the ventricular arrhythmias seen in these heart failure patients.[27]

Congestive Heart Failure

Low serum magnesium levels are often seen in congestive heart failure, and such lower levels have

QT interval prolongation, sometimes leading to ventricular tachycardia, is recognized as one of the most dangerous cardiovascular toxic effects of a number of anticancer drugs, and the recommended treatment for it is the infusion of magnesium.

been independently shown to increase the risk of this condition.[28-30] Impaired relaxation of the heart muscle after contraction (diastolic dysfunction) is consistently seen in established heart failure, and it is also a consistent feature of the pathophysiology leading to it. Along with many other cardiovascular disease risk factors, diastolic dysfunction has an inverse relationship to serum magnesium – dysfunction increases as the serum levels decrease.[31] Magnesium supplementation in diabetic mice prevented the otherwise anticipated diastolic dysfunction from developing, while also improving mitochondrial function and reducing increased intracellular oxidative stress (increased IOS) [32]

Logically, restoring magnesium levels to normal or near-normal would be expected to prevent or slow the development of heart failure, since low levels are consistently associated with it. Left ventricular function relates to the ability of the heart to contract with normal force, which is the primary defect in heart failure. One study examined left ventricular function and the effect of supplementation of a wide array of nutrient agents, including magnesium, administered in a double-blind fashion over a nine-month period. Statistically significant increases in the ejection fraction with significant decreases in left ventricular size were seen. Significant improvement in quality-of-life scores were seen as well.[33] However, since less than 1% of the body's magnesium resides in the blood, serum magnesium levels are not a reliable measurement of overall magnesium status. Normal serum levels often coexist with depleted intracellular magnesium levels. Chronically low serum magnesium levels will reliably reflect low cellular levels, but normal serum magnesium levels might not, especially when present for a shorter period of time, and in the absence of magnesium supplementation. Unlike many

Another study was able to demonstrate that increasing dietary magnesium intake was significantly associated with a reduced risk of heart failure, as well as stroke, diabetes, and all-cause mortality.

water-soluble agents, body-wide magnesium levels can increase or become depleted without being reflected in serum levels, at least in the short-term. Normal serum magnesium levels should never deter the clinician from supplementing the heart failure patient with magnesium.[34]

This really applies to magnesium supplementation in all patients with any chronic disease, but it is especially important in the heart failure patient who, due to diuretic treatment, is likely depleted of magnesium to an even greater degree.

Along with lowered intracellular magnesium levels, chronic heart failure patients commonly have a decreased heart rate variability. Heart rate variability is the amount by which the heart rate varies from beat to beat. A normal heart rate variability is generally reflective of a healthier heart capable of responding more promptly to a variety of external stresses. Magnesium supplementation in a group of heart failure patients compared to heart failure patients who did not receive magnesium resulted in increased serum and intracellular magnesium levels, along with a clear improvement in heart rate variability parameters.[35] Another study was able to demonstrate that increasing dietary magnesium intake was significantly associated with a reduced risk of heart failure, as well as stroke, diabetes, and all-cause mortality.[36]

The traditional drug therapy for congestive heart failure, especially in its more advanced stages with significant edema (swelling) of the feet and ankles due to fluid accumulation, virtually always involves diuretic administration, usually on a daily basis. Most diuretics cause the significant loss of magnesium and potassium in the increased urine output.

AN EXTREMELY IMPORTANT POINT TO REMEMBER

In the clinical management of heart failure patients, the use of diuretics in the treatment actually exacerbates the problem. One of the significant causes of aggravating and sustaining the heart failure is low blood and intracellular levels of magnesium. In heart failure patients on long-term diuretic administration, skeletal muscle biopsies revealed that cellular magnesium content was below normal in roughly two-thirds of these individuals.[37]

Without very vigorous magnesium replacement, then, very few heart failure patients would even have the possibility of any significant reversal in their conditions. Heart failure is basically accepted as a condition that optimally can be stabilized, but no significant long-term improvement is ever anticipated. In a situation that calls for robust doses of magnesium, widely accepted, "standard" protocols generally require daily diuretic administration with no attempt to replace the diuretic-induced magnesium loss. In light of this loss, reasonable clinical stabilization is pretty much the only realistic outcome for heart failure patients when treated by "standard" protocols.[38-40]

Vasoconstriction

Coronary artery spasm, an acute and often focal vasoconstriction of that blood vessel, can occur where there are obvious atherosclerotic narrowings or when an angiogram (a radiographic picture of blood vessels) indicates lesion-free coronary arteries. At times, it can be severe enough to completely block off such a normal-appearing artery to the point of causing a myocardial infarction before relenting. Baseline low-grade vasoconstriction is often present in those arteries that go into

The treatment and prevention of coronary artery spasm with magnesium has also produced consistent and dramatically positive outcomes.

acute spasm, similar to the pathology chronically seen with elevated blood pressures (hypertension) throughout the arterial system.

Increased intracellular calcium levels in the muscle cells of an artery with increased vascular tone are consistently seen, and these vessels tend to keep this elevated muscle tone as long as the underlying cytosolic calcium levels remain elevated. Furthermore, other provocative factors can acutely escalate this elevated tone, resulting in spasm or substantial further vasoconstriction. On the other hand, measures that can decrease cytoplasmic calcium levels in vascular muscle cells can normalize vascular tone, and even cause vascular relaxation, or vasodilation, when these levels are sufficiently lowered.

Magnesium deficiency has been established as an important factor that facilitates and causes coronary artery spasm.[41] Coronary artery spasm can occur following coronary bypass surgery, and significantly low magnesium levels were seen in nearly 90% of the patients following such surgery in one study. The authors in this study reported that correcting the magnesium levels during and after subsequent bypass surgeries eliminated the occurrence of coronary artery spasm.[42]

The treatment and prevention of coronary artery spasm with magnesium has also produced consistent and dramatically positive outcomes. During the angiography of patients diagnosed with coronary spasm-related angina, coronary artery spasm was induced with an infusion of acetylcholine directly into the coronary artery. After the spasm subsided, magnesium was infused into the coronary artery, and the acetylcholine challenge was repeated. A clear alleviation of the degree of spasm was seen in 10 of 14 patients, with none of 8 control patients showing alleviation from a placebo infusion of isotonic intracoronary glucose.[43] Another study that examined 15 patients with vasospastic angina reported that 41 episodes of spasm-related chest pain were promptly relieved by a dose of magnesium administered intravenously.[44]

Magnesium administration for vasospastic angina, or for most other conditions clearly caused or aggravated by a deficiency of magnesium, should not be based solely on the normalcy of serum magnesium levels. As more than 99% of the magnesium content of the body is inside the cells, "normal" serum magnesium levels are not assurances that intracellular levels are normal. Certainly, a chronic and significantly depressed serum magnesium will indicate a body-wide deficiency of magnesium most of the time. However, a normal serum magnesium level cannot be regarded as a clear-cut indication of a normal intracellular magnesium level, or a normal body-wide content of magnesium.[45]

In a study that examined red blood cell levels of magnesium in patients with vasospastic angina versus normal controls, substantially lower cellular magnesium

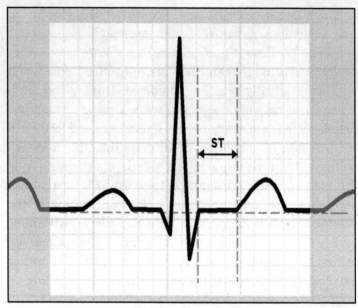

Figure 3.2: the ST Interval

levels were seen in the patients with frequent episodes of angina versus those that had no episodes. And the normal group had higher cell levels of magnesium. Yet no significant difference was seen between the groups with regard to serum magnesium levels.[46]

A case report documented similarly impressive findings, with a 51-year-old man with vasospastic angina and ST segment elevation on electrocardiogram responding well to an infusion of magnesium sulfate. An ST segment elevation is a section on an electrocardiogram (see Figure 3,2) that indicates an acute current of injury that proceeds to myocardial infarction if not promptly relieved. The patient's red blood cell magnesium levels were documented to be low. Ergonovine, a spasm-causing agent, could not provoke any new spasm via intracoronary infusion after the magnesium had been infused. Of note, high doses of prescription calcium channel blockers and nitrates were **_not_** able to relieve the spasm, even though they are able to relieve the increased muscle tone seen in hypertension. This indicates that

Two cases were described where aggressive treatment with calcium channel blockers failed to help at all, but a dramatic relief of symptoms was achieved with intravenous magnesium.

when intracellular magnesium levels are severely depressed, it is not enough to just block the pro-vasocon-striction effects of new calcium entering the cell. Rather, magnesium must be supplied to the cell as well to relieve the more advanced vasoconstrictive state of spasm.[47]

Localized areas of vasoconstriction like coronary artery spasm can occur elsewhere, and the pathophysi-ology behind it is basically the same. A condition known as reversible cerebral vasoconstriction syndrome, some-times accompanied by a low serum magnesium level, can present with refractory (unresponsive to treatment) headache, persistent vasospasm, and some subarachnoid hemorrhage (bleeding into the subarachnoid space of the brain).[48,49] Two cases were described where aggressive treatment with calcium channel blockers failed to help at all, but a dramatic relief of symptoms was achieved with intravenous magnesium. As noted elsewhere, when intracellular magnesium levels are very low, magnesium is the only reliable agent to relieve the vasoconstriction. Once the levels have been raised a bit, calcium channel blockers can then afford additional relief as well as prophylaxis against future episodes of vascular spasm.[50]

Hypertension (High Blood Pressure)

Hypertension along with blood pressures that are slightly elevated but not yet within the parameters of defined hypertension (prehypertension) is extremely common, with over a billion people affected by it worldwide and an incredible two-thirds of the American population being affected.[51] For long-term treatment and control of hypertension, magnesium has not proven to be a good monotherapy for optimal blood pressure control, although some consistent lowering of both systolic and diastolic blood pressures is seen with regular supplementation. Also, greater intake has resulted in an improved blood pressure-lowering effect.[52]

Essential hypertension, a common form of body-wide high blood pressure that is generally chronic in nature and lacks an evident cause, is another arterial vasoconstriction syndrome. It is marked by increased cytosolic levels of calcium in the arteries, as it is the common pathological denominator in all cases of hypertension, which is why magnesium has such a powerful anti-hypertensive impact when sufficiently-dosed. Calcium channel blocker treatment is very effective in most cases of hypertension, including essential hypertension, as intracellular calcium levels are brought down and intracellular magnesium levels rise.[53] One large meta-analysis found that a greater dietary intake of magnesium lessened the risk of hypertension, and another meta-analysis found that higher magnesium levels correlated with a lower incidence of it.[54,55]

Magnesium has also been shown to play a significant role in modulating a number of the risk factors for hypertension. Prostacyclin and nitric oxide help open blood vessels (vasodilators) and thereby lower the internal pressure in blood vessels. Magnesium potentiates (makes more active and/or effective) these natural vasodilators. A deficiency of magnesium exacerbates the vascular inflammatory response, while decreasing the expression and activity of multiple important antioxidants. And magnesium is also essential for maintaining the elasticity and structural integrity of the blood vessels.[56]

Consistent with these observations, syndromes that involve spontaneous muscular contractions are often attributable to significant deficiencies of magnesium, and they typically respond well to magnesium therapy.[57-59]

Hypertensive patients were shown to have significantly lower levels of magnesium inside the lymphocytes versus a control group. Of note, there were no significant differences between these two groups in either plasma magnesium levels or the levels of free magnesium inside platelets. While the levels of free magnesium within platelets (effectively cell fragments) provide a better reflection

Magnesium has also been shown to play a significant role in modulating a number of the risk factors for hypertension.

of total body magnesium than just the plasma levels, it still falls short of consistently and accurately reflecting how much magnesium is contained in the entirety of the intact cells throughout the body. A relatively small amount of intracellular magnesium (about 5%) is free, and the rest is bound or contained in the intracellular organelles (especially the mitochondria), serving as a buffer to replenish cytosolic depletion of magnesium.[60]

Essentially, then, this suggests that the most accurate indicator of total body magnesium depletion is to be found when measuring the entirety of the cellular content of magnesium and not just what is free in the cytoplasm of cell fragments like platelets. In this study, even though the free magnesium levels in the intracellular space of the lymphocytes was not lower than that seen inside the platelets, the total magnesium content of the lymphocytes was significantly lower in the hypertensive patients.[61]

Measurements of the total body stores of magnesium generally use one of three methods. Their relative accuracy, in descending order, is as follows:

✓ Total cell content (most accurate)
✓ Cytosolic or free intracellular levels
✓ Serum level (least accurate)

When the serum level of magnesium is consistently very low over a prolonged period of time, body-wide depletion can be implied most of the time. But when serum magnesium levels are in the "normal" or reference range, substantial deficiencies of total magnesium content can still exist inside the cells, and frequently do.

The reason normal cytosolic magnesium levels often fail to reflect the actual body-wide magnesium status is that the intracellular space can "leach" magnesium from the intracellular organelles. This "stolen" magnesium maintains the appearance of a normal level and will do so until the "buffers" in these organelles become significantly depleted. Therefore, when cytoplasmic magnesium levels are low, the total cell magnesium content is always depressed and always indicates a body-wide depletion. But, when free magnesium levels in the cytoplasm are "normal" a body-wide deficiency can still be present.[62]

But when serum magnesium levels are in the "normal" or reference range, substantial deficiencies of total magnesium content can still exist inside the cells, and frequently do.

The reality that serum magnesium readings can fail to detect magnesium deficiencies was demonstrated by a study on cancer patients being treated with cisplatin. This chemotherapy drug has substantial toxicity and generally increases urinary excretion of magnesium. In order to track magnesium status, serum levels were measured and skeletal muscle biopsies were examined for total magnesium content. While a significant lowering of total magnesium content was seen in the muscles, serum magnesium levels failed to register this depletion until total body stores reached a more critical level of deficiency. The total quantity of magnesium in the plasma is only roughly 0.3% of total body magnesium while the majority of magnesium content is in the bone. However, the skeletal muscles hold about 30% of the total magnesium in the body, and therefore it provides an important magnesium reservoir/buffer for the blood.[63]

One cell study found that the mitochondria serve as a major site of magnesium stores in the cell, and the mitochondria appear to serve very effectively in releasing magnesium into the cytoplasm when circumstances require it.[64] Basically, then, for serum magnesium levels to be reflective of body magnesium content, the level (low or very low) must have been present for an extended

A normal serum magnesium level can be sustained for a very long period of time in the face of significant body-wide depletion.

period of time. A normal serum magnesium level can be sustained for a very long period of time in the face of significant body-wide depletion.

Hypertension also complicates roughly 10% of pregnancies worldwide. When the condition is severe enough to result in protein spilling in the urine or other evidence of organ damage, a condition known as preeclampsia has evolved. And when seizures develop in a pregnant woman with preeclampsia, the diagnosis of eclampsia is then applied. Regardless of the stage of the disease, however, the underlying pathology of low intracellular magnesium and elevated intracellular calcium is present. This pathology causes increased vascular tone eventually leading to significant vasoconstriction. In its pathological expression, eclampsia is very similar to reversible cerebral vasoconstriction syndrome. And the effect of magnesium on eclampsia and preeclampsia is similarly effective.

In postpartum women, it was shown that intravenous magnesium was more effective for preventing preeclampsia from evolving into eclampsia with seizure activity than a prescription calcium channel blocker that had specific cerebral vasodilator activity.[65] Although it is not feasible for the daily treatment of regular chronic hypertension, it is likely that intravenous magnesium would offer superior blood pressure control over any other anti-hypertensives.

In conjunction with its vasodilating, anti-hypertensive effects, magnesium has a marked anti-adrenergic (similar to a beta-blocker) effect further facilitating its ability to lower blood pressures. This means that magnesium helps to suppress catecholamine release from the adrenal medulla, which serves to acutely increase the blood pressure seen in high-stress, "fight-or-flight" situations. Interestingly, calcium, to which magnesium serves as an antagonist in multiple settings, works in opposite fashion to stimulate catecholamine release as its levels increase in the adrenal medulla cells.[66,67]

Vascular Thrombosis

Vascular thrombosis, or blood clots forming in the blood vessels, is another condition where low magnesium levels play a key role.[68] It also tends to occur more in a setting of preexisting vascular disease rather than an isolated phenomenon. A low serum magnesium level is independently associated with the risk of thrombosis and other major adverse cardiac events following coronary stent implantation.[69,70] Stent coatings that incorporate magnesium alloy reduce this blood-clotting tendency as well.[71]

Inflammation is both pro-atherogenic (stimulates the development of fatty plaques in the blood vessels) as well as supportive of an increased risk of blood clotting. It is increased IOS that ultimately triggers the inflammatory response. Because magnesium is a natural calcium antagonist, it also serves as a natural anti-inflammatory agent since it helps to lower the elevated intracellular calcium levels that cause the increased IOS.[72]

Low magnesium levels also promote endothelial cell dysfunction, which is another important factor in setting the stage for inflammation, atherosclerosis, and thrombosis.[73] Endothelial cells in culture demonstrated an enhanced synthesis of nitric oxide with higher magnesium levels, a factor that would make increased blood coagulability (tendency to clot) and thrombosis less likely to occur.[74,75] In an animal study magnesium sulfate administration demonstrated clear antithrombotic activity *in vivo*.[76] In animal studies where thrombosis was deliberately caused, intravenous magnesium demonstrated an ability to significantly reduce blood clot size. It also appeared that this effect occurred without compromising the normal flow of blood (hemostasis) or causing an increased bleeding tendency.[77,78] This is consistent with the idea that magnesium helps to stabilize hemostasis in the body, making both a hypercoagulable state or a bleeding tendency state to proceed towards normalization.

In a study on stable coronary artery disease patients, oral magnesium administration was found to inhibit platelet thrombosis by 35%. This effect appeared to be independent of platelet clumping and activation. Furthermore, the inhibitory effect was additive to the effect of aspirin.[79,80] This finding was consistent with another study that showed low intracellular magnesium levels promoted platelet thrombosis in patients with coronary artery disease.[81]

Insulin's Powerful Partner

Magnesium and Diabetes Mellitus

Metabolically and pathophysiologically, diabetes, coronary artery disease, and hypertension are closely related, each one serving as a risk factor for the others, and with all three conditions often occurring together in many patients. A majority of diabetic patients have hypertension, and the development of hypertension often coincides with the appearance of hyperglycemia.[1,2]

Furthermore, the major cause of ill health and death in diabetes is cardiovascular disease, which is worsened by hypertension. All three diseases share multiple risk factors, including endothelial dysfunction and vascular inflammation.[3] Many of the signs of metabolic syndrome (abdominal obesity, increased triglyceride and blood sugar levels, hypertension, low HDL lipoproteins) are shared in these three conditions as well. Lower magnesium levels, in both the serum and inside the cells, are associated with an increased prevalence of metabolic syndrome and diabetes.[4,5] On the other hand, oral magnesium supplementation has been shown to improve metabolic syndrome specifically by lowering blood pressure, glucose levels, and

In fact, low magnesium levels appear to be a direct cause of insulin resistance.

triglycerides.[6] Magnesium deficiency is a major factor in both setting the stage for diabetes as well as in making it more difficult to effectively manage. In fact, low magnesium levels appear to be a direct cause of insulin resistance. So it is very likely that magnesium replacement is as important or **even more important** than simply increasing insulin dose for optimal long-term blood sugar control. In a large prospective study, a low magnesium level was shown to be independently associated with an increased risk of developing diabetes in women.[7] Low magnesium levels, along with low phosphate levels, also appeared to significantly correlate with abnormal nerve conduction in diabetic patients. This finding is consistent with the peripheral neuropathy often seen in these patients.[8]

Conversely, magnesium supplementation and even high dietary intake of magnesium were shown to decrease the array of cardiovascular risk factors typically seen in diabetics. These risk factor improvements include enhanced insulin-mediated glucose uptake.[9-12] High dietary intake of magnesium also appeared to decrease the risk of diabetes in a Japanese community[13] and in a pooled analysis of three U.S. cohort studies.[14] Similarly, a higher dietary magnesium intake is also associated with a lower prevalence of coronary heart disease in diabetic patients.[15] An animal study showed that magnesium not only decreased insulin resistance, it also increased the numbers of insulin receptors and glucose transporters. These are all factors that would strongly promote optimal insulin function.[16-18]

A vicious cycle of intracellular magnesium deficiency increasing insulin resistance, and of insulin resistance causing magnesium deficiency is present in many diabetics.[19,20] As a rule, a positive clinical response in treating many diabetics is optimized when a magnesium deficiency is properly addressed ***before*** just increasing insulin dose.[21] Much of the time, when this deficit is properly corrected, little to no change in insulin dose is necessary, and sometimes optimal glucose control is achieved with an even lower insulin dose.

In studies on the magnesium content in platelets

A vicious cycle of intracellular magnesium deficiency increasing insulin resistance, and of insulin resistance causing magnesium deficiency is present in many diabetics.

in diabetic children, it was found that insulin clearly increased platelet magnesium levels. However, it was also shown that the magnesium content in the platelets of diabetic children who were substantially insulin-resistant would initially drop, further supporting the idea that decreased intracellular magnesium content underlies the initial biochemical pathophysiology leading to insulin resistance.[22,23] Regardless, magnesium supple-

Gestational diabetes, where non-diabetic women develop elevated blood sugars during pregnancy, is characterized by significant depletions of both extracellular as well as intracellular magnesium.

mentation should be an integral part of the treatment protocol for just about any diabetic patient of any age. Chronically lower magnesium levels clearly promote insulin resistance, and persistent supplementation clearly raises both serum and intracellular magnesium levels in diabetics.[24]

An additional aspect of this magnesium-insulin-glucose relationship is that insulin and glucose have opposite mediating or regulating effects on free intracellular magnesium levels. Research with human lymphocytes clearly demonstrates that insulin increases intracellular magnesium, while glucose decreases it. By implication, independent of its own ability to increase cellular magnesium, insulin further enhances cellular magnesium levels by decreasing magnesium-suppressing glucose.[25]

Gestational diabetes, where non-diabetic women develop elevated blood sugars during pregnancy, is characterized by significant depletions of both extra-cellular as well as intracellular magnesium, as reflected in the blood and inside the red blood cells. In one investigation, non-pregnant women had the best **total** magnesium levels, normal pregnant women had less, and pregnant women with gestational diabetes had the least. Also, the women with gestational diabetes had substantially lower **intracellular** magnesium levels than either the non-pregnant or the normal pregnant women.[26] In another study, supplementation with magnesium in tandem with vitamin E significantly improved glucose control and blood lipids in women with gestational diabetes.[27]

Just as insulin increases magnesium levels inside the cells, magnesium also plays an important role in the regulation of insulin secretion from the pancreatic beta cells. Additionally, it primes the insulin recep-

Consistent with these findings, diabetic patients who have low magnesium levels demonstrate a more rapid progression of their disease, along with an increased risk of the various complications seen in diabetes.

tors for optimal binding with insulin.[28,29] Magnesium supplementation has been shown to improve the ability of the pancreatic beta cells to supply insulin as needed in non-diabetic individuals.[30] Similarly, in non-diabetic individuals, low magnesium levels have been shown to suppress insulin secretion.[31] Consistent with these findings, diabetic patients who have low magnesium levels demonstrate a more rapid progression of their disease, along with an increased risk of the various complications seen in diabetes.[32]

Mind and Mood Manager

Magnesium and Neurological Diseases

In the nervous system, magnesium serves a vital role in optimizing nerve conduction and in neuro-muscular coordination. It also helps to protect from neuronal over-stimulation (excitotoxicity) that leads to increased neurological pathology and cell death.[1] Consistent with these effects, magnesium deficiencies have been identified in multiple neurological diseases, and magnesium administration has generally proven to be a positive intervention in lessening the pathology of these diseases.[2]

Depression and Anxiety

Statistically, depression accounts for roughly 40% of neuropsychiatric disorders in the United States. Anxiety is often seen as an accompanying condition to depression, and is considered by many as features of the same clinical syndrome.[3] In both animal model studies and human studies, a magnesium deficiency has been linked to anxiety and depression, both separately and as a single clinical entity.[4-11]

Consistent with the association between magnesium deficiency and the syndrome of anxiety/depression, magnesium supplementation has consistently been shown to positively impact this condition. A randomized controlled trial of magnesium supplementation in the treatment of depression showed clear benefit in adults with mild-to-moderate depression.[12] Another double-blind, placebo-controlled trial of magnesium supplementation in depressed patients with low serum magnesium levels also showed clear benefit not only in depression status but also in the improvement of those depressed serum magnesium levels.[13]

Some patients with clinical depression become classified as treatment-resistant when they do not respond in a significantly positive way to prescription drugs given for this condition. Even in this subset of patients who are extremely unresponsive to management by traditional approaches, magnesium has proven to be of significant benefit. This has been demonstrated in treatment-resistant depression in both an established animal model as well as in patients.[14,15]

Magnesium supplementation has also been shown to clearly augment the benefits of traditional agents for the treatment of depression, sometimes in a synergistic rather than just additive fashion.[16,17] Furthermore, magnesium in combination with certain natural, non-prescription agents has also shown added benefits to that of magnesium alone.[18,19]

Other medical syndromes that are associated with magnesium deficiency also have associated depression, anxiety, or both. In a group of pediatric migraine patients treated over a six-month period with magnesium as a preventative measure, less migraine attacks along with fewer symptoms related to anxiety and depression were seen.[20] Depression in post-stroke

Consistent with the association between magnesium deficiency and the syndrome of anxiety/depression, magnesium supplementation has consistently been shown to positively impact this condition.

patients occurs commonly and both conditions are strongly associated with low serum magnesium levels.[21]

Two other conditions, postpartum depression and preeclampsia, also appear to be often associated, with both frequently responding to magnesium supplementation.[22] Addiction is a state that appears to be related to magnesium deficiency and responsive to magnesium supplementation, and both anxiety and depression appear to be regularly associated with addiction and the factors leading to it.[23]

Insomnia often coexists with depression and anxiety. A large meta-analysis showed that insomnia is significantly associated with an increased risk of depression.[24] Another meta-analysis that looked at insomnia treatments indicated that an effective impact on insomnia often resulted in a lessening of depression that was present in those patients as well. Alleviating insomnia appeared to mediate a later remission from depression.[25,26] And alleviating anxiety and depression appears to lessen insomnia and related symptoms.[27]

Whether one condition actually causes another is not clear. A common provocative factor, like decreased body stores of magnesium, would seem more likely to be the main link between these three conditions. Regardless, just as in anxiety and depression, magnesium supplementation is beneficial. A double-blind, placebo-controlled clinical trial of supplementing insomnia patients with magnesium appeared to improve subjective measures of insomnia.[28] Another study found that a supplement containing melatonin and zinc along with magnesium clearly improved the quality of sleep in a nursing home population.[29] In a study on alcohol-dependent patients, magnesium appeared to result in clear-cut improvement in sleep parameters with less insomnia-related symptoms.[30] Another study on patients with insomnia and restless legs syndrome also showed magnesium administration helped both conditions.[31]

Epilepsy and Seizure Disorders

A seizure is an event triggered by uncontrollable electrical activity in the brain, which can manifest in an array of symptoms or just result in a clear-cut physical convulsion. Seizures can occur for multiple reasons, including brain tumors, certain types of poisoning, neurological development problems, infectious diseases, and high fevers. However, roughly 50% of patients with seizures do not have a diagnosed reason. When seizures are recurrent and remain undiagnosed, a diagnosis of epilepsy is generally applied.

Pathophysiologically, all seizure activity begins with the unstable electrical activity generated by the increased intracellular calcium levels in the affected neurons.[32] Furthermore, the long-term maintenance of the epileptic state without any significant resolution or control of seizure frequency appears related to a more permanent loss of the mechanisms that normalize

Pathophysiologically, all seizure activity begins with the unstable electrical activity generated by the increased intracellular calcium levels in the affected neurons.

calcium concentrations at the cellular level. This physiological change makes the ability to reduce intracellular calcium levels with standard pharmacological interventions increasingly problematic.[33,34] Individuals with much less frequent seizure activity have more temporary, but large elevations of intracellular calcium levels, and they tend not to keep the calcium levels at such elevations.[35]

In status epilepticus, a clinical emergency with either continuous seizure activity or rapid and recurrent seizures without the regaining of consciousness between seizures, calcium levels inside the affected cells become very elevated and tend to stay at those elevated levels.[36] Additionally, neurons tend to further accumulate calcium during seizure activity, making prompt calcium-lowering interventions mandatory to mitigate/stop seizure activity, and also to prevent the cell damage and cell death that results when these accumulations remain unaddressed.[37]

In general, then, cellular calcium influx in a neuron increases electrical excitability and instability, and cellular magnesium influx has the opposing, calming effect.[38] In fact, in cell and tissue models looking at the induction of seizure activity, one way researchers reliably induce seizure activity in cell and

In fact, in cell and tissue models looking at the induction of seizure activity, one way researchers reliably induce seizure activity in cell and tissue models is by exposing the cells or tissue to low magnesium concentrations.

tissue models is by exposing the cells or tissue to low magnesium concentrations.[39,40]

Because of the relationship between seizure activity and elevated intracellular calcium levels,[41] calcium channel blocking drugs can exert an anti-seizure effect on the involved neurons. In cell studies, the ability of verapamil to block calcium flow across the cell membrane appeared to be the primary reason for its anti-seizure properties.[42] Magnesium also has calcium antagonist and calcium channel-blocking properties, and this is reflected in a number of clinical studies.

Magnesium not only has been shown to protect against seizures, it appears to enhance the effects of standard anti-seizure drugs as well as to raise the seizure threshold in animal and human studies.[43,44] Also, higher doses of magnesium appear to provide greater protection than lower doses.[45,46] In patients with seizures resistant to traditional drugs, oral magnesium supplementation resulted in a significant drop in seizure activity, and 2 out of 22 patients became seizure-free.[47] In treating two patients with the most advanced degree of epilepsy, status epilepticus, that was unresponsive to a combination of anti-epileptic drugs, intravenous magnesium resulted in prompt clinical improvement, permitting a rapid removal of the endotracheal tube of both patients.[48]

A low plasma level of magnesium has been shown to be associated with epilepsy, and the mean magnesium levels in a group of epileptic patients were significantly lower than in a healthy control group.[49] A study on children with seizures associated with high body temperature also showed both low serum levels of magnesium levels and lower intracellular levels compared to control patients.[50] Conversely, a higher dietary intake of magnesium was found to be associated with a lower incidence of epilepsy in a 22-year follow-up study on 2,442 men.[51]

Best Epilepsy Treatment Protocol Ignored?

It remains difficult to understand why magnesium is not a part of all treatment protocols of epilepsy patients. It is also difficult to fathom why it is not the *first* agent to be used, giving it the chance to completely resolve the seizures without going to further measures, as it has been reported to do at times in seizure patients unresponsive to the usual prescription medicines. Furthermore, traditional anti-seizure medicines have many side effects, and they do not reverse the underlying pathology or repair cellular damage as is seen with magnesium. Starting the seizure therapy with magnesium would prevent many side effects in many patients from ever occurring. For neurological diseases in general, the literature collectively indicates that in addition to improving the clinical picture of these diseases, magnesium also reduces the progressive neurodegeneration seen with them. Conceivably, a high enough dose of magnesium at an early enough stage of some neurological diseases might result in an actual reversal of disease-associated pathology.[52]

Parkinson's Disease, Alzheimer's Disease, and Dementia

These three neurological disorders are all chronic neurodegenerative diseases with progressive loss (death) of the affected neurons. This results in a gradual reduction of brain mass over time, along with an array of intracellular metabolic abnormalities in the remaining viable cells. Progressive dementia can often be indistinguishable from Alzheimer's disease in its later stages, while Parkinson's disease appears to affect more prominently other areas of the brain. However, variable degrees of dementia are also common in Parkinson's patients.

Generally, diseases of the brain and nervous system are associated with magnesium depletion as is seen with most other chronic diseases. Also, different neurological diseases can present with greater depletions of magnesium in one area of the brain versus another. Oftentimes, an excess of a neurotoxic metal, such as aluminum, will also be seen where the magnesium depletion is greatest, which generally means that more than just magnesium repletion is necessary for optimal treatment of the neurological condition. This is likely the case with Alzheimer's disease.[53,54] Autopsy-derived brain tissue in patients with senile dementia of the Alzheimer type revealed concentrations of aluminum in the nuclei of a high percentage of neurons with a microscopic feature known as neurofibrillary tangles.[55,56] Certainly, increased intracellular oxidative stress (IOS) is present inside all of the affected neurons in any neurological disease, accompanied with/caused by increased cellular calcium levels. However, due to a number of factors, the most effective treatments for reducing elevated IOS are not as straightforward as in the rest of the body outside of the nervous system. Nevertheless, the reduction of the pathophysiology leading to and sustaining the increased IOS in the affected neurons is still the goal.

Much of the literature addressing the pathology and treatment of neurological diseases centers on cell culture and animal model studies. In a rat model for Parkinson's disease, the involved neurons were exposed to increasing magnesium concentrations. Higher magnesium exposures had a "significant and striking" effect in the prevention and lessening of the typical neuronal pathological changes.[57]

Another similarly-structured study found that the improved viability of the affected cells directly related to increased cytoplasmic magnesium levels. These increases resulted from magnesium release from the mitochondrial stores, along with an increased uptake of magnesium across the cell membrane.[58]

In an animal model for Alzheimer's disease, ~~the~~ mice were treated with magnesium threonate and the brain levels of magnesium were successfully increased. The authors concluded that such an elevation of brain

The authors concluded that such an elevation of brain magnesium was able to prevent synaptic loss with some reversal of cognitive defects as well.

magnesium was able to prevent synaptic loss with some reversal of cognitive defects as well. They also showed that magnesium had positive impacts on affected neuronal tissue slices.[59] Magnesium threonate is a form of magnesium now available for supplementation that appears to better access the brain and nervous systems than other commonly-used forms in animal studies.[60] In a rat Alzheimer's model, the abdominal injection of magnesium appeared to protect cognitive function and synaptic integrity.[61]

The association of low serum magnesium levels and these neurological diseases is not as clear-cut as with many other diseases outside of the central nervous system. Some studies not only correlated low serum magnesium levels with Alzheimer's disease, but they also suggested that lower serum magnesium levels were related to the clinical degree of Alzheimer's disease.[62,63] Another study reached the conclusion that low and high serum magnesium levels were associated with an increased risk of dementia.[64] A recent meta-analysis found increased circulating magnesium levels in

Parkinson's patients.[65] Yet, a study in a cell model of Parkinson's demonstrated that more magnesium clearly supported lowered degrees of IOS.[66] Consistent with this significant lack of agreement in correlating magnesium levels and neurological disease status, a number of studies have shown magnesium in the serum to have a poor penetration across the blood-brain barrier.[67]

A methodology known as phosphorus magnetic resonance spectroscopy now exists that can measure *in vivo* the free cytosolic magnesium concentrations in different tissues. New studies utilizing this technology will probably better resolve seemingly conflicting data on magnesium status in the body in the future.[68]

Although the serum magnesium levels do not correlate as well as with neurological diseases as with diseases elsewhere in the body, the increased IOS resulting from excess cytoplasmic calcium still appears to be a consistent state of pathophysiology in all diseases, including those in the nervous system.

Some studies not only correlated low serum magnesium levels with Alzheimer's disease, but they also suggested that lower serum magnesium levels were related to the clinical degree of Alzheimer's disease.

Magnesium levels were found to be significantly lower in the cerebrospinal fluid of Alzheimer's patients compared to controls, even when there was no significant difference in the serum magnesium levels between these two groups.[69] In another study comparing Alzheimer's patients to controls, serum total magnesium levels showed no differences, but serum ionized magnesium levels were significantly lower in

Magnesium levels were found to be significantly lower in the cerebrospinal fluid of Alzheimer's patients compared to controls.

the Alzheimer's group and those lowered levels were directly related to cognitive function.[70] In a study that quantified magnesium content in nervous tissue, it was found that in normal brains there were significantly different amounts of magnesium in different parts. And in the diseased areas of Alzheimer's patients, magnesium content was lower than in those same areas as in normal patients.[71] Nevertheless, it appears that improving the magnesium status in such diseased cells in order to counteract the calcium excess remains a significant therapeutic goal, even if it not realized as readily as elsewhere in the body. New supplemental approaches, including liposome-encapsulated magnesium threonate that is now available, might make this therapeutic goal more achievable.

In a study extending over a 10-year follow-up period, the use of magnesium oxide (a common laxative) appeared to significantly reduce the risk of developing dementia.[72] And in patients already diagnosed with dementia or Alzheimer's, magnesium supplementation has been shown to improve learning and to result in improvement in other related symptoms.[73]

In addition to magnesium deficiency, other minerals appear to be important factors in different forms of dementia and Alzheimer's. It has been hypothesized that a group of patients with ALS (amyotrophic lateral sclerosis) associated with dementia or parkinsonian features resulted from long exposure to low magnesium along with excess aluminum and manganese in the drinking water and soil.[74] Lead excess in brain tissues also appears to be a common finding in a form of presenile dementia.[75]

Many cell, animal, and human studies strongly support the concept that the presence of excess cellular calcium and impairment in the mechanisms that regulate calcium are primary metabolic common denominators in the pathology and eventual cell death in neurological diseases and in neurodegeneration in general.[76-81] This further gives support to the thesis that

In patients already diagnosed with dementia or Alzheimer's, magnesium supplementation has been shown to improve learning and to result in improvement in other related symptoms.

the inversely-related magnesium levels in the affected cells are low as well, and that finding a way to increase those magnesium levels is a primary way to lessen the calcium excess. However, many diseases, especially the neurological ones, have their increased IOS pathology attributable to multiple oxidation-inducing toxins, including iron and copper, which appear to be major additional factors in the cause and maintenance of a disease such as Parkinson's.[82] In fact, it appears that increased iron content in diseased cells is further enhanced by increased iron uptake via the use of the transmembrane calcium channels (see Figure 5.1), further explaining the positive impact of calcium

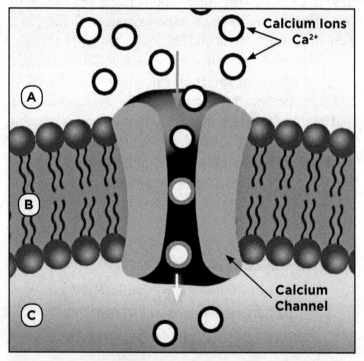

Figure 5.1 Calcium Channel
Calcium channels are pore-like structures implanted in cellular membranes (B) that allow calcium ions — as well as toxins like iron and copper — to travel from the extracellular space (A) into the intracellular space or cytosol (C). Calcium channel blockers prevent that movement.

channel blockers on the evolution of the pathophysiology of these neurological diseases.[83]

Prescription calcium channel blockers appear to lessen the development of the pathological changes in Parkinson's.[84,85] Two meta-analyses found that the use of these drugs resulted in a significantly decreased risk of developing this disease compared to a group not taking them.[86,87] Another study found that the use of the dihydropyridine calcium channel blockers in treating hypertension also appeared to result in a reduced risk of Parkinson's disease.[88] Magnesium administration, a natural calcium channel blocker and calcium antagonist, would also be expected to positively impact this pathophysiology in neurological diseases, as long as the magnesium reached the target tissues in adequate amounts.

Outside of the circumstances of excess intravenous magnesium administration and/or varying degrees of renal failure, clearly and persistently elevated levels of magnesium in the blood are quite rare. One subset of patients to keep in mind that could have a significant percentage of such hypermagnesemic patients are the very elderly, especially those in nursing homes and extended-care facilities. This group of patients often become reliant on magnesium-containing cathartics to keep the bowels moving. Furthermore, the very presence of the constipation for which the cathartics are being given assure that the magnesium stays in the GI tract for a longer period of time, permitting an even higher degree of absorption than is usually seen with regular magnesium supplementation. With or without renal dysfunction, these cathartics can potentially push magnesium levels high enough to be fatal.[89]

Stroke

A stroke occurs when insufficient blood flow or a complete loss of blood flow results in injury and/or death to neurons. It is generally classified as ischemic in nature, due to a severe decrease in blood flow to an area of the brain, or as hemorrhagic. The hemorrhagic, or bleeding, form results in a secondary loss/death of neurons due to loss of blood supply in one area and/or compression from blood accumulation resulting in cell death in another area.

Regarding magnesium and stroke, the greatest benefit offered by magnesium appears to be in stroke prevention from increased magnesium intake, including from dietary sources. One meta-analysis of prospective studies found that dietary magnesium intake was inversely associated with risk of ischemic stroke.[90] Another meta-analysis of cohort studies came to the same conclusion.[91] Other studies have found that lower dietary magnesium was associated with increased stroke risk, as well as with higher blood pressure.[92,93] These two conditions often coexist. Consistent with these findings, another study found that many hospitalized ischemic stroke patients presented with low serum magnesium levels, and that these decreased levels were independently associated with greater in-hospital mortality.[94] It was also reported that low levels of serum magnesium in acute ischemic stroke patients appeared to be a risk factor for developing cognitive impairment after one month.[95]

When patients presenting with acute ischemic stroke were given a substantial dose of intravenous magnesium over the first 24 hours of hospital admission, there was not seen a statistically significant degree of stroke recovery compared to a control stroke group.[96] It would seem that in the case of neurological damage from stroke, low magnesium increases the risk of it occurring, higher levels decrease the risk of it occurring, but after-the-fact magnesium administra-

A meta-analysis of five clinical trials has also demonstrated this neuroprotective effect of magnesium on the salvage of damaged but still viable nervous tissue.

tion appears to do little for reducing the neurological damage sustained.

When the stroke is not "complete," however, and there is evidence of the neurological defect showing some capability of resolution, there does appear to be a beneficial role for magnesium administration. In an animal model of transient focal ischemia, where the vascular blockage is undone before permanent damage takes place, the resulting shock from a quick return of blood flow to the nervous tissue is lessened synergistically by a combination of magnesium and a nonsteroidal anti-inflammatory agent.[97] A meta-analysis of five clinical trials has also demonstrated this neuroprotective effect of magnesium on the salvage of damaged but still viable nervous tissue. In patients who suffered subarachnoid hemorrhage-related brain injury, magnesium administration was shown to reduce the risk of poor outcome clinically while also reducing the occurrence of delayed brain ischemia events.[98] In several animal models of brain injury, magnesium increases the recovery of cognitive brain function following such injury.[99,100]

Magnesium, in combination with a calcium channel blocker, has also been shown to be of significant benefit in patients who have sustained a subarachnoid hemorrhage. In a prospective and randomized, double-blind clinical trial on 120 such patients, intravenous magnesium along with oral nimodipine was shown to decrease the consequences of the cerebral vasospasm commonly occurring with such an injury. A clear reduction in post-event cerebral ischemia with associated death of brain tissue (cerebral infarction) and neurologic deficits was seen.[101] Low serum magnesium was also found to be independently associated with hemorrhagic complications following stroke.[102] Further evidence of the apparent ability of magnesium to lessen bleeding was demonstrated in a study on 299 patients with acute spontaneous intracerebral hemorrhage. Higher serum magnesium levels were seen to be independently related to lower volume of blood accumulation (hematoma size) on admission.[103]

Take a Deep Breath

Magnesium and Pulmonary Diseases

Asthma and Bronchospasm

Magnesium intake has been associated with the support of good lung function in multiple studies. Dietary magnesium is independently related to lung function and the occurrence of wheezing (bronchospasm). More dietary magnesium intake relates to better lung function and dietary deficiency is associated with impaired function.[1,2] Serum magnesium levels positively correlate with better symptom control in asthmatic adults.[3] It appears to improve, or help to prevent, the loss of lung function as measured by multiple parameters. Magnesium has at least three significant ways in which it positively impacts lung function:[4]

1. It has both a strong vasodilator and bronchodilator effect,
2. It helps to regulate the release of acetylcholine and histamine (bronchoconstrictors),

3. And it has anti-inflammatory (decreased oxidative stress) effects.

In patients with chronic asthma and low serum magnesium levels, multiple pulmonary functions were significantly less normal than compared to chronic asthmatic patients with normal magnesium levels.[5] Lower serum magnesium levels in chronic asthma patients also correlate with a worsened clinical status.[6] Not surprisingly, intracellular magnesium levels in asthma patients were significantly depressed. These lower intracellular levels also correlated with increased bronchial reactivity, or tendency to bronchospasm.[7]

It is true that higher levels of magnesium make asthma less likely to develop or for it to be less symptomatic if it does manifest. It is also true that low magnesium levels appear to make preexisting asthma worse. However, the effectiveness of magnesium therapy for asthma is less clear-cut. Acute asthma attacks are generally treated in the emergency room

In patients with chronic asthma and low serum magnesium levels, multiple pulmonary functions were significantly less normal than compared to chronic asthmatic patients with normal magnesium levels.

with inhaled as well as intravenous agents. Multiple studies have consistently shown that intravenous magnesium has a definite, but not necessarily dramatic, effect in improving lung function and lessening symptoms in acute asthma. Furthermore, the inhaled route of magnesium administration (nebulization) has consistently showed little to no significant benefit in alleviating acute attacks.[8-12] Chronic oral supplementation of magnesium along with standard asthma treatments in asthmatic adults and children only suggested a limited benefit in a recent review and meta-analysis.[13] Nevertheless, as with so many other chronic diseases, regular magnesium supplementation still appears to be advisable, although a significant body-wide deficiency of magnesium can make a clear benefit slow to appear. Furthermore, such supplementation can be expected to decrease the incidence of many other diseases and/or lessen their associated symptoms.

COPD

Chronic obstructive pulmonary disease (COPD) is pathologically quite different from asthma, with a gradual destruction of lung tissue over time. In the chronically compromised patients, exacerbations of the inability to breathe are often precipitated by infections and environmental/chemical irritants. An exacerbation of COPD, with increased difficulty breathing, often has associated bronchoconstriction as well. One systematic review of four randomized clinical trials found that intravenous magnesium appeared to potentiate the effect of bronchoconstriction-relieving agents, although the degree of this effect was not felt to be substantial.[14] In a double-blinded, placebo-controlled study, intravenous magnesium was felt be a beneficial adjunct to standard bronchodilators in COPD exacerbation patients.[15] Another study on treating exacerbations of COPD patients found that the intravenous administration of magnesium had no significant bronchodilating effect by itself, and it did not reduce the length of hospital stay.[16] One study found that nebulized magnesium, which appeared to have no impact on asthmatic bronchoconstriction, does favorably impact the breathing parameters in exacerbations of COPD.[17] However, as noted with asthma patients, regular magnesium supplementation would still appear to be good idea for COPD patients. Lower magnesium levels in COPD are associated with a decreased quality-of-life even in the absence of worsened pulmonary function.[18]

Bone, Joints, and Muscles

Magnesium and Musculoskeletal Diseases

Roughly 60% of the total body content of magnesium is stored in the bones, and roughly 40% more is contained in the skeletal muscles and soft tissues. Less than 1% of the bodily content of magnesium is found outside of the cells, in the blood and extracellular fluid.[1,2] Magnesium is known to stimulate the proliferation of osteoblasts (bone-forming cells).[3] Furthermore, a magnesium deficiency results in decreased bone formation and eventual osteopenia (earliest stage of osteoporosis), as this state not only inhibits the activity of osteoblasts, it also promotes the activity of osteoclasts (bone-destroying cells).[4,5] In studies looking at new bone formation along with healing, an animal study showed having magnesium impregnated into titanium implants placed into bone sites both promoted rapid bone formation as well as the expression of different bone-forming markers.[6]

115

Osteoporosis

A fractured bone is the worst clinical outcome of osteoporosis. In a long-term prospective cohort study, low serum magnesium levels were found to be strongly and independently associated with an increased risk of fractures.[7] Another study on 3,765 patients over an 8-year period showed that both men and women with the highest dietary intake of magnesium had substantially fewer fractures than those with the lowest dietary intake.[8] Conversely, magnesium supplementation in a group of menopausal women over a 2-year period was shown to both decrease the chances of fracture while significantly increasing bone density.[9] Not surprisingly, higher dietary magnesium intakes also appeared to slow the skeletal muscle deterioration seen with aging and increasing osteoporosis.[10]

Having and maintaining normal calcium and phosphate metabolism in the body is critical to healthy bone. Furthermore, having normal assimilation of vitamin D

Conversely, magnesium supplementation in a group of menopausal women over a 2-year period was shown to both decrease the chances of fracture while significantly increasing bone density.

and maintaining normal levels of this vitamin in the body is vital to keeping calcium/phosphate metabolism properly regulated. Magnesium also plays an important role in the activation of vitamin D in the body.[11,12] In both humans and animals magnesium deficiency is associated with lowered vitamin D levels as well.[13] In addition to playing a role in the metabolism of vitamin D, magnesium also plays an essential role in its synthesis.[14]

A study in postmenopausal women with osteoporosis demonstrated that serum magnesium levels were lower in these individuals than normal controls. Bone mineral density also correlated directly with magnesium levels.[15] These findings strongly indicate that magnesium stores in the bone (and throughout the body) are vital to maintaining bone health, and that quality magnesium supplementation is important for prevention as well as treatment of bone disease in general.

Osteoarthritis

In general, magnesium deficiency has been recognized as a major risk factor for the development and progression of osteoarthritis, as its deficiency has been associated with cartilage damage, increased inflammatory mediators, and defective formation of new cartilage-forming cells.[16] Lower magnesium intake, as reflected in deficiencies in both diet and supplementation, was found to be associated with increased knee pain in patients with radiographic evidence of osteoarthritis.[17] Another study demonstrated that dietary magnesium intake is inversely associated with X-ray evidence of osteoarthritis and joint space narrowing.[18] Similarly, it was shown that lower serum magnesium levels inversely correlate with radiographic evidence of osteoarthritis.[19]

Other studies also lend support to the importance of a magnesium deficiency provoking osteoarthritis, or of increased magnesium intake, including by intra-articular injection, lessening the symptoms and evidence of osteoarthritis.[20,21] The inflammatory marker CRP has been found to be inversely related to increased dietary magnesium intake and serum magnesium levels in patients with early X-ray evidence of osteoarthritis.[22] Chondrocalcinosis, a condition of calcium deposition in cartilage, is often seen with osteoarthritis and felt by many to be part of the pathophysiological spectrum of osteoarthritis evolution. This condition has been shown to increase in prevalence the lower the serum magnesium levels goes.[23] Magnesium chondroitin sulfate has been synthesized and found to successfully treat parameters of osteoarthritis (increased proliferation of chondrocytes and decreased destruction by apoptosis).[24]

Muscular

Like all the other cells and tissues of the body, the skeletal muscle needs optimal magnesium content for optimal muscle health and function. While there is not a great deal of literature directly addressing magnesium status and muscle health, what there is indicates it is just as important for muscles as all other cells and tissues.

In an animal study a dietary deficiency of magnesium resulted in greater calcium content and oxidative stress in the skeletal muscle tissue, which would logically lead to muscle tissue lesions and deterioration.[25] Along with insufficiencies of other dietary nutrients, low dietary intake of magnesium correlated with increased sarcopenia (loss of muscle mass).[26] In a review of studies looking at exercise and physical performance in athletes, magnesium was considered to have "quality evidence" supporting its role in improving such performance.[27]

Key to Vitality

Magnesium and Organ Systems

Liver

The relationship between magnesium intake and liver disease has not been extensively studied. One large study did examine the association between magnesium intake and the risk of mortality from liver disease. It concluded that for every 100 mg increase in daily magnesium intake there was a 49% reduction in mortality risk from liver diseases. The study also found that this inverse relationship between magnesium intake and mortality from liver disease was even more striking among alcohol drinkers and individuals with hepatic steatosis (fatty liver disease).[1]

In a hepatic cell study, it was found that a magnesium compound helped protect those cells from the type of injury seen in non-alcoholic fatty liver disease.[2] A mouse study demonstrated that magnesium could protect the liver from a sepsis-related toxin.[3] In another study on rats, magnesium was also shown to protect against the injury that would otherwise result from a surgically blocked bile duct, a model of what happens when a gallstone blocks the duct.[4] In rats exposed to carbon tetrachloride, a liver-damaging toxin, magnesium was shown to lessen the otherwise-anticipated

...for every 100 mg increase in daily magnesium intake there was a 49% reduction in mortality risk from liver diseases.

injury, with a dramatic reduction in elevated liver enzymes and a substantially reduced liver cell death.[5] Another animal model study also demonstrated that magnesium could protect against the liver damage caused by oxaliplatin, a chemotherapy drug.[6]

In a study on patients diagnosed with compensated liver cirrhosis, a condition where there are sufficient healthy liver cells present that can compensate for the scarred portion of the liver, it was found that better intracellular and serum magnesium levels correlated positively with better cognitive performance. These findings suggested that magnesium could lessen the chances or degree of hepatic encephalopathy, a condition where a diseased liver causes changes in mood, movement, personality, or consciousness.[7] In another study, magnesium administration was shown to significantly improve cognitive and motor functions in rats with induced hepatic encephalopathy.[8] The collective studies appear to underscore the fact that magnesium, by lessening the levels of intracellular oxidative stress (IOS) in the liver and elsewhere, strongly supports the liver's vital role of detoxification by freeing it to properly process and negate new toxin exposures.

Pancreas

In an animal study, magnesium was shown to protect against the liver injury induced by acute pancreatitis, limiting its impact on multiple liver damage parameters.[9] In another animal study, magnesium supplementation was shown to decrease the severity of an artificially-induced experimental model of pancreatitis, while a nutritional magnesium deficiency was shown to increase susceptibility to inflammation-inducing stimuli.[10] An investigation of non-diabetic individuals demonstrated that magnesium supplementation improved the metabolic responsiveness of the insulin-secreting capacity of the pancreas (beta cells) compared to the metabolic responsiveness of those cells in individuals with

An investigation of non-diabetic individuals demonstrated that magnesium supplementation improved the metabolic responsiveness of the insulin-secreting capacity of the pancreas.

significantly low serum magnesium levels.[11] In rats with induced diabetes, magnesium supplementation prevented the otherwise-anticipated pathological changes in the pancreas.[12]

Reproductive System

Currently, magnesium is commonly used as a tocolytic agent (inhibitor of uterine contractions) in higher risk pregnancies to prevent preterm labor and preterm delivery.[13] Prescription calcium channel blockers, which share this property with magnesium, are also commonly used in these circumstances. Such intervention has also been shown to be a likely neuroprotective agent, diminishing the chances of cerebral palsy and cerebral hemorrhage.[14,15]

During pregnancy, especially as the pregnancy proceeds, levels of many nutrients, vitamins, and minerals – including magnesium – are reduced by the increased metabolic demands of the pregnant state. The literature has also suggested that the women who most significantly deplete their body stores of magnesium are the ones who are most prone to preeclampsia. Leg cramping and pre-term birth are also significantly more common in this magnesium-depleted group.[16] This is certainly consistent with the fact that intravenous magnesium is the agent of choice for such patients

The literature has also suggested that the women who most significantly deplete their body stores of magnesium are the ones who are most prone to preeclampsia.

as blood pressures rise in pregnancy. It has also been suggested that sudden infant death syndrome is largely due to the fetal consequences of a significant enough magnesium deficiency in the mother.[17]

In fact, magnesium is regarded as an ideal agent for "controlled hypotension," which really means a high enough dose can make the blood pressure go as low as is desired.[18,19] This also means that the main negative "side effect" of too much magnesium

It has also been suggested that sudden infant death syndrome is largely due to the fetal consequences of a significant enough magnesium deficiency in the mother.

is making the blood pressure too low to sustain life. Excess calcium channel blockage from magnesium is pharmacologically similar to a prescription calcium channel blocker overdose (often as a result of attempted suicide), presenting to the emergency room as hypotensive shock. Because of this, prescription calcium channel blockers are considered to be drugs with a narrow therapeutic index (the minimum toxic concentration is less than two times the minimum effective concentration).[20] Both magnesium and calcium channel blocker drugs are nevertheless widely considered as safe agents in patients, pregnant or otherwise, but in need of appropriate monitoring during the periods of their administration.[21,22]

Kidney

In individuals with no known kidney disease, lower magnesium levels correlated with an accelerated deterioration or loss of renal function, as reflected in lowered estimated glomerular filtration rate. In a study involving 2,056 participants and spanning a median of 7 years, the lowest serum magnesium levels correlated with the most substantial loss of renal function. Furthermore, the decline in function was even more

And in patients with established chronic kidney disease or with end-stage renal disease, low serum magnesium levels were significantly associated with increased cardiovascular and all-cause mortality.

pronounced in those individuals with diabetes.[23] And in patients with established chronic kidney disease or with end-stage renal disease, low serum magnesium levels were significantly associated with increased cardiovascular and all-cause mortality.[24] When magnesium levels are maintained in the slightly elevated range, lower mortality and less calcification has been seen in chronic kidney disease patients.[25]

Hearing

There is a substantial amount of literature demonstrating the importance of magnesium in both the protection of hearing capacity as well as in the recovery of hearing capacity after damage from noise as well as from other causes. Magnesium deficiency states have long been shown to increase susceptibility to noise- and toxin-induced auditory damages.[26] In a placebo-controlled, double-blind study on 300 healthy military recruits facing two months of basic military training, one group received 167 mg of magnesium aspartate in a drink daily while the other group received a placebo drink. At the end of the training period, it was demonstrated that the magnesium-treated group had developed significantly less noise-induced permanent hearing losses.[27]

Magnesium also works well as a treatment for hearing damage that has already occurred. In a prospective and randomized trial that was double-blind and placebo-controlled, patients with a sudden onset of sensorineural (involving the nerves) hearing loss were given steroids with magnesium. Another group was given steroids with a placebo. The magnesium group had a significantly higher proportion of patients with improved hearing across all frequencies tested, and the degree of improvement was significantly greater as well.[28]

Aside from magnesium supplementation, it also appears that better dietary magnesium intake strongly supports auditory health. In an analysis of cross-sectional data in 2,592 adults aged 20 to 69, hearing thresholds were measured over a 3- to 4-year period. Dietary magnesium intake, along with the dietary intakes of vitamin C and beta-carotene were estimated, and it was found that higher intakes of these agents were associated with a lower risk of hearing loss.[29]

In two different strains of guinea pigs, hearing damage (ototoxicity) due to a toxic exposure to gentamicin (an antibiotic) was significantly lessened by the addition of magnesium and vitamins to the diet.[30] Another guinea pig study actually analyzed the magnesium content in the cochlea after hearing loss due to acoustic trauma. The study showed that the greater the magnesium content, the lesser the hearing loss.[31] Still another study in guinea pigs with hearing loss from exposure to gunshot noise showed that magnesium-induced improvement was only temporary, but

The magnesium group had a significantly higher proportion of patients with improved hearing across all frequencies tested, and the degree of improvement was significantly greater as well.

that when the magnesium was continued for a month the improvement appeared to represent resolution of the damage.[32]

In patients with moderate to severe tinnitus (ringing in the ears), it was found that a 3-month period of supplementation with oral magnesium resulted in a significant reduction of the degree of this condition.[33] Another hearing loss disorder interwoven with symptoms of Meniere's disease (daily vertigo, headache, and vomiting) over a 6-month period in a 5-year-old girl completely resolved with magnesium and riboflavin supplementation and a diet regimen recommended for migraine patients.[34]

Splitting Headache Relief

Magnesium and Migraines

About 16% of the U.S. population has experienced one or more migraines.[1] This debilitating, commonly experienced condition can fall into more than one pathological category. Some regard it as a "primary" headache or neurological disorder while others would consider it to be a vascular disorder. More than likely, the underlying cause has to do with the tone of the smooth muscle tissues in the blood vessels (vascular tone). As vascular tone increases, the diameter of the vessel decreases. In the case of migraines, it appears that chronically increased vascular tone sporadically and somewhat unpredictably constricts to such a point that it results an array of symptoms, including severe headaches. The sequence of events in the evolution of a migraine is not fully understood at present. For certain, however, most clinicians feel that this syndrome involves a significant disturbance of normal vascular status and function in the brain.[2]

Much of what is experienced as symptoms in a migraine is probably due to the "washout" that results from the rapid restoration in blood flow that occurs when severely constricted vessels suddenly dilate. This is similar to what is seen when a completely blocked artery is opened up, as after an acute heart attack when the initially blocked coronary artery is opened up with an angioplasty or a clot-dissolving drug. New heart arrhythmias nearly always appear as the downstream damaged cells seek to re-normalize their metabolism. It is logical that as the migraine syndrome evolves, the body attempts to re-normalize damaged brain cells in a similar fashion as to when blood flow is restored to a previously completely blocked coronary artery. But since brain cells are affected and not heart cells, there are no arrhythmias that result. Rather, there is a wide array of different symptoms that can appear with (or without) the migraine headache, including visual and auditory abnormalities, as well as transient neurological deficits. Multiple studies have shown that magnesium significantly reduces the oxidative stress injury observed in laboratory animals when blood flow is restricted or prevented for a time and then restored (ischemia/reperfusion injury models). This observation certainly fits into the vascular model proposed for severe migraine.

In a study that was able to measure blood volume in the cerebrum it was demonstrated that an infusion of magnesium resulted in a vasodilation effect with increased cortical blood volume.[3]

Magnesium naturally relaxes constricted blood vessels (vasodilation) **and** reduces oxidative stress. Because of this dual ability, it is expected that the administration of magnesium would have a greater positive impact on a migraine than a vasodilator drug that has no impact on prooxidant activity.[4-9]

Migraines often develop in pregnancy, clearly worsening as the pregnancy proceeds, much like the

Magnesium supplementation has been shown to not only decrease the frequency and intensity of migraine attacks in pregnant women, it also appears to decrease the chances of hospitalization.

progressive vasoconstriction seen in the evolving preeclampsia of many pregnancies.[10] Magnesium supplementation has been shown to not only decrease the frequency and intensity of migraine attacks in pregnant women, it also appears to decrease the chances of hospitalization.[11]

Regardless of the precise nature of the underlying causes, much research has shown that a magnesium deficiency is a factor clearly associated with the development of migraine.[12] Serum magnesium levels were not only observed to be consistently low in migraine patients compared to healthy individuals, the levels were even lower during the migraine attacks.[13] This suggests the possibility that severely depressed cellular magnesium levels might be the primary reason for the onset of a migraine attack.

Much of the migraine literature cites the positive contributions of magnesium to both preventing and treating this condition, but it seems to consistently avoid the clear-cut conclusion that magnesium, adequately-dosed, is the *agent of choice* for migraine. Some of the agents that have been used and continue to be used in the treatment and prevention of migraine include: metoclopramide, acet-

---

Much of the migraine literature cites the positive contributions of magnesium to both preventing and treating this condition

---

aminophen, butalbital, opioids, diphenhydramine, topiramate, propranolol, nadolol, metoprolol, amitriptyline, gabapentin, ketorolac, caffeine, sodium valproate, candesartan, butterbur, feverfew, riboflavin, coenzyme Q10, carnitine, niacin, vitamin D, vitamin B6, vitamin B12, alpha lipoic acid, and melatonin.[14-16]

This very large and growing list further underscores the lack of understanding of the pathophysiology of this condition. It also shows an alarming lack of appreciation for the symptom and pathology relief that magnesium has to offer for this condition.

In a subset of advanced migraine patients with the most severe and unremitting of pain continuing for 72 hours or more, known as status migrainosus, the intravenous administration of magnesium resulted in a significant pain reduction in 54% of these patients. 44% had such complete pain relief that intramuscular pain medications did not have to be administered.[17] In studies on migraine attacks of less severity but requiring emergency intervention, intravenous magnesium has been consistently effective in pain relief. In a meta-analysis of 21 randomized controlled clinical trials, intravenous magnesium significantly relieved acute migraine as promptly as 15 minutes after administration.[18]

In another study in the emergency room setting, intravenous magnesium not only relieved migraine pain promptly, it was clearly more effective than ketorolac, a commonly administered prescription drug for migraine symptoms and pain relief.[19] A similarly structured study showed that intravenous magnesium completely eliminated migraine pain within two hours of administration. Intravenous caffeine resulted in some migraine pain relief in the same time frame but was unable to relieve it completely.[20] One case report in a 5-year-old girl diagnosed with Meniere's disease (inner ear equilibrium disorder) with a 6-month history of daily episodes of headache, vomiting, and vertigo was able to become symptom-free after a 6-week regimen that incorporated magnesium and

...intravenous magnesium not only relieved migraine pain promptly, it was clearly more effective than ketorolac, a commonly administered prescription drug for migraine...

riboflavin supplementation.[21]

Oral magnesium has also been shown to be effective in migraine prophylaxis, although complete elimination of attacks is not generally seen.[22-24]

Clinicians who treat migraine either do not read the pertinent literature or do not fully understand it, or they simply choose to ignore the clear-cut data indicating that magnesium should always be the primary agent in their treatment protocols. The case for its consistent use in migraine patients is very straightforward, but as with just about every other positive non-pharmacological intervention, the conclusions of so many studies after overwhelming positive outcomes is that the tested agent "might" be indicated, and that more studies are needed. Nevertheless, it has been suggested in the literature that magnesium treatment is warranted in all migraine patients.[25]

Considering the dramatic effects of magnesium given intravenously in the treatment of acute migraine attacks in the emergency setting, it seems likely that complete control or near-complete control of subsequent attacks might be obtained with a larger daily dosing of magnesium than has been given in these studies. This might be achievable by taking enough of a quality liposome-encapsulated form of magnesium to better raise intracellular magnesium levels, along with other forms and routes of magnesium administration. Also, it is always best when a multi-pronged approach to the support of metabolism and hormone balance is undertaken along with the administration of magnesium for optimal results. Such a regimen resulted in the complete elimination of migraine in a study on 30 patients.[26]

Powerful Poison Antidote

Magnesium as an Antitoxin

At a minimum, decreased intracellular antioxidant capacity, if not increased intracellular oxidative stress (increased IOS), is always the final common pathophysiological state seen in any toxin- or poison-induced cellular damage. This is equally true inside the cells affected by any chronic disease. Even though magnesium by itself is not a direct electron-donating antioxidant (like vitamin C and others), it nevertheless has a powerful antioxidant impact as its presence in the body, and especially inside cells, increases.

Not surprisingly, as an agent that can substantially decrease and even normalize increased IOS, magnesium (along with potent antioxidants such as vitamin C and glutathione) has a substantial positive clinical effect in reversing toxin impact or in preventing it in the first place. As mentioned elsewhere, probably the primary reason magnesium has this antitoxin effect is that it is a uniquely powerful natural calcium antagonist – as magnesium levels inside the affected cells increase, calcium levels drop and thereby alleviate IOS. This is why any acute or chronic cases of poisoning or extreme toxin exposure should always include intrave-

This is why any acute or chronic cases of poisoning or extreme toxin exposure should always include intravenous or oral magnesium administration as part of the treatment protocol.

nous or oral magnesium administration as part of the treatment protocol.

In assessing the ability of magnesium to serve as a powerful antitoxin, it is important to remember that

all diseases, medical conditions, infections, or direct toxin and poison exposures result in the same intracellular pathophysiology.

No pathology exists anywhere in the body if intracellular levels of oxidative stress inside the cells are "normal," as in a degree reflecting the results of normal metabolism. As such, magnesium will always be helpful in the remediation of any disease or toxic condition that might present itself (except in the extremely rare event of magnesium excess or overdose (see Chapter 18 for specific details). And in the case of infection-induced toxicity, magnesium has the additional benefit of having a powerful anti-pathogen impact to go along with its powerful antitoxin impact. As such,

> **Magnesium is the natural partner
> with vitamin C in the treatment of
> all medical conditions.**

Toxin Impact and the QT Interval

Many drugs cause abnormalities in the electro-cardiogram (ECG), even when they are being employed in therapeutic doses within blood level target ranges. A considerably larger list of drugs, along with many known poisons, reliably cause these abnormalities when ingested to excess. When an overdose of any of these drugs or poisons results in a fatality, the cause of death is often due to a cardiac arrhythmia caused by an abnormality know as a prolonged QT interval (see Figures 10.1 and 10.2). Sometimes this abnormality evolves into a highly unstable heart rhythm known as torsade de pointes, and sometimes it evolves into a dangerous, but usually somewhat less unstable, ventricular tachycardia.

Generally, it appears that the more prolonged the QT interval, the greater the chance of developing torsade de pointes.[1] One study showed that poisoned patients presenting to the emergency room with QTc prolongation had a threefold increased risk of cardiac arrest and all-cause mortality for the first 30 days.[2] If the QT interval cannot be effectively treated (shortened), abnormal heart rhythms can eventually degenerate into ventricular fibrillation, promptly resulting in death.

The QT interval is that part of the ECG that reflects the repolarization, or recovery phase, of the heart muscle cells after the much more rapid depo-

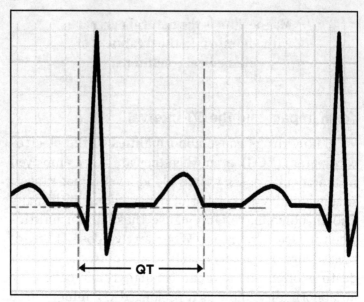

Figure 10.1: ECG with Normal QT Interval

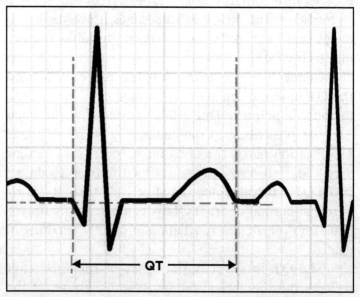

Figure 10.2: ECG with Prolonged QT Interval

larization, or contraction phase, of those cells. As this phase of recovery is prolonged, reflected in a longer or prolonged QT interval on the ECG, the heart muscle cells become increasingly unstable electrically and

Acutely shortening the QT interval in poisoned patients while the body works to excrete the toxin is often the critical factor in determining survival.

much more prone to abnormal heart depolarizations and contractions, along with any of a number of abnormal, unstable heart rhythms. Even though a low **serum** calcium level is often noted when there is a sufficient toxin effect to prolong the QT interval, it appears that agents with cardiac toxicity often promote movement of calcium from intracellular calcium storage sites to the cytoplasm.[3]

This induces a state of calcium excess in the cytoplasm even though the blood calcium levels might be noted to be low. In many of these prolonged QT states caused by excess toxin or drug ingestion, magnesium has been shown to be an effective agent in accelerating the return of this prolonged QT state to a normal or near-normal duration, probably accomplishing this by its calcium antagonist effect, blocking the uptake of new calcium into the cell, while also blocking the release of calcium stores from the sarcoplasmic reticulum (calcium storage site) into the cytoplasm.[4-7] Acutely shortening the QT interval in poisoned patients while the body works to excrete the toxin is often the critical factor in determining survival.

Very many drugs with a narrow risk/benefit ratio with regard to safe dosing and many frankly toxic (poisonous) agents have been documented to prolong the QT interval as a critical part of their toxic impact.[8] Furthermore, many of the acute presentations of overdosing on these agents are monitored as to whether a treatment is effective by the degree or promptness to which the QT interval begins to shorten and eventually reach a normal, electrically stable duration. QT prolongation following an overdose has been correlated with the serum concentration of the overdosed agent.[9] Here is a partial listing of the agents that have been documented to prolong the QT interval, especially when taken in especially large doses or frank overdoses:

- ✓ Tiamulin (antibiotic)[10]
- ✓ Propafenone (antiarrhythmic)[11]
- ✓ Aconitine (cardiotoxin, neurotoxin)[12]
- ✓ Wild mushroom[13]
- ✓ Marijuana (psychoactive)[14]
- ✓ Methadone (opioid)[15,16]
- ✓ Ibogaine (hallucinogen)[17]
- ✓ Amitriptyline (antidepressant)[18]
- ✓ Glyphosate (herbicide)[19]
- ✓ Paraquat (herbicide)[20]
- ✓ Cocaine (stimulant, anesthestic)[21]
- ✓ Mad axe plant (*Hyoscyamus reticulatus*)[22]
- ✓ Oxycodone (narcotic analgesic)[23]
- ✓ Ethanol (nervous system depressant, animal study)[24]

✓ Indoramin (alpha-blocker for enlarged prostate)[25,26]

✓ Lithium (bipolar disorder)[27]

✓ Organophosphate (pesticide)[28]

✓ Dosulepin (antidepressant)[29]

✓ Fluoride (toxic mineral)[30]

✓ Lead (heavy metal)[31,32]

✓ Pyrilamine (antihistamine)[33]

✓ Rhododendron honey ("mad honey")[34]

✓ Risperidone (antipsychotic)[35]

✓ Escitalopram (antidepressant)[36]

✓ Cesium (mineral)[37]

✓ Sulpiride (antipsychotic)[38]

✓ Amantadine (antiviral and for Parkinson's)[39]

✓ Trazodone (antidepressant)[40]

✓ Azithromycin (macrolide antibiotic)[41]

✓ Carbon monoxide[42]

✓ Venlafaxine (antidepressant)[43]

✓ Arsenic (pesticide, acute and chronic)[44,45]

✓ Amisulpride (antipsychotic)[46]

✓ Citalopram (antidepressant)[47]

✓ Moclobemide (antidepressant)[48]

✓ Diphenhydramine (antihistamine)[49]

✓ Thioridazine (antipsychotic)[50]

✓ Quetiapine (antipsychotic)[51]

✓ Bupropion (antidepressant)[52,53]

✓ Nefazodone (antidepressant)[54]

✓ Sotalol (antiarrhythmic)[55]

✓ Buflomedil [vasodilator)[56]

✓ Pimozide (antipsychotic)[57]

✓ Astemizole (antihistamine)[58]

✓ Amiodarone (antiarrhythmic)[59]
✓ Haloperidol (antipsychotic)[60,61]
✓ Thiometon (insecticide, animal study)[62]
✓ Pervitin (amphetamine)[63]

Antitoxin Mechanisms

Magnesium serves as a highly effective anti-toxin via multiple mechanisms. For many of the acute poisonings or other intoxications that present with arrhythmias and/or a prolonged QT interval, as outlined above, magnesium serves to stabilize the heart rhythm and accelerate the shortening or normalization of this critical ECG parameter. When the chance of death from acute arrhythmia can be eliminated, many overdoses can then be approached in a much less urgent manner.

Magnesium has long been used successfully in the treatment and stabilization of overdose patients with prolonged QT interval and torsade de pointes. Both magnesium boluses (concentrated single doses injected into the bloodstream) and infusions have been shown to be effective.[64] In organophosphorus poisoning, which often prolongs the QT interval, magnesium infusions were shown to decrease hospital length of stay and/or mortality, even when there was no attention paid to QT interval status.[65-67] In another study, intravenous magnesium sulfate not only clearly decreased the mortality from acute organophosphate poisoning, it was demonstrated to be dramatically more effective as the dosage was progressively increased. While the study size was small, the highest doses used completely prevented deaths from the poison exposure.[68] In a case report of organophosphate poisoning, intravenous magnesium sulfate clearly resolved the life-threatening appearance of torsade de pointes arrhythmia.[69]

In tricyclic antidepressant poisoning, one study showed that intravenous magnesium reduced mortality from 33.3% to 13.9% in a treated group of patients compared to a control group of the same size (36). Although QTc (length of QT interval adjusted for heart rate) prolongation was not discussed, it was noted that the main cause of fatality from this type of poisoning resulted from cardiac arrhythmias.[70]

A Conspiracy of Inconclusion

Unfortunately, medical politics continues to play a major role in whether magnesium is administered in poisoned patients with drug-induced QT prolongation. This should not be surprising considering the very limited roles that insulin for non-glucose-regulating indications and vitamin C play in current treatment protocols, in spite of the mountains of clinical and laboratory data that indicate they should play leading roles in nearly all protocols. A survey of medical toxicologists revealed that 59% of them would not recommend intravenous magnesium to a poisoned patient with a very prolonged QT interval. Yet 90% believed that 1 or 2 boluses of intravenous magnesium would be completely safe to administer to such a patient.[71] Consider the voluminous data supporting magnesium having a safe as well as strongly positive role in such patients, one can only speculate as to why it remains so unused. Literally, the collective medical literature can be considered a **_conspiracy of inconclusion_**. It doesn't matter how definitive the study, there can never be sufficient data to merit the conclusion that a new therapy or a new clinical approach should be taken for a given medical condition.

For agents such as magnesium, vitamin C, and insulin, the conclusion remains something like:

"A positive effect might be present. Further studies and larger studies are needed."

This has gone on for roughly 80 years for each of these three incredibly powerful, inexpensive, and safe therapeutic agents.

In acute organophosphorus poisoning, a large meta-analysis also indicated that the calcium antagonist properties of magnesium are likely very important in lessening symptoms and mortality, as prescription calcium channel blockers appear to have a similar positive impact.[72] This is consistent with the fact that acutely poisoned cells consistently have excessive cytoplasmic levels of calcium, which ultimately result in lethal levels of increased IOS when calcium levels increase beyond a certain point. Also, magnesium chloride was shown *in vitro* to activate the toxin-inactivated enzyme needed for exporting calcium out of the cells.[73-75]

Different forms of oral magnesium could also be useful for many orally-ingested toxins and poisons, as some can adsorb (bind) the agent, promote its elimination, and prevent greater amounts from being absorbed.[76] And even if a given form of oral magnesium is not able to bind the toxin, all of the oral forms can still promote accelerated evacuation of the gut while facilitating the absorption of magnesium to perform its toxin-neutralizing effects body-wide. Such oral applications would serve to augment the toxin-binding effect of activated charcoal, not replace it.

One of the most common toxins in society today is alcohol, which can also prolong the QTc interval in high enough doses. Both acute and chronic administrations of alcohol effectively block magnesium accumulation in the body. In addition, alcohol consumption is recognized as a major cause of magnesium loss from various tissues. This is reflected in very large increases of urinary magnesium excretion. In fact, one animal study documents the increase to be 200% to 300% more than normal.[77] Magnesium treatment appears to alleviate the toxic damage of alcohol in alcoholics as reflected in lowering liver enzyme levels.[78]

Organophosphorus pesticide poisoning is a major

In addition, alcohol consumption is recognized as a major cause of magnesium loss from various tissues.

public health concern in some developing countries. An IV infusion of only 4 grams of magnesium sulfate over a 30-minute period, when administered within 24 hours of admission to the ICU, has been of great benefit in enhancing the impact of the atropine and oxime therapy typically given for this type of poisoning. The magnesium has been shown to decrease the atropine

Intravenous magnesium administered to patients with acute aluminum phosphate poisoning cut in half their chances of death relative to poisoned patients not given magnesium.

requirement and the need for intubation, while shortening the ICU stay.[79]

It has been extensively demonstrated in the scientific literature that antioxidants in general, and vitamin C most significantly, are the most powerful antitoxins and anti-poisoning agents in existence, including those available only by prescription.[80] It bears repeating that magnesium, while not technically an antioxidant, and not having electrons available to directly quench toxins or to repair oxidized biomolecules, exerts a very powerful ***antioxidant effect***.

Intravenous magnesium administered to patients with acute aluminum phosphate poisoning cut in half their chances of death relative to poisoned patients not given magnesium. This study was conducted without any attention to cardiac arrhythmias or QTc prolongation, although two case reports showed that magnesium was able to successfully treat the ventricular and supraventricular tachycardia associated with this type of poisoning.[81,82]

Aluminum poisoning is especially cardiotoxic and frequently fatal.[83,84] In a series of children poisoned with aluminum phosphide, magnesium administration was associated significantly with improved survival.[85] Another study suggested that magnesium improved survival in patients poisoned with this agent, in the absence of a "specific antidote."[86]

Ironically, magnesium does a great deal of benefit for many poisoned patients while getting no credit. Although still not administered frequently enough, magnesium is often given for the "arrhythmia" aspect of many poisonings, and there appears to be no awareness that such magnesium administration also blocks and reverses much of the oxidative damage that otherwise would result in death or long-term morbidity to very many patients.

In another study, patients with this type of poisoning who demonstrated ECG abnormalities were all (18 of 18) found to have low serum magnesium levels. Inflammation of the heart muscle was also seen at autopsy independent of ECG changes. ECG changes were most common when magnesium levels were lowest.[87] Multiple experimental and clinical studies have shown that a wide array of agents that are either directly or indirectly antioxidant in nature alleviate the impact of this type of poisoning.[88] If all poisonings were sufficiently studied, it would likely show that all treatments that are capable of decreasing oxidative stress will partially or completely block the clinical impact of those poisonings. Magnesium administration

...those studies that were found all support the concept that it should be a major part of any clinical protocol for the treatment of an acute or chronic poison exposure.

consistently decreases oxidative stress throughout the body.

Conversely, deficiency states of magnesium are consistently seen when increased body-wide oxidative stress is present.[89] The ability of magnesium to lessen the intracellular accumulation of calcium results in a synergistically powerful clinical impact by facilitating the intracellular accumulation of vitamin C and gluta- thione in the place of calcium. The net effect is that magnesium is one of the most powerful agents known for lowering elevated intracellular oxidative stress, the hallmark and **primary defining condition** of all diseases and all intoxications/poisonings.

While the studies directly examining the impact of magnesium on intoxications and poisonings are rela- tively limited, those studies that were found all support the concept that it should be a major part of any clinical protocol for the treatment of an acute or chronic poison exposure. Some of these studies (human and animal) include the following:

✓ In a retrospective study looking at patients receiving cisplatin chemotherapy for lung cancer, it was shown that magnesium supplementation reduced the risk of toxic kidney damage often seen with that drug.[90] Cisplatin-induced kidney injury is seen is roughly 30% of the patients who receive this drug. Also, an animal study (mice) showed that magnesium supplementation blocked cisplatin-induced injury and even improved the cisplatin-mediated tumor killing.[91] Another magnesium salt was also shown to help protect the liver from the toxicity of another chemotherapy drug, oxaliplatin, in mice and in cultured human liver cells.[92]

✓ Intraperitoneal injections of magnesium into rats prevented and reversed the laboratory and microscopic evidence of kidney toxicity when cadmium (a toxic metal) was injected at the same time.[93] In another study on cadmium toxicity in the rat, magnesium was shown to be able to prevent and reverse damage to the testis.[94] Magnesium has also been shown to protect against cadmium toxicity in the rat liver.[95] Another rat study showed that the parameters of increased oxidative stress in the plasma induced by cadmium were lessened by magnesium administration.[96]

✓ In rats exposed to endotoxins, greater magnesium deficiencies were associated with increased toxin-related lethality. The study also showed that magnesium replacement therapy provided significant protection against death from endotoxin exposure.[97] In mice, pretreatment with magnesium protected the liver from the acute injury mediated by lipopolysaccharide (an endotoxin) in a model of sepsis.[98] A cell study showed that magnesium could prevent lipopolysaccharide-induced cell death.[99] Conversely, in another cell study, a deficiency of magnesium was shown to increase the inflammation-inducing capacity of lipopolysaccharide exposure, while a high magnesium concentration at least partially inhibited the inflammatory response.[100,101]

✓ A magnesium salt was shown to attenuate the toxic effects of carbon tetrachloride on the livers of rats.[102]

✓ In both animal (rat) and cell models, a magnesium salt (isoglycyrrhizinate) was found to reduce liver-related toxicity from the Chinese herb, triptolide. It was also noted that this magnesium compound is used clinically in China to treat both chronic viral hepatitis and acute drug-induced liver injury.[103]

✓ In pregnant rats, a magnesium compound was shown to protect against liver damage caused by paracetamol and ethanol.[104]

✓ In carbon monoxide-poisoned rats, magnesium sulfate administration not only effectively treated the associated ECG abnormalities, but it also decreased the degree of cell death (necrosis) in the animal hearts.[105] In another rat study, magnesium reduced necrosis and oxidative stress in carbon monoxide-poisoned animals compared to controls who did not receive magnesium.[106]

✓ A dog acutely poisoned with barium (heavy metal) and that presented with generalized flaccid muscle paralysis and an irregular heart rhythm was treated effectively with magnesium sulfate, along with potassium chloride (presentation included a very low potassium level) and supportive care.[107]

✓ Oral magnesium sulfate was effective in helping some mice to survive after they were given known lethal doses of sodium fluoride, and a higher dose was more effective than a lower dose.[108]

✓ Magnesium (with zinc) decreased the toxic effects of lindane (insecticide) poisoning on the liver and brain in exposed rats.[109]

✓ In plants as well, magnesium has been shown to exert protective effects against toxins and heavy metals. One study demonstrated that magnesium relieved the adverse effects of lead on growth and the effectiveness of photosynthesis on plant seedlings.[110]

Conclusions

All of the positive effects of magnesium ultimately relate to its ability to reduce oxidative stress throughout the body, especially in the intracellular space. The

different ways in which magnesium results in this
effect include the following:

1. Magnesium is a powerful calcium channel
   blocker and calcium antagonist in general. As
   increased intracellular levels of calcium are
   the direct cause of the increased intracellular
   oxidative stress seen in all toxin-inflicted
   damage, anything that reduces or normalizes these calcium levels will improve or even
   completely resolve the clinical syndrome
   arising from the toxin or poisoning.
   Magnesium works to normalize intracellular
   calcium levels by at least three mechanisms:
   ✓ Blocking the transmembrane calcium
     channels that allow the uptake of calcium
     into the cell
   ✓ Inhibiting the transfer of calcium from
     storage sites in the cells into the cytoplasm
   ✓ Supporting the normal enzyme function
     needed to actively push calcium out of the
     cells

2. Magnesium directly works to shorten the
   abnormally prolonged QTc intervals seen
   with many poisonings and accounting for
   many deaths seen early-on. The positive
   impact on magnesium on the cardiac cells
   also results in a prompt lessening or elimination of any cardiac arrhythmia or abnormal
   heart contractions resulting from the acutely
   poisoned state. Magnesium also appears to
   have its rhythm-stabilizing effect when QTc
   prolongation is not present. QTc prolongation just generally reflects the times when

cardiotoxic effects are most pronounced and dangerous.

3. As magnesium actively lowers cellular calcium uptake and promotes cellular calcium extrusion, the decreased oxidative stress further facilitates the ability of vitamin C to be assimilated into the cell.

4. Without having the mechanisms clearly defined, magnesium has been repeatedly demonstrated to decrease oxidative stress related to many different toxin exposures in man, animals, test tube, and plants. Some studies show that oxidative damage is not only prevented, but repair of oxidative damage is also supported and accelerated.

5. Magnesium supports the immune system and increases phagocytic capacity, making it especially important in resolving the clinical syndromes resulting from toxins produced by pathogens (see Chapter 11).

6. In poisonings by orally-ingested toxins, oral magnesium administration can sometimes bind toxins (certain forms) and prevent further absorption. All oral forms can accelerate the elimination of unabsorbed toxins into the stool (cathartic effect), while allowing some magnesium to be absorbed systemically as well.

7. Magnesium interferes as well with the accumulation of some toxins.[111]

8. Magnesium supports and improves the effect of Nrf2 (a nuclear factor that increases the expression of multiple antioxidant enzymes in the cell).[112]

There is absolutely no sound scientific reason for not routinely including magnesium administration in the optimal treatment of all poisonings and intoxications, whether acute or chronic in nature. Quite the contrary, the information in the medical literature indicates that a treating physician is medically negligent not to include magnesium (and vitamin C) in all patients suffering from any degree of toxin exposure.

Infection Protection

Magnesium and Pathogens

Magnesium and Polio

While magnesium remains greatly underutilized in the treatment of a wide range of medical conditions, it is gradually becoming a more common nonspecific positive "health tonic" added to an increasing number of intravenous infusions given around the world. And as the theme of this book has repeatedly emphasized, getting as much magnesium to accumulate inside the cells over time is a highly desirable goal, short of the limited number of scenarios where magnesium assimilation can be pushed to toxic levels (see discussion of these scenarios in Chapter 18).

As has been discussed, an infectious disease does its damage by ramping up oxidative stress throughout the body. Virtually everything associated with an infection's progression increases the presence of pathogen-related toxins, both in the extracellular and intracellular spaces. ***These toxins are always pro-oxidant.***

Except for the possible structure-altering characteristics of some infections (like focused oxidation that
eventually erodes into a blood vessel with hemorrhagic
and even fatal consequences), an infection only inca-

*When elevated IOS can be restored to
normal levels, intracellular physiology
normalizes, and the cell can be
essentially regarded as cured.*

pacitates to the degree that it depletes available antioxidants. This means that vitamin C levels can drop to the
point of being extremely low and even immeasurable
with standard urine testing. Interestingly, magnesium
levels appear to drop in concert with the vitamin C
decline, which suggests a strong therapeutic synergy
between vitamin C and magnesium in the normalization of previously elevated intracellular oxidative stress
(IOS). When elevated IOS can be restored to normal
levels, intracellular physiology normalizes, and the
cell can be essentially regarded as cured. This is true
whether it was an infection or another toxin source
that elevated the IOS in the first place. Furthermore,
at the point that the IOS has been normalized, it can
reliably be assumed that the immune system has effectively neutralized and/or killed the infecting pathogens.
That's because the normalization of IOS cannot really
be achieved and maintained as long as active pathogen
proliferation is taking place.
Vitamin C can attack pathogens directly by
increasing their internal oxidative stress to the point

of pathogen rupture or inactivation via upregulation of the Fenton reaction inside the cells. As already discussed, vitamin C also enhances the capacity of all the immune cells by concentrating inside them and allowing them to supply a greater immediate antioxidant delivery to areas of focal infection and inflammation. In a more indirect way, magnesium can combat infections by increasing the phagocytic (engulf and destroy) capacity of the scavenging white blood cells.

Regarding magnesium's pathogen-fighting qualities, a review of some older literature reveals that magnesium chloride *alone*, given orally several times daily, has cured acute polio, even when significant paralysis had already developed (see below).[1,2] The physician reporting these stunning results, Dr. Auguste Neveu, also found magnesium chloride to be highly effective against other infections as well, including in animals.[3,4] Another author also wrote on the effects of magnesium chloride on infectious diseases in animals and humans.[5]

Almost certainly, this anti-pathogen effect occurs

In a more indirect way, magnesium can combat infections by increasing the phagocytic (engulf and destroy) capacity of the scavenging white blood cells.

because, like vitamin C, magnesium can independently and promptly normalize the ever-present pathology of increased IOS present in toxin exposures of any origin, including from infectious diseases. For this reason, it has already been suggested that magnesium and vitamin C would make great therapeutic partners. The additions of insulin and hydrocortisone to such a combo should further accomplish the goal of

Protocols featuring various combinations and doses of these agents, especially when sex hormone and thyroid hormone statuses are completely normal, might well prove to be profoundly more effective than any other anti-infection and antitoxin protocols to date.

rapidly normalizing IOS, largely due to their ability to get more vitamin C and magnesium inside the cells, while lowering elevated intracellular calcium levels. Protocols featuring various combinations and doses of these agents, especially when sex hormone and thyroid hormone statuses are completely normal, might well prove to be profoundly more effective than any other anti-infection and antitoxin protocols to date.

For many infections, it seems likely that the synergy of vitamin C and magnesium is largely achieved because it accomplishes the desired goal of decreasing elevated IOS by different mechanisms. Vitamin C, as the premier antioxidant in the body, directly lowers IOS the more it can be delivered inside the toxic/damaged/infected cells. Magnesium, even though it is not known as having a direct antioxidant effect, promptly brings down elevated cytoplasmic calcium levels inside damaged or infected cells, which in turn promptly lowers IOS as well.

Magnesium-Polio Case Report Summaries

1. The first case of polio treated by Dr. Neveu was a four-year-old boy in September of 1943. It was noted that the infection was of rapid onset. The child was crying, would not eat, and he was unable to stand on his left leg. Dr. Neveu mixed 5 grams of magnesium chloride in 250 cc of water. 80 cc doses were given orally at 1 pm and again at 4 pm. At the time of the second dose, the state of leg paralysis was already considered to be "complete." Another dose was given 3 hours later. The next morning both the paralysis and the fever that had been present were resolved. There was no return of symptoms. This represented a complete cure with less than 24 hours of receiving magnesium chloride treatment, as there was no report of relapse or continued illness.

2. Dr. Neveu treated his second case of polio two years later. He saw an 11-year-old boy with headache, discomfort in the neck and the back, and an inflamed throat with reported difficulty in just swallowing saliva. He reported that his legs had no feeling, and that they seemed as if they were made of wool, with a complete inability to stand up. He had upper arm pain, and his eyes were very sensitive to light. Rectal temperature was 102°F.

   - Dr. Neveu prepared a solution of magnesium chloride with 20 grams dissolved in a liter of water. The child had been stricken suddenly that morning and was receiving his first dose of magnesium chloride, 125 cc orally, early that afternoon, with follow-up doses every six hours. Evening temperature had increased to 103°F.

- The next day morning temperature was 100.1°F and evening temperature was 101°F. The child had slept well the first night, all symptoms had generally lessened, and he was able to stand up when he awoke. He asked for food the second night.

- The following day (48 hours after onset of symptoms) morning temperature was 99.3°F and evening temperature was 99.8°F. Overall condition was clearly improved, and the magnesium dosing frequency was decreased to 125 cc every eight hours.

- The next day it appeared that the child had been largely cured of his condition, although it was noted that he was still slightly sensitive to light. Dosing was continued at 125 cc every eight hours.

- The next day (four days after being stricken) recovery was deemed complete, and magnesium therapy was discontinued. The following day showed a morning temperature of 98.6°F and an evening temperature of 99.4°F.

3. The third case reported on by Dr. Neveu was a 47-year-old woman who presented with complete paralysis in the right lower leg and in the lower back. A **complete cure** was observed

on the magnesium therapy, but it required 12 days of treatment.

4. A 13-year-old boy had an abrupt onset of chills with shivering and headache. Temperature was 40°C (104°F). The next day the temperature was 38.8°C, and there was severe pain in the head, neck, and back. His eyes could not tolerate light (photophobia). The temperature rose back to 40.4°C. The boy's physician (not Dr. Neveu) told his mother that he suspected the child contracted polio, and that he would check back in two days. The following morning the mother said all symptoms were even more severe. She had seen an article about Dr. Neveu and his magnesium therapy and convinced him to see her son at home. Dr. Neveu termed the child's condition a "swiftly progressing poliomyelitis," and he gave the child his first dose of 125 cc of the magnesium chloride solution (20 grams in one liter of water), to be repeated every six hours. Temperature was still 39.6°C at that time. The following morning the head, neck, and back pain had subsided. Morning temperature was 37.1°C and evening temperature was 37.8°C. The child began to engage in normal activities. On the following day only two doses of the magnesium were taken, and the return of slight head discomfort was noted, along with a temperature back up to 38.2°C. Three doses were taken the next day, and the following day the magnesium was discontinued with morning temperature of 37.2°C and evening temperature of 37°C. There

was no return of symptomatology, as a complete cure had been achieved.

5. A 9-year-old boy presented with right lower leg paralysis. He was completely cured by Dr. Neveu with one week of magnesium therapy.

6. A 13-year-old girl presented with stiffness in the back and with lower limb nervous trembling. The magnesium administration resulted in a rapid clinical response. The parents decided to discontinue the magnesium, and Dr. Neveu later restarted it, but the child ended up keeping a paralysis of the extensor muscle of her left big toe, probably because of the interruption in the treatment.

7. A 20-year-old woman presented with a persistent headache that progressed to vomiting and a stiff neck and back. The family physician suspected polio. The pain became so severe that the patient threatened to commit suicide. After the first dose of magnesium given by Dr. Neveu, the woman had enough pain relief to allow her to sleep. A complete cure was realized with 12 days of magnesium therapy.

8. A 3-year-old girl had been hospitalized for polio and was later discharged to home with paralysis in both legs. Magnesium therapy was started a full **25 days** after the polio was contracted. After two weeks of treatment, a great deal of leg mobility had returned. Following physical rehabilitation, she remained with a slight limp.

9. A 20-year-old male farmer presented with paralysis in both legs and in the right arm.

Magnesium was started *32 days* after the initial polio attack. He responded well, and he was able to walk with crutches after four months of treatment. Two years later he could walk with just the assistance of a cane.

10. A 19-year-old woman who first saw Dr. Neveu *four months* after the initial polio attack. Her left leg was not only paralyzed, it had also begun to atrophy (muscle wasting). She was treated for 15 days with the magnesium and demonstrated marked improvement of the leg. She was eventually able to ride a bicycle and walk with a limp.

11. A 2-year-old girl who received magnesium treatment 17 days after the initial polio attack. When first seen she was unable to stand and could not move her right arm. While her legs regained completely normal function, her right shoulder remained paralyzed.

12. A 4-year-old girl with right arm and right leg paralysis who received magnesium treatment 10 days after the initial polio attack. She eventually had a dramatic return of arm and leg function, but with only roughly 60% of normal strength.

13. A 2½-year-old boy was started on magnesium therapy 10 days after diagnosis. The abdominal paralysis improved significantly after two days, and a complete recovery was seen after 2½ months.

14. A 20-month-old male infant was diagnosed with polio that was confirmed by spinal tap 12 days after onset of the clinical syndrome. His left foot was completely paralyzed, but he responded to

magnesium well and was nearly normal after five months, but required the support of orthopedic shoes.

15. A 12-year-old girl presented to Dr. Neveu immediately after the onset of sore throat and stiff neck. Magnesium was started, but the stiffness increased and went down the spine at first. However, with continuation of the magnesium, the stiffness had resolved by the next morning. The sore throat was gone the following morning.

Magnesium and Medical Politics

If taken at face value, believing that Dr. Neveu is competently and accurately relating his experiences with magnesium chloride and the treatment of polio, the potential public health impact of his work

Just as vitamin C has effectively treated many diseases and has reliably cured polio and many other infectious diseases, it would appear that magnesium chloride has perhaps as great, or possibly even greater, a role in the treatment of such diseases as vitamin C.

is enormous. There are few agents as cheap and as widely available as magnesium chloride. However, whenever evaluating whether a therapy will be adopted, no matter how incredibly effective and safe it might be, its potential economic impact on other traditional therapies is really the primary factor to be considered. Incredibly rich pharmaceutical companies will not just step aside and permit or facilitate the use of something

Also, while all forms of magnesium are of benefit to the general health of the body and the treatment/prevention of a wide array of diseases, the anti-pathogen capabilities of magnesium have been best documented with magnesium chloride.

that can end up costing them hundreds of millions to billions of dollars as their many toxic and expensive drugs go unprescribed. The ignoring and even active suppression of such highly effective therapies as vitamin C has been going on for nearly 80 years now, in spite of it being one of the most highly researched and publicized therapeutic agents on the planet. This is discussed in great detail in another book.[6]

It should come as no surprise that something as cheap and effective as magnesium chloride has been ignored and dismissed for an even **longer** period of time. Just as vitamin C has effectively treated many diseases and has reliably cured polio and many other infectious diseases,[7-12] it would appear that magnesium chloride has perhaps as great, or possibly even greater, a role in the treatment of such diseases as vitamin C. However, as all diseases and toxins consume vitamin C, there is no good reason not to approach all medical conditions, infections, and infectious diseases with a protocol that includes both magnesium chloride and vitamin C, regardless of whatever else is being used to treat the patient.

Also, while all forms of magnesium are of benefit to the general health of the body and the treatment/ prevention of a wide array of diseases, the anti-pathogen capabilities of magnesium have been best documented with magnesium chloride. Even though other forms *might* do as good a job against pathogens, this has not been clearly established in the literature. For example, one article showed that magnesium sulfate protected the measles virus from heat-induced inactivation, while magnesium chloride enhanced the inactivation of the virus at all temperatures tested.[13] It would appear that the anion (sulfate or chloride, in this instance) plays an important role in the anti-infection capacity of a magnesium compound. This is also seen with sodium associated with chloride, as many sodium compounds do not have a substantial antibacterial activity, while sodium chloride (as in a throat gargle for sore throat) does.

It is also very important to realize that cell studies can be *very* misleading, as magnesium chloride has an astoundingly positive clinical impact in cases of polio, as noted above. Yet, the ability of some viruses (poliovirus, echovirus, coxsackievirus) to kill cells in agar models *in vitro* is enhanced by the presence of magnesium chloride.[14] Obviously, the clinical study remains the most significant, as the resolution of an infection is the criterion of most importance regardless of what a cell study might show. Sometimes cell studies are of enormous practical value, but they should never take priority over a contradictory, positive result in a clear-cut clinical outcome study.

Magnesium and Pathogens

Although Dr. Neveu wrote books about his expe-

Dr. Delbet found that magnesium chloride left tissue undamaged while effectively destroying pathogens and greatly enhancing the phagocytic capacities of the immune system.

riences with infections and magnesium chloride, it does not appear that he published any papers that were published in a peer-reviewed fashion, or at least such studies were not found. Pierre Delbet, MD, a professor of clinical surgery, was one of Dr. Neveu's teachers, and it appears that he was Neveu's inspiration to using magnesium chloride and writing about its stunning clinical impact.

Dr. Delbet began his work with magnesium chloride in the early 1900s during World War I, as he was looking for an agent that would effectively clean and treat the wounds of the soldiers. Common wound treatments at that time were known to damage tissue along with the antiseptic effect. Dr. Delbet found that magnesium chloride left tissue undamaged while effectively destroying pathogens and greatly enhancing the phagocytic capacities of the immune system. After

World War I, Dr. Delbet began looking at the effects of ingested magnesium chloride as well.

Dr. Delbet, in collaboration with a Dr. Karalanopoulo, submitted a paper to the French Academy of Sciences in September of 1915 entitled *Cytophylaxis*. The paper addressed the abilities of phagocytic white blood cells to effectively destroy pathogens in the blood. Using his own *in vitro* technique, Dr. Delbet mixed pathogens and white blood cells of defined numbers in a variety of solutions. Many of the solutions damaged the cells as well as the pathogens. Eventually, he found that sodium chloride was one of the best solutions for pathogen killing while leaving the immune cells undamaged. He then used a magnesium chloride solution and found it to be much more effective in killing pathogens. He found magnesium chloride to be an effective wound treatment solution, and he also found that magnesium

...magnesium chloride injected into a dog caused the phagocytic cells that were later harvested to have an enhanced pathogen-killing capacity by 100% to nearly 400%, depending on the experiment.

chloride injected into a dog caused the phagocytic cells that were later harvested to have an enhanced pathogen-killing capacity by 100% to nearly 400%, depending on the experiment.[15,16]

Dr. Neveu proceeded to use magnesium chloride for a wide variety of infections and medical conditions. While there are no papers to specifically cite, Dr. Neveu found that magnesium chloride was very effective in treating all infections he encountered in his practice, including diphtheria as well as polio. Dr. Neveu's wife continued his work with magnesium chloride after he passed. Anecdotally, the "Delbet-Neveu" magnesium chloride protocol was found to be effective in treating meningitis, tetanus, toxin exposures, tuberculosis, asthma, bronchitis, pneumonia, tonsillitis and pharyngitis, the common cold, pertussis, measles, rubella, mumps, scarlet fever, osteomyelitis, and infected wounds.

Raul Vergini, MD also worked a great deal with magnesium chloride for a wide variety of conditions.[17] He used a great deal of magnesium chloride intravenously (and he emphasized it had to be magnesium *chloride*, not any other form). The intravenous "formula" was to use a 25% solution of magnesium chloride hexahydrate (25 grams in 100 cc distilled water, sterilized). Doses of 10 to 20 cc were given intravenously slowly, over a period of 10 to 20 minutes, once or twice a day). Intramuscular administration was not advised, due to the pain of the injection. The oral approach was as follows (2.5% solution, 25 grams in 1000 cc of water):

Adults and children over 5 years:125 cc
4 years: . . . . **100 cc**
3 years: . . . . **80 cc**
1 to 2 years: . . . . **60 cc**
6 months to 1 year: . . . . **30 cc**
Under 6 months . . . . **15 cc**

✓ For chronic diseases, this oral route was often administered twice daily for months or even years.

✓ For acute diseases and infections, administration was every six hours.

Multiple other studies using different forms and applications of magnesium agents, especially in the context of bone infections and implant-related infections, have consistently shown the broad anti-pathogen properties of magnesium.

✓ For disease prevention, administration was once a day, indefinitely.[18]

While clinical studies that directly try to measure the impact of magnesium chloride and other forms of magnesium on infection and infectious diseases have not been found, there is a modest amount of research from which some logical assertions can made about the therapeutic impact of magnesium on pathogens, aside from the extensive anecdotal evidence presented above.

In animals, pure magnesium granules implanted into models of osteomyelitis accelerated new bone growth while lowering the pathogen count in the bone.[19] Multiple other studies using different forms and applications of magnesium agents, especially in the context of bone infections and implant-related infections, have consistently shown the broad anti-pathogen properties of magnesium.[20-25] It should also be noted that acute and chronic bone infections are especially resistant to effective treatment.

Magnesium is a known cofactor in natural killer cell and T-cell reactivity, and it appears important in preventing infections from getting started, as low serum magnesium levels were found to be associated with an increased risk of infection after kidney transplantation.[26] Similarly, patients with low magnesium levels on admission to the hospital had an increased risk of developing septic shock.[27] In an animal model of pneumococcal meningitis, magnesium chloride improves animal survival and clinical condition, lessening the impact of the infection-related toxin, pneumolysin.[28]

Magnesium has also been shown to be effective against different types of pathogens. Not surprisingly, in light of the response of polio cases to magnesium chloride therapy, different forms of magnesium have proven to have antiviral effects. Magnesium has demonstrated significant antiviral activity or viral protection against enterovirus, the virus of hoof-and-mouth disease (animals), hand, foot, and mouth disease (children), and Epstein-Barr virus.[29-32] Magnesium has also been demonstrated to be anti-pathogenic against protozoa, yeasts, and other bacteria.[33-35]

RECAP

1. While not extensively documented in the medical/scientific literature, magnesium, especially in the form of magnesium chloride, appears to be a powerful anti-pathogen agent,

both independently and in combination with other agents. Anecdotally, it appears to be significantly effective against nearly all acute infectious diseases.

2. Magnesium chloride has been reported to be enormously effective in consistently curing polio, as well as in dramatically reducing the severe side effects (such as muscular paralysis) when given as long as months after the infection was acquired.

3. Magnesium appears to strongly support the phagocytic capacity of white blood cells.

4. There are simple and very inexpensive protocols for administering magnesium chloride either intravenously or orally, both for the treatment of infection and diseases, as well as for infection and disease prophylaxis.

Dynamic Cellular Defense

Dealing with Oxidative Stress

The medical dictionary definition of inflammation calls it "a protective response elicited by injury or destruction of tissues, serving to neutralize the injurious agent while attempting to repair, or allow to be repaired, the injured tissue." This definition does not clarify how the injurious agent is inflicting its damage, or how the protective response is nullifying that agent or repairing the tissue damage.

Inflammation is a hot topic, much continues to be written about it, and many research studies examine its relationship to a wide variety of medical conditions and diseases. Nevertheless, little effort has been made to define what is happening at the molecular level when inflammation is present.

The physiology of inflammation at the molecular level will be discussed here. Protocols designed to relieve inflammation based on that physiology along with specific therapeutic agents will be addressed in a separate chapter.

Increased Oxidative Stress

Increased oxidative stress is a state of imbalance that occurs when the number of electrons being stolen from biomolecules (oxidation) is growing faster than available free electrons can replace them (reduction). In the same way that rust (oxidation) compromises the integrity of iron, the oxidation of biomolecules impairs or prevents them from performing their normal biochemical functions. When enough biomolecules are oxidized, a disease or medical disorder exists. The clinical identity of the disease depends entirely on where the oxidized biomolecules are located, the percentage of them that are oxidized in a given tissue, how long they have been oxidized, and, of course,

In the same way that rust (oxidation) compromises the integrity of iron, the oxidation of biomolecules impairs or prevents them from performing their normal biochemical functions. When enough biomolecules are oxidized, a disease or medical disorder exists.

which types of biomolecules have been oxidized (sugar, protein, fat, structural molecule, enzyme, RNA, DNA, and all the associated "support" molecules). In other words, it is no exaggeration to boldly state:

Excess oxidation IS disease.

Many scientific articles assert that excess oxidation, or increased oxidative stress, causes disease, and to a significant degree this is true. However, it is much more accurate to regard disease of all varieties as **BEING** the increased oxidative stress and not just resulting from it. This understanding also completely explains why diseases occur, what diseases occur, what alleviates diseases, and even what might completely resolve some diseases (including many diseases for which little or no effective therapy exists today).

Increased oxidative stress always exists when the production of oxidizing agents (free radicals and other unstable electron-depleted molecules) exceeds the antioxidant capacity of the body to neutralize (reduce) them, or to prevent their production/accumulation in the first place.[1] In other words, increased oxidative stress occurs when the physiological state of a given area of the body is being oxidized at a greater rate than it is being reduced. This is the foundational concept in Redox (Reduction-Oxidation) Physiology. Some very important basic redox facts include the following:

1. Pro-oxidants take electrons away from biomolecules (oxidation)
2. Antioxidants donate electrons back to oxidized biomolecules (reduction)
3. Oxidized biomolecules are either unable or have reduced ability to perform their normal biochemical function.
4. Reduction of oxidized biomolecules restores their normal biochemical function.

5. All toxins are pro-oxidants, or at least cause oxidation to occur indirectly.

6. All negative physiological and clinical effects of toxins are due to the location and the quantity of oxidized biomolecules, which types of biomolecules have been oxidized, and how long they have been oxidized.

7. Infections and areas of pathogen growth are the greatest sources on ongoing toxin (pro-oxidant) production/exposure.

8. Any food or supplement is only beneficial to the body to the degree that it ultimately results in antioxidant (electron-donating) capacity at the molecular level. Conversely, to the degree that oxidized molecules are assimilated from food or supplementation, a toxic effect is realized as those molecules seek to have their electron quota restored.

Vitamin C (ascorbate) is the premier antioxidant in the body and the primary player in redox biology in and around all of the cells of the body. Because of this, the complete understanding of the biochemistry of vitamin C facilitates the formation of a solid foundation for appreciating most of the basic physiological concepts essential to administering optimal clinical protocols for any disease. And as electrons are literally, not figuratively, the primary fuel on which every cell of the body runs, vitamin C also stands out as the most important nutrient in the body. All antioxidants have a nutrient/electron-donating value, but the chemical structure of vitamin C allows for its unique contribution to the overall health of the body. This contribution largely occurs because of the following considerations:

1. Vitamin C is a small molecule very close to glucose in structure (and competitively shares the insulin-facilitated transport mechanisms into cells with glucose). In vitamin C-producing animals, glucose is enzymatically converted into vitamin C.

2. Vitamin C accesses all the tissues and cells of the body (including the nervous system; the blood-brain barrier does not effectively impede the access of vitamin C to the nervous tissues)

3. Each vitamin C molecule is capable of donating two electrons rather than the single electron provided by many other antioxidants.

4. When vitamin C has donated only one electron, it forms the ascorbyl radical, which is relatively stable, and can eventually proceed to donate the other electron or be restored by electron donation from another electron back to its fully reduced form. This intermediate state of vitamin C can effectively be viewed as an electron buffer state, able to provide a more rapid source of electrons for new toxin-induced oxidative stresses.

5. Vitamin C, when present in sufficient concentrations in and around the cells of the body, can directly promote healthy microcurrents, which further optimize cellular health. A microcurrent is nothing

more than a flow/exchange of electrons to a degree that voltage differences can be measured across the cell membranes.

6. The combination of all these qualities of vitamin C make it the ultimate nonspecific antitoxin for literally any type of poisoning (toxin overdose). No toxin has been discovered that vitamin C has failed to neutralized when properly administered, either *in vivo* or *in vitro*.[2]

Probably the best way to view inflammation is to regard it as the physiological state resulting from the immune response to areas or tissues of the body with substantially increased levels of oxidative stress. As with any other compensatory mechanism, the response is designed to relieve the state it is reacting to as best as possible. In other words, the goal of the immune system response to inflammation is to alleviate that increased oxidative stress if at all possible. When the factors precipitating the increased oxidative stress are ongoing and unrelenting, the compensatory response will never completely repair the oxidized biomolecules in the affected tissues. Therefore, the chronic immune response becomes equally unrelenting and that response then becomes an integral part of the clinical disease or condition. Unfortunately, this reality is often missed because the vast amount of scientific literature rarely uses consistent language in its definitions. From a practical point of view, however, it can be asserted that:

**Chronic focal vitamin C depletion
assures the presence of a
chronic inflammatory immune response.**

**Chronic inflammation assures the
inflamed area is severely
depleted of vitamin C.**

Conceptually, then, the literature is much easier to understand by applying the following generalizations:

**Focal inflammation is focal scurvy.
Focal scurvy is focal inflammation.**

As vitamin C deficiency becomes more widespread or even body-wide, a state of generalized inflammation will always be present as well.

Laboratory and clinical findings strongly support these definitions and generalizations. It has been shown that extremely low plasma levels of vitamin C are consistently present in hospitalized patients with significant infections and following trauma.[3,4] And in addition to the depressed vitamin C levels, the blood levels of C-reactive protein (CRP), a reliable index of generalized inflammation in the body, are consistently elevated.

In areas like the coronary artery endothelium, or lining, where atherosclerosis eventually develops after the onset of inflammation, a severely diminished to measurably absent vitamin C presence will be the rule, as pathogen colonization in the endothelium is a strongly pro-oxidant factor that will quickly consume any vitamin C stores that might be present.

The presence of the DNA of multiple pathogens, generally consistent with an oral cavity origin, is nearly always present. In one study, pathogen-related DNA was present in 38 out of 38 specimens from atherectomy procedures on known coronary artery disease patients. Control material from postmortem patients without coronary artery disease contained no detectable pathogen DNA.[5] Other researchers have also consistently found oral pathogen DNA in both coronary and carotid artery atherosclerotic plaques.[6-9] Indeed, in pathology specimens, early investigators found no detectable vitamin C at all in some arteries that had been blocked off by blood clots.[10]

SECTION TWO:

Applying Magnesium's Unparalleled Curative Power

Curative Treatment

General Principles

The recurrent theme throughout this book centers upon increased oxidative stress – especially inside the cells – as the singular cause of all disease and all medical conditions. Elevated levels of cytoplasmic calcium are not only the primary cause of increased intracellular oxidative stress (increased IOS), but they are **always** present during this state. And as the evidence presented throughout this book has shown, **increased magnesium is the natural antidote** for elevated cytoplasmic calcium levels.

This chapter presents a series of treatment principles that all share the goal of addressing this universal causation of disease through the lowering or normalization of increased IOS. In fact, with virtually no exceptions, all effective clinical protocols that truly arrest and/or reverse a disease process must ultimately decrease elevated IOS. This must be accomplished with an increased antioxidant capacity – to restore (reduce) oxidized biomolecules – and/or by slowing the rate of biomolecule oxidation (less new toxin exposure).

Often, prescription drugs that provide symptom relief are only effective because they oxidize or otherwise block biochemical pathways that lessen or temporarily prevent the manifestation of those target

Often, prescription drugs that provide symptom relief are only effective because they oxidize or otherwise block biochemical pathways that lessen or temporarily prevent the manifestation of those target symptoms.

symptoms. With very few exceptions, they do not reverse the underlying cellular pathology in diseases and medical conditions. Prescription calcium channel blockers are the most significant exception to this sad reality. However, as mentioned previously, these drugs might decrease sex and thyroid hormone levels, meaning these levels must be regularly monitored, with ongoing replacement therapy administered as indicated.

Since the objective is to attack the underlying cause of disease (IOS) there are multiple ways to achieve true disease alleviation and even disease reversal. This is possible when:

1. antioxidant/nutrient agents can fully access the oxidized biomolecules
   — and when —

2. daily exposure to new oxidizing agents, or toxins, can be stopped or markedly reduced.

While there is an enormous amount of complexity to the many nuances and details of biology, medicine, and disease, the underlying cause of disease is straightforward, and the essence of the most effective treatment protocols is just as clear-cut.

The overriding message of this book is that:

1. All disease results from increased IOS,
2. accompanied with and caused by increased intracellular calcium levels, and
3. strongly opposed and mitigated by increasing magnesium assimilation,
4. as well as by any other intervention that can increase the antioxidant capacity inside the cells, especially vitamin C and glutathione,
5. and is always further aggravated by the appearance of new pro-oxidants (toxins).

Therefore, any agent that can directly or indirectly **lower elevated IOS** will be a primary agent for resolving disease and promoting healing.

Cellular Pathology

All cellular pathology originates and develops from the presence of increased IOS concurrent with rising levels of intracellular calcium. As has been demonstrated conclusively,[1] this increased is always caused by or worsened by elevated levels of intracellular calcium. When this oxidative stress escalates or becomes chronic, intracellular magnesium levels reciprocally decline while the two most important intracellular antioxidants – glutathione and vitamin C – are consumed (oxidized) by the elevated IOS. Therefore, all effective health-restoring treatment protocols, regardless of the disease or condition being treated, are conceptually quite simple. The goal is to lessen, and optimally to normalize, elevated levels of IOS by:

1. Decreasing elevated intracellular calcium levels
2. Directly increasing antioxidant levels inside those affected cells
3. Lessening the ongoing exposure of the body to new oxidation-inducing toxins

When the oxidative status of the diseased cells of the body is restored to normal or near-normal, a lessening of disease pathology and even a return to a normal clinical status can be seen, especially when the onset of the increased IOS, or disease state, was relatively recent. Optimal magnesium administration would be expected to help achieve this goal in most individuals.

Many chronic diseases, including those that have never before been treated from this perspective, can be expected to improve with this approach. However, when years or even decades have passed since the onset of the disease, countless "layers" of oxidative damage can result in gross structural damage that will likely never resolve.

A heart valve that has deteriorated due to the mechanical breakdown of the valve tissue itself along with supporting connective tissues cannot be expected to repair itself, at least not with any contemporary approaches. Perhaps in the future stem cells and other reconstructive approaches that are capable of generating new tissues might overturn this "rule." At that point in time, the essence of aging itself might be effectively addressed and significantly slowed. Even then, the need to reduce intracellular IOS through the use of antioxidants and by limiting toxin and pro-oxidant exposures will always be very important.

Treatment Principles

Because all pathophysiology develops as a result of increased IOS, every aspect of an optimal treatment protocol should aim to lessen this oxidative stress, either directly or indirectly. Furthermore, such an optimal protocol should include measures to stop or substantially lessen the ongoing exposure to, or production and dissemination of, new pro-oxidant agents (toxins, poisons, radiation) throughout the body. Simplified, then, an optimal treatment protocol should both:

PREVENT

and

REPAIR

Conventional medicine protocols are not designed to accomplish either of these goals. And integrative/complementary medicine too often only strives to repair. Any intervention that can even partially satisfy either or both of these goals can be expected to improve, at least to some degree, the pathophysiology of the affected cells in a patient. However, until both goals are met in as complete a manner as possible, an optimal response cannot occur and should not be anticipated. Therefore, an optimal treatment protocol seeks by whatever means/mechanisms possible to:

1. Stop/lessen the exposure to new toxins
2. Neutralize and/or excrete existing toxins and repair (reduce) as many of the damaged (oxidized) biomolecules as possible
3. Lower or normalize elevated intracellular calcium levels
4. Increase intracellular and extracellular antioxidant capacity (improved extracellular capacity feeds more intracellular capacity)
5. Normalize the levels of the main oxidation-modulating hormones (sex, thyroid, cortisol)

Minimizing Toxin Exposures

Preventing New Damage

New toxin exposures can emanate from either external or internal sources. External toxins are present in a person's environment and impact the body when they are inhaled, ingested, or come into contact with the skin. Internal toxins are those produced or accumulated inside the body from localized infections or from substances that have concentrated to toxic levels in various areas in the body such as in the intestines, lungs, fat stores, or teeth (such as mercury in amalgam fillings).

External Sources

As every patient has a fairly unique array of external toxin exposures, a thorough history should be taken in order to identify and then minimize toxin exposure from air, food, water, and any other significant environmental sources. The amount of effort expended to avoid a certain source of toxins will largely depend on the motivation and economic status of the patient, as well as the relative clinical impact of a given toxin source as determined by the treating physician. For a number of reasons, a given toxin source can be enormously consequential in the clinical status of one patient, while being relatively inconsequential in

An initially surprising yet major source of external toxins comes by way of dietary supplements.

another. This is where the guidance and clinical expertise of a qualified integrative medical practitioner can be invaluable.

An initially surprising yet major source of external toxins comes by way of dietary supplements. While most quality supplements have no real downside even when generously dosed, there are three notable exceptions. Excesses of these three can contribute greatly to increased body-wide oxidative stress and inflammation, as well as to increased all-cause mortality. A good way to view them is that they are "toxic nutrients," meaning their assimilation is absolutely critical for maintaining good health, but only at a level that is substantially lower than the level currently being promoted world-wide, especially to the supplementing population.

These toxic nutrients are:

✓ Calcium
✓ Iron
✓ Copper

All three of these agents, above a minimal intake level, *reliably increase IOS*, which has already been discussed as a clear-cut common denominator in both causing and sustaining poor health and chronic disease. Increased cellular calcium levels have been shown to always co-exist with increased levels of IOS, as both a *cause and an effect* of that abnormal metabolic state. Increased levels of calcium ingestion via excess dairy, along with just about any degree of regular calcium supplementation have been definitively linked to increased all-cause mortality. This is discussed and analyzed at great length elsewhere.[1]

Similarly, iron supplementation should never be taken by anybody who does not have a documented iron deficiency anemia (very low ferritin level with hypochromic, microcytic red blood cells on microscopic examination). Even though iron plays an important role as a cofactor in the activation and normal function of many enzymes throughout the body, this role requires a relatively tiny presence of iron, and supplementation is *never* needed to fulfill this enzymatic function.

*Increased cellular calcium levels have been shown to always co-exist with increased levels of IOS, as both a **cause and an effect** of that abnormal metabolic state.*

However, much larger amounts of iron are needed to allow the ongoing synthesis of a normal level of hemoglobin in the blood. Because of this, it should be realized that if enough iron is present to allow the production of normal amounts of hemoglobin, then there is much more than enough in the body to sustain its other functions. More is nearly always better with substances that have nutrient value, but this is never the case with iron.

Copper increases oxidative stress throughout the body, but especially inside the cells, in a similar fashion to iron. But unlike iron, which can certainly become deficient in some individuals, a state of copper deficiency in the body is so rare as to be virtually nonexistent. Because of this, any amount of supplemented copper is too much, and it will reliably increase the level of body-wide oxidative stress to some degree, depending on the level of increased exposure to this agent.

The truly sad aspect of these three toxic nutrients is that so many people take them to make themselves healthier. And, in spite of this noble goal, they are making themselves sicker and more prone

*Supplementing these agents is very much a "self-inflicted" wound to the body as they **always** increase oxidative stress, which is a state that must always be avoided or minimized at all costs.*

to the development and worsening of all the chronic degenerative diseases, including the big killers: heart disease and cancer. Supplementing these agents is very much a "self-inflicted" wound to the body as they

always increase oxidative stress, which is a state that must always be avoided or minimized at all costs. Statistically speaking, these toxic nutrients are probably second only to oral cavity focal infections and

The "threat" of an iron deficiency
epidemic was exchanged for a rampant
"plague" of chronic iron overdose.

toxins in their detrimental impact on the public health.

Iron, in particular, has been thrust upon the "developed" populations of the world for over 70 years in the most unbelievable and insidious of fashions. In the 1940s, the public health authorities of the United States finally decided that the babies and children (and apparently, the rest of the overall well-fed US population) needed protection against what was perceived as an epidemic of iron deficiency around the world. However, this "epidemic" was only occurring in the most malnourished of populations. Nevertheless, it was decided that the population of the United States needed protection against this "grave" threat of iron deficiency. Beginning in 1941, virtually all of the grains in foods sold in the United States had iron and three B vitamins added to them.[2] This was termed "enrichment" or "fortification" of these food products. And this enrichment has continued to this day, unabated. The "threat" of an iron deficiency epidemic was exchanged for a rampant "plague" of chronic iron overdose.

Iron, in general, increases oxidative stress wherever it is found. Any chronic increase in iron intake beyond the regular amounts found in good food chronically inflames the gut and aggravates the stomach lining. In multiple animal studies iron supplementation has been shown to reliably increase oxidative stress and inflammation in the gut and elsewhere.[3-7]

In pregnant women, it has been shown that pregnancy itself is associated with increased oxidative stress, which is further worsened by iron supplementation.[8,9] Even in pregnant women with an anemia due to iron deficiency, iron supplementation should be closely monitored and minimally-dosed. Just minimal iron supplementation can readily provoke and sustain an increased oxidative stress that elevates the risk of maternal complications such as gestational diabetes. In other words, administration of iron in any amount can exert a harmful toxic impact even in the face of a clear-cut diagnosis of iron deficiency anemia.[10,11]

Iron supplementation should never be started nor continued indefinitely in any woman, pregnant or not, in order to "prevent" an iron deficiency anemia from developing. And it should never be a routine supplement to any degree in men.

Once an iron deficiency anemia has been resolved, all iron supplementation should promptly be discontinued.

Even with the existence of all of this research unequivocally documenting the toxicity of iron, it continues to be routinely supplemented in pregnant women, even when they are not anemic. It also remains in many multivitamin supplements dosed on a daily basis solely for the purpose of promoting good health. Old medical habits die hard, and often not at all, in

Just minimal iron supplementation can readily provoke and sustain an increased oxidative stress that elevates the risk of maternal complications such as gestational diabetes.

spite of mountains of evidence supporting a needed change in practice.

It is rarely advisable to give any agent, much less one with known toxicity above certain levels of intake, to 100% of the population. Adding iron to mainstay foods such as grains, flours, and cereals (always labeled with "enriched" or "fortified") exposes nearly everyone to iron overload. There are literally millions of individuals around the world who have medical conditions caused by, associated with, or simply aggravated by excessive iron ingestion.[12-14] The last thing these individuals need is any additional iron intake, regardless of its form. Many other individuals who do not already have defined disorders due to iron excess but are also not iron deficient are still put at risk by additional sources of supplemented iron for a wide variety of medical conditions. These include heart disease, endocrine disorders, infectious disease, cancers, bone disease, pulmonary disease, and neurological conditions.[15]

Sadly, this obsession with getting more people to ingest more iron has even resulted in foods such as rice being genetically engineered to contain more iron. As long as these new rice forms are ingested by just

To make matters even worse for the promotion of body-wide increased oxidative stress and inflammation, the form of much of the government-recommended iron enrichment has been, and **continues to be***, metallic iron filings.*

extremely poor, malnourished populations, possibly more good than harm to the public health could be anticipated.[16,17] However, the otherwise well-nourished populations should stick with unenriched rice, optimally grown in an organic fashion.

Not surprisingly, excess iron is also well-documented to have the same association with increased intracellular calcium that it has with body-wide increased oxidative stress in general. In a cell study, the administration of iron resulted in a striking increase in intracellular calcium levels.[18] Iron has also been shown to feed the increased calcium levels seen in diseased neuronal cells.[19-21]

The best approach for treating increased intracellular calcium levels caused by iron excess and to promptly lessen the symptoms of an associated disease process is to decrease iron intake while supporting iron elimination. Simultaneously, restoration of depressed magnesium levels inside calcium-toxic cells should still be done to lessen cytoplasmic oxidative stress as rapidly and completely as possible.

To make matters even worse for the promotion of body-wide increased oxidative stress and inflammation, the form of much of the government-recommended iron enrichment has been, and **continues to be**, metallic iron filings (go to YouTube: type in "Iron in cereal"). In case there is any uncertainty, it is never an appropriate or even remotely healthy practice to ingest any metal in its elemental form, much less the highly pro-oxidant iron. It is the role of plants to convert such metals or elements into a biologically available, ingestible food form. Iron simply should never be consumed in its unaltered and completely reduced metallic state.

It is also important to realize that iron can be readily overdosed in all of its supplemental forms

Iron in the form of metallic iron filings simply magnifies the iron-fueled inflammatory reaction of the gut to an even greater degree than would be seen with iron in its other supplemental, medicinal, or food forms.

as well, even when it is not in a completely reduced, metallic form. However, ingesting iron in its metallic form on a regular basis just makes a toxic practice even more toxic.

Iron in the form of metallic iron filings simply magnifies the iron-fueled inflammatory reaction of the gut to an even greater degree than would be seen with iron in its other supplemental, medicinal, or food forms. Even in a prescription form, iron has been shown to induce cellular inflammation. However, isolated "pieces" of metallic iron greatly compound the injury by adding a foreign body reaction to the assault. And chronic inflammation of the gut lining ultimately leads to – and becomes indistinguishable from – the gut pathology seen in the leaky gut syndrome. Once the gut becomes leaky, then all of the different forms of food allergy and auto-immune reactions are unleashed by the incompletely digested food that is able to escape complete digestion and pass through the excessively permeable gut.

Furthermore, since this chronic iron-induced trauma to the gut is rarely recognized and remedied, it becomes a life-long condition and rarely improves or even lessens except through the adoption of some-major dietary changes. And those changes are often made inadvertently because of suspected gluten intolerance or just a desire to eat a healthier organic diet. It just so happens that a gluten-free and/or organic diet is **nearly always iron-free**.

Anecdotally, one case of gluten sensitivity (mild, not advanced) was observed to completely resolve after about six months of avoiding enriched foods and eating only the gluten-free foods that also rarely have iron added to them. One explanation for this loss of gluten sensitivity is that a mildly inflamed or leaky gut can have the ability to heal completely when the daily exposure to excess and needless iron is discontinued. Once the gut is healthy, gluten can then be properly digested, like any other protein.

Unwittingly Buying, Consuming Toxic Waste

Interestingly, there is a striking analogy between the addition of fluoride to the water supply and the addition of iron filings to foods. Iron filings, even the ones added to the food supply, are typically the waste byproduct of the grinding, filing, or milling needed to make finished iron products. This means that money is being *made* on the sale of these filings rather than being *spent* on their proper disposal. This is no different than *paying* your neighbors for the privilege of removing *their* trash.

Similarly, about 90% of the water supplies in our country are fluoridated with a hazardous waste product purchased from companies that produce chemical phosphate fertilizers. Hydrofluosilicic acid is an unstable, poisonous, and corrosive acid that is generated in the chimneys of plants that produce these fertilizers. Literally millions of gallons of this lead-, arsenic-, and mercury-containing hazardous waste is produced on a regular basis.[22] Rather than having to pay huge sums of money to process and dispose of this toxic material, these companies sell it to cities for the fluoridation of their water supplies at a large profit.

Even now, most water fluoridation proponents are not aware of the true source of the fluoride they seek to put into the water supplies of the public. However, the analogy is strong: Iron filings and hydrofluosilicic acid are both waste products. They are both toxic. Without another way to get rid of them, money would have to be spent to process them and dispose of them. Yet both are sold and put into our food and water supplies. Profit goes to the waste producers, while the public pays to consume their toxic debris.

While excess iron, copper, and calcium should always be avoided, statistically speaking, the two toxic nutrients with the most negative impact are iron and calcium. Copper could certainly "become" as toxic as iron and calcium, but the supplemental exposure to copper is nowhere close to the enormous and excessive dietary and supplemental exposures to iron and calcium. Practically speaking, then, just completely avoiding supplements containing copper largely solves the potential problem with excess copper. However, iron is a different story, as noted above. And a chronic excess exposure to calcium is possibly even more difficult to avoid than an excess exposure to iron.

The difficulty in avoiding excess calcium exposure is especially aggravated by the fact that calcium continues to be extolled as a wonderful supplement essential for good bone health, and even health in general. In fact, over the past 10 years or so, calcium supplementation worldwide has been on the rise as more pharmaceutical companies have entered the dietary supplement market and have even had a special focus on the promotion of calcium as a good supplement.[23]

To make matters worse, there's a constant drumming of the message that calcium-laden dairy products are "good" for you, in any amount. These assertions remain believed by most of the public as well as an overwhelmingly large percentage of healthcare practitioners today. Calcium remains one of the most popular supplements on the planet.

In addition to "deliberate" calcium supplementation (taking a supplement containing only or nearly only calcium), two more major sources of additional calcium supplementation/ingestion occur on a regular basis. Many multivitamin and/or multimineral supplements have a very large amount of calcium in them. Also, the massive antacid market is dominated by calcium-containing products, especially calcium carbonate. Much of the public regularly overdoses on these calcium-containing antacids – oftentimes in amounts far exceeding their "deliberate" calcium supplementation, including the calcium intake from regular milk drinking. When this "unintentional" calcium supplementation is combined with the deliberate intake, the total calcium supplementation that regularly takes place in many people is enormous.

To make matters worse, there's a constant drumming of the message that calcium-laden dairy products are "good" for you, in any amount.

Also, with regard to dairy, the calcium overdose awaiting the uninformed consumer is aggravated by another factor. Different milk products are sometimes "fortified" with additional amounts of calcium. Nearly all the non-dairy milks (almond, cashew, rice, coconut, etc.) have calcium added – a serving of these alternatives often delivers as much or **more** of a calcium overdose as in drinking a glass of regular milk. Now orange juice with a greater content of calcium than is

Several large studies have clearly demonstrated calcium intake above a certain level increased the chances of cardiovascular and all-cause mortality.

found in regular milk is available. The dairy industry, with the help of most doctors, is focused on getting as many people as possible to ingest as much calcium as possible, and it continues to be very successful in achieving this goal. And like the heavily-researched topics of magnesium or vitamin C, there appears to be no mountain of evidence high enough to stop or slow this onslaught of toxic calcium intake, at least not yet.

The case for the toxicity of excess calcium intake is strong, and it is intellectually difficult to refute when the totality of all the studies looking at calcium and its relation to different chronic diseases is taken as a whole.[24] Several large studies have clearly demonstrated calcium intake above a certain level increased the chances of cardiovascular and all-cause mortality.[25-27]

The bottom line, however, is that excess calcium is progressively more toxic the more that it is ingested, although the toxicity can be partially mitigated when assimilated from a quality dietary source containing significant amounts of vitamin D. Even though it is possible to find a study that may confuse or try to negate the warnings against excessive calcium intake, the preponderance of evidence suggests that anyone who insists upon taking a calcium supplement, a calcium-containing antacid, or regularly drinking milk as a beverage, is doing so at a great risk to their health and longevity.

Many studies indicate that increased IOS is due to an increased intracellular calcium concentration and a deregulation or breakdown of cellular calcium metabolism in general.[28] This is what makes the natural abilities of magnesium to block calcium channels and to antagonize the actions of calcium so therapeutically significant. A clear example of this therapeutic, antagonistic relationship between intracellular magnesium and intracellular calcium was documented in essential hypertension (persistent and pathological high blood pressure) patients. Prior to treatment, intracellular calcium levels were elevated and intracellular magnesium levels were depressed. Increasing the levels of extracellular magnesium increased intracellular

In neurons, for example, elevated intracellular calcium levels initiate cell injury that can lead to neuron death if left unchecked.

magnesium levels and decreased intracellular calcium levels in a reciprocal fashion.[29]

In neurons, for example, elevated intracellular calcium levels initiate cell injury that can lead to neuron death if left unchecked. In fact, it has long been recognized that this calcium overload inside such neurons is an essential pathological state that causes the neuronal injury due to lack of blood flow to the brain (ischemia).[30] An increase in intracellular calcium has been identified as one of the early events in the development of ischemic stroke.[31]

While it should be clear that chronic excess calcium intake will eventually be reflected in increased intracellular calcium levels with increased IOS, other mechanisms increasing intracellular calcium levels exist. Some toxins induce a significant and sustained elevation of free cytosolic calcium by causing a rapid depletion and shift of calcium out of the mitochondrial pool into the cytoplasm. This cytosolic calcium increase can be further fueled by the impairment of the cell's ability to extrude calcium from the cell. Such an impairment appears to be important in sustaining the initial elevation of calcium in the cytoplasm.[32] Other

Some toxin-exposed cells can poison themselves "from within" by a redistribution of its calcium stores into the cytoplasm from organelles such as the endoplasmic reticulum and mitochondria.

studies have also demonstrated that toxins cause a prompt rise in intracellular calcium levels.[33,34]

Studies have shown that agents capable of preventing cytosolic calcium levels from rising in the face of different toxins also block the effects of those toxins on the cells.[35,36] These observations add further support to the fact that toxins consistently provoke increases in cytosolic calcium. In addition, the positive systemic effects of antioxidants on cells always results in a lowering of intracellular calcium levels.[37]

The maintenance of normal cellular calcium metabolism is an important function of the mitochondria.[38] In fact, an interference with mitochondrial metabolism impairs cellular calcium metabolism, and vice versa.[39] Viral infection of cells, another source of significantly increased cellular oxidative stress, has also been documented to significantly increase intracellular calcium concentration.[40]

In another cell-toxin study model, removal of extracellular calcium in the presence of a toxin known to induce increases in cytoplasmic calcium levels did not prevent those increases or eventual cell death, thus showing that the increase in calcium levels did not originate from outside the cell. However, an intracellular calcium chelator was able to substantially reduce cytoplasmic calcium levels and prevent the otherwise anticipated outcome of cell death.[41,42]

Although all toxins increase cytoplasmic levels of calcium, there are two different mechanisms that produce this increase. Some toxin-exposed cells can poison themselves "from within" by a redistribution of its calcium stores into the cytoplasm from organelles such as the endoplasmic reticulum and mitochondria. Other toxins increase cytoplasmic levels by facilitating the uptake of new calcium from the extracellular space via the calcium channels in the cell membrane.[43] The logical conclusion is:

> **Any mechanism that raises cytoplasmic
> calcium levels produces a toxic effect.**

Internal Sources

Internal sources of toxins generally come as a result of being freshly generated, as from a focal infection or a constipated gut. The other substantial internal sources of toxins result as toxins accumulate beyond a certain degree in different areas of the body. While a significant antioxidant presence might compensate for such accumulations over an extended period of time, a variety of mechanisms can start mobilizing these accumulations and thereby expose "new" areas of the body to "old" toxins.

Many detoxification protocols can be so effective at freeing up toxins that the intended chelation/elimination processes become overwhelmed. This means that a large amount of mobilized toxins remain unchelated and/or uneliminated, subjecting new tissues to the challenge of those toxins being redistributed. In any detoxification protocol, which can be very important in the recovery of some patients, the detoxification will always result in some degree of retoxification. The protocol needs to be designed to allow for a slow and steady release and excretion of toxins such that important normal laboratory tests (like the lipid panel) are not rendered abnormal, and such that the patient remains comfortable and feeling well during the detoxification process.

Rarely is rapid, large quantity detoxification better than slow and steady. It can literally be the difference between clinical recovery and a clinical decline that might be irreversible. A good example of an agent that can inflict such harm if not administered with expertise is DMPS (dimercaptopropane sulfonate). Generally, giving large doses of vitamin C (25 to 75 grams intravenously) is advisable at the time of a DMPS injection. Depending on patient response and the degree of detoxification-related symptoms, such vitamin C dosing can be repeated daily for one or more additional days. In spite of the potential downside, a powerful detoxification agent such as DMPS can still be occasionally indicated, especially when a very large amount of stored toxins is felt to be present, and clinical improvement on a comprehensive treatment protocol remains minimal or absent in the face of that large store.

When the patient is demonstrating a satisfactory positive detoxification response (clinically and/or as indicated by laboratory testing), this slower and safer approach can be continued. Some relatively common

Rarely is rapid, large quantity detoxification better than slow and steady. It can literally be the difference between clinical recovery and a clinical decline that might be irreversible.

prescription agents that pull toxins out less vigorously than DMPS include DMSA (dimercaptosuccinic acid), BAL (dimercaprol), EDTA (ethylenediaminetetraacetic acid), penicillamine, deferoxamine, and deferasirox.

However, such prescription agents should not be utilized unless it appears that the treatment protocol, along with the administration of multiple non-toxic and

Regardless of the agent utilized to promote increased toxin excretion, the clinician should always be on the alert for the need to give additional antioxidant support during the excretion/elimination process, such as can be afforded by intravenous vitamin C.

non-prescription detoxification agents, have failed to improve the status of the patient.

Non-toxic supplements and nutrient chelators include ALA (alpha lipoic acid), IP6 (inositol hexaphosphate, or phytic acid), whey protein, NAC (N-acetylcysteine), S-acetyl glutathione, and a quality liposome-encapsulated glutathione. Many of these natural agents work to improve intracellular glutathione levels while stimulating glutathione-related enzymes, which helps to optimize the natural toxin-eliminating pathways in the toxin-burdened cell.

Regardless of the agent utilized to promote increased toxin excretion, the clinician should always be on the alert for the need to give additional antioxidant support during the excretion/elimination process, such as can be afforded by intravenous vitamin C. Nevertheless, eliminating pro-oxidant toxins while restoring intracellular glutathione levels are two important ways to help achieve the goal of decreased IOS.

Possibly the best long-term way to deal with the excretion of toxins in a slow but steady and minimally toxic manner is by using a far-infrared sauna on a regular basis. While all saunas offer the ability to sweat out toxins, the far-infrared sauna appears to be especially adept at it, facilitating a sweat that has an even higher concentration of toxic solutes in it than is achieved with a regular sauna or an exercise-induced sweat. Good nutrient supplementation is even more important when regularly using the sauna, as significant amounts of magnesium and potassium will reliably be lost through the sweating process as well.

Focal Infection Sources

Focal infections capable of promoting a generalized body-wide increase in inflammation can exist in many different areas of the body.[44] These include, but are not limited to:

✓ Pulmonary sources (chronic bronchitis with bronchiectasis)[45]

✓ Gastrointestinal tract ulcers; infections in hemorrhoids, diverticula, and appendix[46,47]

✓ Lymph nodes, including in the mesentery

✓ Gallbladder and liver

✓ Fallopian tubes, uterus, prostate, urethral tract, seminal vesicle

✓ Skin and nails (boils, furuncles, toenails)

✓ Heart (endocarditis)

✓ Kidney (often initiated from an oral cavity
   focus)[48]
✓ Joint (arthritis often initiated from an oral
   cavity focus)
✓ Inflamed or infected veins[49]
✓ Inflamed or infected bone

Of note, nearly all of the articles dealing with focal
infection are quite old, and very little contemporary
research even addresses this topic. However, if you
take the time to examine any of these "old" papers, you
will find the observations of some very astute physicians and researchers. This early focal infection literature connects many different medical conditions with
oral cavity infections, especially with regard to the
chronic infection found in all root canal-treated teeth.
This diligent, high-quality research as a whole has been
repeatedly disparaged as being poorly done and long-
since "proven" to be irrelevant and even completely
wrong.

The Fallacy of Discarding Research
Solely Based on Age

The word "old" should never even be
mentioned with regard to scientific research. Using
the publishing date of any research as a criterion
for validity leads to some ludicrous conclusions.
Should Nobel Prize winners in medicine give back
their awards after their research extends beyond
a certain age, since research that old could not
possibly have been done in a qualified and compe-
tent fashion? Banting and Best discovered insulin

in 1921. The research that facilitated that discovery is now extremely old. However, it is doubtful that any diabetic wants to give up his or her access to insulin because the research is "no longer valid" or "clearly proven" wrong because of its great age. The truth is, the scant research cited to "disprove" focal infection research was often performed by people or groups that had financial fortunes that were in jeopardy should the research become widely accepted.

But with regard to the notion that oral cavity infections have little to do with body-wide medical conditions and diseases, nothing could be more outlandish or further from the truth. Any dentist who maintains that the focal infection literature has been proven false and irrelevant is either incapable of straightforward logical thought, or too blindly interested in maintaining a lucrative income to consider the evidence. Root canal procedures *are* big business; over 25 million root canal procedures annually easily justify the blanket assertions of safety by dental associations and in dental journal editorials. These at-risk fortunes also largely block an objective review of the preponderance of current literature that more than validates the earlier root canal research.[50,51]

This is not to say that all root canal procedures are automatically bad for the patient. This is definitely not the case and has been addressed elsewhere.[52] However, quality and unbiased prospective studies are still needed to track patients with root canal-treated teeth, concentrating on such parameters as serial X-ray appearances, clinical outcomes such as heart disease, and serial measurements of laboratory data that correlate with increased systemic inflammation, such as CRP, reverse T3, fibrinogen, glucose, lipids, and sex hormone levels. Algorithms could then be developed that could help a dental provider determine the actual health risk at any given time. It would be quite valuable to know whether a given root canal-treated tooth is not likely to have a substantial negative impact on general health, or likely to cause a heart attack, or whether the tooth is at an intermediate level of concern warranting closer monitoring. Ultimately, it would be good to have trustworthy data that can help both patient and doctor decide whether such a tooth gets extracted or stays put a while longer. And even when the data generated raises no alarms or concerns, regular follow-up needs to continue indefinitely, since a root canal-treated tooth could "deteriorate" at some point in time, even though it might not have had a significant negative impact on general health for years or even decades prior to such deterioration.

In fact, although the list of potential sites of focal infection as noted above is lengthy, the oral cavity is the site of the focal infection(s) and toxins that significantly increase body-wide inflammation well over 95% of the time. These oral cavity sites/sources include the following:

✓ Chronically infected but asymptomatic teeth (chronic apical periodontitis, or teeth with apical abscesses; statistically a very large factor worldwide)
✓ Root canal-treated teeth, also usually asymptomatic (all infected, but not

all disseminating that infection; also
statistically a very large factor worldwide)
✓ Acutely abscessed and painful teeth
(ironically a tiny minority of all infected
teeth)
✓ Chronic periodontal (gum tissue) infection
and inflammation (a very large factor)
✓ Cavitational osteonecrosis (wet gangrene
accumulations at sites of old extractions—
very common)
✓ Chronically infected tonsils (typically
appearing externally normal—very
common in mouths that have or have had
root canal-treated teeth or other infected
teeth)
✓ Chronically infected sinuses (often
originating from infected teeth in the
maxilla)
✓ Infected dental implants
✓ Infected lymph nodes in and close to the
oral cavity
✓ Toxic and biologically incompatible metals
and other restorative materials

A more detailed discussion of dental infections and
toxins and their cause-and-effect relationships with
many chronic degenerative diseases, especially heart
disease and breast cancer, along with the supporting
dental, medical, and scientific literature is available
elsewhere.[53-55]
Another source of internally generated toxins that
can strongly support a body-wide state of increased
inflammation comes from a poorly functioning gut.
The less complete and slower that digestion occurs, the

greater the proliferation of pathogens with their associated toxins. While having fewer bowel movements might seem a relatively inconsequential problem, it can have an enormously negative impact on the health of the body because of the haven of proliferating pathogens that results from such gastrointestinal stasis. To minimize the percentage of food that rots and putrefies rather than digests normally, at least one and preferably two (or more) bowel movements should take place daily.

For many constipated individuals, simply avoiding certain food combinations that slow gut transit time, while taking in more oral vitamin C powder and magnesium can completely remedy the sluggish gut. This matter is discussed at greater length elsewhere.[56,57]

Healing
Hormones

*Lowering Body-Wide
Oxidative Stress*

The proper balance of sex hormones, thyroid hormone, and cortisol plays a critical role in keeping inflammation and excess oxidation in check throughout the body, thereby directly supporting good healing and healthy cells. Below-normal levels of estrogen in women and testosterone in men make it difficult for any otherwise positive treatment protocol to have anywhere close to optimal impact on keeping intracellular oxidative stress (IOS) and intracellular antioxidant concentrations at normal (physiological) levels. And when thyroid function is even minimally low in the cells throughout the body, maintaining an inflammation-free body with a normal redox status inside the cells is virtually impossible. Both low and high cortisol levels negatively impact the oxidative status of the body as well.

Insulin is another hormone that strongly promotes the body-wide normalization of cellular oxidative stress and offers strong support of good healing. It exerts a powerful health impact in both a focal fashion when applied topically and throughout the body when administered systemically.

Estrogen

This hormone is well-known for its ability to maintain the health of the reproductive and sexual organs and to determine the normal secondary sexual characteristics in women. However, it does far more than that, as it is critical in regulating calcium metabolism throughout the body and not just in promoting bone health as an anti-osteoporosis hormone.

Estrogen has a powerful anti-inflammatory effect that has been demonstrated in many cell, animal, and human studies.[1-7] Of course, the ability to positively regulate calcium metabolism is likely a primary reason why estrogen is such a potent anti-inflammatory agent. The action of estrogen as an antagonist to calcium has also been suggested as a reason for its cardiovascular disease protective effect.[8]

In vitro studies on animal and human cell lines

Estrogen has also been shown to protect toxin-exposed cells from death by lessening cellular calcium uptake through calcium channels.

show that estrogen functions as a calcium channel blocker and a calcium antagonist in general.[9,10] Estrogen has also been shown to protect toxin-exposed cells from death by lessening cellular calcium uptake through calcium channels.[11] Even some estrogen-related agents (phytoestrogens) have been shown to be calcium channel blockers in a study on human platelets.[12]

And in addition to decreasing elevated intracellular calcium levels, estrogen has also been shown to effectively raise intracellular magnesium levels.

And in addition to decreasing elevated intracellular calcium levels, estrogen has also been shown to effectively raise intracellular magnesium levels. These alterations in the mineral composition of the cell and its cytoplasm are two essential manifestations of the decrease in IOS seen when inflammation is resolved or lessened.[13-15]

Estrogen also significantly promotes increased magnesium levels in the body by stimulating its active reabsorption into the cells of the distal convoluted tubules of the kidney. Magnesium is extruded back into the bloodstream from these tubules, avoiding much of its elimination in the urine.[16] In rats that had their ovaries removed, an injection of estrogen (estradiol) resulted in an early and persistent increase in cytoplasmic magnesium in the vaginal epithelial cells. This again underscores the important role that estrogen plays in magnesium metabolism and in the control of IOS.[17] Healthy estrogen levels are also clearly vital to longevity in general. Because estrogen helps optimize intracellular levels of magnesium and calcium, it is able to stabilize or reverse this most important pathophysiological marker/cause of disease.

Estrogen deficiency in the form of lowered levels of estrone (one of the three major endogenous estrogens in the body) was linked to increased all-cause

Women who began their menopause before age 40, losing their natural estrogen protection at a much younger age than usual, demonstrated a higher rate of all-cause mortality.

mortality in post-menopausal women with known coronary artery disease or at high risk of it.[18] In a large group of Swedish women, hormone replacement therapy resulted in a substantial decrease in all-cause mortality in each of the 12 categories of cause of death except for injuries.[19] Another study looking at estradiol-based hormone replacement therapy also showed a dramatic lowering of deaths from all causes.[20] A cohort of 1,458 women who participated in randomized, placebo-controlled clinical trials over periods averaging about 10 years also showed a dramatic decrease in all-cause mortality on various hormone replacement protocols that were only given over a 2- to 3-year period.[21] Women who began their menopause before age 40, losing their natural estrogen protection at a much younger age than usual, demonstrated a higher rate of all-cause mortality.[22]

There is another connection between estrogen effect and magnesium status. Metabolic syndrome classically involves at least three of the following:

- ✓ abdominal obesity
- ✓ increased triglycerides
- ✓ low HDL lipoproteins
- ✓ high blood pressure
- ✓ elevated fasting blood sugar

Magnesium levels have been clearly shown to be lower in adults with this condition than in normal controls.[23] Magnesium supplementation in metabolic syndrome patients with low magnesium levels effectively treats the laboratory and clinical abnormalities present in such patients.[24] Another study, a meta-analysis of nine articles, showed that higher consumption of magnesium resulted a lower risk of developing this syndrome.[25] In animal studies, estrogen reversed the abnormalities of metabolic syndrome.[26,27] In women, not only has estrogen replacement been shown to improve the laboratory abnormalities seen in this syndrome,[28] but studies also show that low estrogen increases the risk of developing it in the first place.[29-31] One fairly clear-cut interpretation of all of these studies together is that the ability of estrogen to increase intracellular magnesium levels would appear to be a primary, or at least a very important, mechanism by which estrogen replacement lessens metabolic syndrome abnormalities. The optimal ways to administer and dose estrogen are discussed in greater detail elsewhere.[32]

RECAP
The qualities of estrogen that reduce (or
cause to be reduced) increased IOS

1. Lowers intracellular calcium concentrations, acting as a calcium channel blocker
   and calcium antagonist
2. Serves as a potent anti-inflammatory agent
3. Raises intracellular magnesium levels
4. Helps to reabsorb magnesium that would
   otherwise be excreted by the kidneys
5. Hormone replacement dramatically
   decreases all-cause mortality
6. Lessens metabolic syndrome parameters, probably by increasing intracellular
   magnesium levels

Testosterone

Like estrogen, testosterone is also an anti-inflammatory agent.[33] This is mediated at least in part
by its ability to act as a calcium channel blocker and
lower intracellular calcium levels.[34-37] In cell studies,
testosterone has demonstrated its anti-inflammatory
properties. In human neutrophils from healthy male
subjects, physiological concentrations of testosterone
were shown to suppress superoxide production while
enhancing the production of nitric oxide.[38,39] These
facts support the important role of testosterone in
modulating the immune response to inflammation.

In fact, a reliable generalization about the effect
of any hormone, but especially about estrogen, testosterone, insulin, cortisol, and thyroid hormone, is that
they all function to lower body-wide oxidative stress
and thereby normalize and optimize cellular function.

Even though the biochemical pathways that are affected will vary significantly from one hormone to the next, they all work to optimize biochemical pathway

Normalizing testosterone levels reliably reduces insulin sensitivity and improves glucose tolerance, whereas low levels have been clearly linked to increased oxidative stress, impaired mitochondrial function, and the laboratory abnormalities leading to atherosclerosis and heart disease.

efficiency while minimizing energy consumption in the process.

Testosterone is well-documented to play a key role in the metabolism of carbohydrate, fat, and protein. It has been specifically shown to have a major impact in optimizing both body fat composition and muscle mass in men. Factors associated with metabolic syndrome have also been shown to be consistently impacted in a positive manner when testosterone deficiencies are properly restored. Normalizing testosterone levels reliably reduces insulin sensitivity and improves glucose tolerance, whereas low levels have been clearly linked to increased oxidative stress, impaired mitochondrial function, and the laboratory abnormalities leading to atherosclerosis and heart disease.[40,41]

Multiple studies have consistently shown that low serum testosterone levels correlate with increased all-cause mortality, a result that is not surprising in light of the many other studies documenting the clinical and laboratory abnormalities seen in male patients with low testosterone.[42-46] An increased all-cause mortality rate is also seen in men with a greater rate of age-related decline in testosterone levels, independent of the baseline levels of testosterone.[47] Conversely, and very significantly, the normalization of testosterone levels from replacement therapy is associated with a significant *reduction* in all-cause mortality, along with heart attack and stroke.[48]

One recent study even showed a definite decrease in all-cause mortality with testosterone therapy even when clear-cut improvement in cardiovascular disease risk factors was not seen. This further underscores the importance of testosterone in facilitating the normal function of all cells in the body.[49] The susceptibility of cells to infection in general also appears to be increased when testosterone levels are low, further showing that testosterone, probably by lessening intracellular

*Conversely, and very significantly, the normalization of testosterone levels from replacement therapy is associated with a significant **reduction** in all-cause mortality, along with heart attack and stroke.*

oxidative stress, protects all cells against disease and infection.[50]

Low testosterone levels are strongly related to insulin resistance.[51] Furthermore, the ability of testos-

terone to reduce insulin sensitivity logically suggests
that this hormone directly facilitates magnesium
uptake into cells or otherwise promotes the optimization of intracellular magnesium levels by other mecha-

...it has been shown that advanced
insulin resistance shows little response to
increased insulin dosing until a significant
administration of magnesium has first
been assimilated by the affected cells.

nisms. As is discussed below in the section on insulin,
it has been shown that advanced insulin resistance
shows little response to increased insulin dosing until
a significant administration of magnesium has first
been assimilated by the affected cells. This would make
testosterone an important "partner" with insulin in its
optimization of glucose metabolism in the body.

When insulin resistance is seen with the laboratory abnormalities of the metabolic syndrome in a
male patient with decreased testosterone levels, there is
really never a good reason for not addressing this deficiency judiciously, regardless of the age of the patient.
"Judiciously" is the key word here, as evidence certainly
exists that giving excessive, supraphysiological doses
of testosterone can increase oxidative stress.[52] Anyone
receiving testosterone replacement must have frequent
enough blood testing to clearly establish that the-key
markers are moving toward or remaining in healthy
reference ranges.

Not surprisingly, considering the critical role that magnesium plays in promoting normal metabolism in every cell of the body, it also appears that magnesium plays an important role in both increasing and

> *...it also appears that magnesium plays an important role in both increasing and sustaining higher free plasma testosterone levels.*

sustaining higher free plasma testosterone levels. These positive effects of magnesium on testosterone levels were seen in both sedentary and individuals who vigorously exercised, with more pronounced increases seen in those who exercised.[53,54] Similarly, it has been shown that men with normal total testosterone levels have significantly higher serum magnesium levels than men with total testosterone deficiencies.[55]

There are relatively few studies that directly address the effects of testosterone on magnesium metabolism, or of magnesium on testosterone physiology. However, there is substantial documentation of testosterone as an anti-inflammatory agent and as a calcium blocking agent, likely indicating that this hormone interacts with and supports some or all of the mechanisms and agents that work to increase intracellular magnesium levels.

Insulin, discussed more in detail below, is known to strongly enhance the cellular uptake of magnesium against the huge concentration gradient that would otherwise serve to translocate magnesium from its high intracellular levels to its very low extracellular levels. Testosterone, by unclear mechanisms, has been shown to have insulin-effects in an *in vitro* study on skeletal muscle cells.[56] There is also evidence that circulating testosterone levels correlate with fasting insulin levels, but without clearly impacting lipoprotein levels. Some research has also suggested that insulin can mediate an elevated level of testosterone production.[57,58] Similarly, it has been shown that relative to placebo, testosterone can significantly increase cortisol levels.[59] Collectively, this information might indicate the downside of too-rapid and too-high dosing of testosterone replacement, especially in elderly individuals. But it is still not an argument against low-dosed and slowly-increased testosterone dosing in this patient group for minimizing morbidity and optimizing lifespan.

Vitamin D, regarded by many as being more a hormone than a vitamin, also appears to have an independent linear association with free testosterone.[60] Although the nature of this association has not been clearly defined, it further highlights the need for a balance of all hormones and hormone-like substances in the body.[61]

RECAP
The qualities of testosterone that reduce (or cause to be reduced) increased IOS

1. Acts as a calcium channel blocker and calcium antagonist to lower intracellular calcium concentrations
2. Serves as a potent anti-inflammatory agent and immune system supporter
3. Helps to optimize function of other hormones

4. Hormone replacement dramatically decreases all-cause mortality
5. Lessens metabolic syndrome parameters, probably by increasing intracellular magnesium levels; lower levels are associated with insulin resistance

Insulin

While insulin is primarily known as the hormone that regulates glucose metabolism throughout the body since its discovery by Banting and Best in 1921, the literature repeatedly documents it as a potent healing agent. It is certainly true that insulin is vital to promoting the proper uptake of glucose into the cells of the body so that the Krebs cycle can generate optimal levels of ATP from the intracellular metabolism of glucose. However, some other, lesser-known functions of insulin are arguably of equal importance.

Almost since its discovery insulin has been shown

Almost since its discovery insulin has been shown to have strong healing properties in both its local and systemic applications.

to have strong healing properties in both its local and systemic applications.[62-64] In diabetic patients, systemic insulin therapy was demonstrated to significantly increase the wound-healing rate of diabetic ulcers.[65] Additionally, topical insulin applied to cutaneous wounds accelerated healing in rats with or without acute diabetes.[66] In a double-blind place-bo-controlled clinical trial, topical insulin cream was

Also, as long as it is not grossly overdosed, insulin is one of the safest agents that can be used either systemically or locally.

found to markedly improve wound healing in diabetic patients.[67] A review examining the results of nine clinical trials in patients and twelve animal studies concluded that insulin is a low-cost growth factor that has clear-cut value in healing wounds more quickly and more thoroughly.[68]

Also, as long as it is not grossly overdosed, insulin is one of the safest agents that can be used either systemically or locally. Combined and separately, insulin and zinc were also shown to substantially accelerate the healing of deliberate, uniformly-inflicted cuts applied to the forearms of both diabetic and non-diabetic volunteers, with one arm serving as the control for the other.[69] Consistent with this accelerated healing, insulin-zinc injections at wound sites have also been documented to stimulate/accelerate local DNA synthesis.[70] Topical insulin has also been shown to accelerate the healing of

✓ Traumatic eardrum perforations in rats[71]
✓ Corneal wounds in diabetic and
   non-diabetic patients[72,73]

✓ Pressure wounds or bedsores, which can be especially resistant to improvement and complete resolution[74]

✓ Large, full-thickness wounds in diabetic patients, with an increase in the formation of connective tissue and new blood vessels[75]

✓ Wounds in non-diabetic patients, with the formation of new blood vessels documented by biopsy after only two weeks[76]

✓ Diabetic wounds by the mechanism of suppressing and/or reducing the persistent chronic inflammation that often inhibits good healing[77]

Another Medical Mystery: Why Isn't Insulin Used for Wound Care?

Incredibly, although these dramatic and safe applications of insulin have been repeatedly documented in the medical literature for well over 80 years now, few wound care centers in the United States or around the world use insulin to both accelerate and improve the quality of wound healing. "More studies and research need to be done" still remains a common mantra at the end of many studies that clearly and unequivocally documented the effectiveness and safety of insulin used in this fashion.

One can only wonder how many "gold standard" studies (randomized, double-blind, placebo-controlled) could ever be done with striking enough outcomes to actually get physicians to start using insulin for wound care. What should be the standard of care remains effectively unused and not even part of the wound healing medical discussion. Insulin treatment for wound care has been neglected in much the same manner as the heavily-researched but little-utilized vitamin C. Why? Insulin is especially puzzling, since many of its variations remain under patent protection and could generate much larger profits for the insulin-producing pharmaceutical companies if the clinical applications were to expand. Vitamin C, of course, remains free of a pharmaceutical-owned patent, which is likely a major explanation for its gross under use.

Two important, and possibly the most important, reasons that insulin is such a reliable healing agent has to do with its ability to raise intracellular vitamin C and intracellular magnesium levels. Increasing the levels of vitamin C and magnesium inside the cells are two of the most direct ways to decrease elevated levels of IOS. As elevated IOS is the cellular pathology causing and sustaining all chronic degenerative diseases, any measures that will lower those elevations will directly and substantially lessen, and sometimes completely reverse, the pathology of any given disease. More vitamin C inside the cells accomplishes this directly, and more magnesium inside the cells facilitates the lowering of the elevated calcium levels inside the cells that elevated the IOS in the first place.

It has also been established that insulin acts to conserve magnesium. In a study on mouse distal convoluted tubule cells (kidney cells that filter the blood to make urine), insulin was shown to stimulate magnesium uptake into those cells, which basically means that insulin bolsters magnesium levels in the body by minimizing magnesium loss and promoting its reabsorption before being eliminated in the urine.[78]

It has been established that insulin actively promotes the cellular uptake of vitamin C in a competitive fashion with glucose. The more glucose is present, the less vitamin C gets into the cell, and vice-versa.[79] Increased glucose without added insulin has also been shown to promptly decrease intracellular vitamin C levels in the leukocytes of normal subjects, further highlighting the competition between glucose and vitamin C for entry into the cells of the body.[80]

Glucose and vitamin C are structurally very similar molecules, and glucose is enzymatically converted to vitamin C in the livers of animals capable of synthesizing their own vitamin C. Their structural similarity probably accounts for their competitive nature in the degree to which insulin promotes

This ability of elevated glucose levels to decrease intracellular vitamin C concentrations is probably the primary reason for all of the pathology and long-term side effects seen in diabetics.

their cellular uptake. This ability of elevated glucose levels to decrease intracellular vitamin C concentrations is probably the primary reason for all of the pathology and long-term side effects seen in diabetics.

In other words, elevated glucose levels result in a state of **intracellular scurvy** (severe vitamin C depletion) in virtually all the cells of the body, with some tissues typically being more severely impacted than others.

Insulin also increases the intracellular accumulation of magnesium, which is a very critical factor in lowering elevated intracellular levels of calcium and oxidative stress, as well as in maintaining those lowered levels.

And the higher and more chronic the glucose elevations, the worse the intracellular scurvy. Conversely, insulin has also been shown to not only increase the uptake of vitamin C in its oxidized state (DHAA) via special transporters (GLUT), it has also additionally been shown to facilitate the reduction of the oxidized vitamin C to its active, reduced form inside the cells (AA). This means that insulin pulls vitamin C into the cell in its spent state and then helps recharge it once it is there.[81]

Insulin also increases the intracellular accumulation of magnesium,[82] which is a very critical factor in lowering elevated intracellular levels of calcium and oxidative stress, as well as in maintaining those lowered levels. Both *in vivo* and *in vitro* studies have demonstrated the ability of insulin to move magnesium from the extracellular to the intracellular space. This has been demonstrated in both human lymphocyte and platelet experimental models.[83-87]

Conversely, intracellular magnesium has been shown to be a positive modulator of insulin and an important factor in lessening insulin resistance.[88] Not surprisingly, then, intracellular levels of magnesium are

Conversely, intracellular magnesium has been shown to be a positive modulator of insulin and an important factor in lessening insulin resistance.

consistently low in patients with type 2 diabetes, along with lowered levels of vitamin C.[89]

In an animal study, magnesium supplementation was shown to upregulate both insulin receptors and glucose transporters, meaning the number of those receptors and transporters is increased, offering at least one clear mechanism for the synergistic effect of magnesium and insulin in reducing elevated IOS.[90]

When one realizes the role insulin plays in moving magnesium **and** vitamin C from the extracellular space to the intracellular space, studies reporting the positive impact of insulin on clinical outcomes make even more sense. They also reaffirm the great importance of including substantial magnesium and vitamin C supplementation as an important part of **any and all** treatment protocols.

Numerous documented non-diabetes-related clinical applications of insulin further support this reasoning.[91] In one large study the use of intensive insulin therapy (an infusion to maintain glucose between 80 and 110 mg/dl) in critically ill surgical

ICU patients receiving mechanical ventilation reduced in-hospital mortality by 34% when compared to conventional therapy. Furthermore, the greatest reduction in mortality was seen in the subset of patients with advanced sepsis.[92,93] Another study showed that when elevated blood sugars in myocardial infarction patients without previously diagnosed diabetes ("stress hyperglycemia") remain uncontrolled, there is also a significantly increased risk of in-hospital mortality.[94]

Considering that many individuals live with diabetes and blood sugars well above 110 mg/dl on a daily basis for years, it would seem that the additional effects of insulin administration – beyond tighter glucose control – might play the primary role in the dramatic decrease in the early mortality rate of these ICU and CCU patients. As more magnesium and vitamin C are moved inside the cells, a larger

*When one realizes the role insulin plays in moving magnesium **and** vitamin C from the extracellular space to the intracellular space, studies reporting the positive impact of insulin on clinical outcomes make even more sense.*

percentage of the sickest cells survive due to the lowering of the elevated IOS seen in many of the cells in patients close to death. Many of these cells can then be repaired back to a normal or near-normal redox state.

Increasing the number of healthy cells always equates to longer survival and less disease-related symptoms.

While not characterized as a calcium channel blocker, insulin has also been suggested to have a calcium regulatory effect. In neurons, insulin appears to lessen the negative impact of increased intracellular calcium levels on the ability of that state to result in cognitive decline due to a phenomenon known as afterhyperpolarization.[95]

RECAP
Insulin qualities that reduce, or cause
to be reduced, increased IOS

1. Primary factor for optimizing glucose metabolism, preventing or lessening the negative impacts of chronically increased glucose levels and their ability to increase body-wide oxidative stress and inflammation, as well as limited energy production via the Krebs cycle inside the cells

2. Directly increases the cellular uptake of vitamin C

3. Directly increases the cellular uptake of magnesium

4. Lessens the negative metabolic impact of increased intracellular calcium levels

5. More insulin receptors and more glucose/vitamin C transporters result from magnesium supplementation, further promoting via positive feedback the sustaining of increased cytoplasmic

magnesium levels (and decreased cytoplasmic oxidative stress)

6. Helps to reabsorb magnesium that would
   otherwise be excreted by the kidneys

Hydrocortisone

Hydrocortisone (cortisol) and vitamin C are the
two most important and most powerful naturally-occurring anti-inflammatory agents. A logical analysis
of available scientific data could conclude that the
primary reason initiating the acute inflammatory
response of the immune system is the absence or
severe deficiency of vitamin C and associated antioxidants. Wherever, focally or systemically, there
exists a severe deficiency of vitamin C, inflammation
ensues. Furthermore, the inflammation never resolves
completely until a sufficient antioxidant presence,
spearheaded by vitamin C, is restored. From a practical
point of view, vitamin C deficiency and inflammation
are essentially the same thing. At the very least, you
will never find one without the other.

When a vitamin C deficiency is not present
throughout the body, it simply represents a state of
what can be considered focal scurvy with focal inflammation. The inflammatory response to an area of infection, for example, occurs because the pathogens have
consumed all of the vitamin C normally present in that
area before infection ensued. When inflammation is
body-wide, the vitamin C deficiency is body-wide as
well, and variable degrees of intracellular scurvy are
also present throughout the body. Low to extremely
low plasma levels of vitamin C are consistently present
when systemic inflammation is present, as in hospital-

ized patients with significant infections and following trauma.[96-98] In addition to the depressed vitamin C levels, the blood levels of C-reactive protein, a reliable index of inflammation in the body, are consistently elevated.[99]

Because of the way the primary immune response in inflammation occurs where vitamin C levels have been depleted, often to immeasurable levels, it can be argued that an important role of the immune system, or conceivably even the *primary* role of the immune system, is to directly supply a concentrated vitamin C/antioxidant delivery to the areas or tissues of the body most acutely depleted of vitamin C.

The first immune cells to reach an area of acute inflammation are monocytes. These are cells that have exceptionally high concentrations of vitamin C (as much as 80-fold, or 8,000% higher than the surrounding plasma). Other immune cells also have very high concentrations of vitamin C.[100-102] Of note, the only other cells having such extraordinarily high concentrations of vitamin C are some neuronal cells, which can have vitamin C concentrations 100-fold higher than the plasma.

Monocytes also appear to have a significantly larger content and concentration of magnesium relative to lymphocytes.[103] This further supports the concept that the monocytes appearing as the first immune cells of an acute inflammatory response at the site of marked vitamin C deficiency are coming to deliver the antioxidant capacity of both magnesium and vitamin C. These appear to be the two most important agents for normalizing or at least lowering the elevated IOS present in the C-depleted cells. It has been suggested that the monocyte magnesium content would be a good indicator of total body magnesium status.[104]

Regarded as the anti-stress hormone, cortisol is normally secreted from the adrenal glands promptly

This further supports the concept that the monocytes appearing as the first immune cells of an acute inflammatory response at the site of marked vitamin C deficiency are coming to deliver the antioxidant capacity of both magnesium and vitamin C.

after any significant form of mental or physical stress is encountered. This acute release of cortisol results in an increase in blood glucose levels. Of significant interest is that in a vitamin C-producing animal, such an increase in blood glucose would subsequently result in a prompt increase in blood vitamin C levels as well, as glucose is the substrate that is converted to vitamin C in the liver of such an animal. Furthermore, in a vitamin C-producing animal, this glucose conversion into vitamin C is rapidly and profoundly increased in the face of substantial stress. However, man is genetically deficient in the last enzyme needed to catalyze the last chemical reaction in the biochemical pathway designed to produce vitamin C on demand. And since man is not such a vitamin C-producing animal, none of the acutely-released glucose gets turned into vitamin C. Subsequently, when such stress becomes chronic, the initial positive anti-inflammatory action of cortisol eventually becomes overwhelmed. Then an immune system-weakening effect begins to develop, as with the chronic immune system suppression seen with high-dose, long-term corticosteroid intake. Additionally, the toxicity of excess, poorly metabolized glucose signifi-

Magnesium supplementation results in a significant lowering of cortisol levels in circumstances of extreme physical stress.

cantly contributes to the negative long-term side effects of excess cortisol, whether taken as a prescription medication or pathologically produced in the body.

Magnesium and cortisol also have similar effects with regard to the lowering of elevated IOS. In an animal study, magnesium supplementation reduced salivary cortisol levels in conjunction with a reduction in stress-related behaviors.[105]

Magnesium supplementation results in a significant lowering of cortisol levels in circumstances of extreme physical stress.[106-108] One explanation for this effect is that such stress increases oxidative stress. This can be largely relieved by magnesium, and the need for the presence of increased amounts of cortisol to deal with the stress is lessened, bearing in mind that one **critical** role of cortisol is to help the cells to take up greater amounts of vitamin C.

Another study found that magnesium supplementation in elderly subjects with primary insomnia, another stressful situation, not only led to better sleep, but cortisol levels were also significantly lowered in the process.[109] This magnesium-cortisol-vitamin C connection is further supported by a randomized double-blind, placebo-controlled trial in young adults showing that 3,000 mg of vitamin C supplementation reduced cortisol levels while reducing subjective responses to acute psychological stress.[110] It would appear that when the "need" for cortisol-induced vitamin C uptake into cells is relieved by the administration of supplemental vitamin C, the cortisol level no longer has a physiological reason to rise. This also supports the idea that the ability of hydrocortisone to increase the intracellular levels of vitamin C is likely one of its **most important** effects when administered acutely and on a limited, short-term basis.

It is also useful to look at the relationship between cortisol and intracellular calcium levels. Like magnesium, cortisol is antagonistic to calcium's role in increasing IOS. Once again, what will be discussed are the effects of cortisol on an acute, limited basis, not those involved with long-term exposure to high doses or high endogenous levels.

Multiple cell studies document the ability of hydrocortisone to dramatically lower intracellular calcium levels. This effect results in an acute lowering of IOS.

Like magnesium, cortisol is antagonistic
to calcium's role in increasing IOS.

Multiple *in vitro* studies examining the cellular uptake of calcium consistently show that hydrocortisone acts as a very effective calcium channel blocker, significantly limiting the influx of new calcium into the cytoplasm. This effect consistently results in a lowering of intracellular calcium levels.[111-116]

Another study showed that the stimulation of glucocorticoid receptors decreases internal calcium

The ability of limited corticosteroid dosing to quell this inflammation, presumably via the mechanisms already discussed, resulted in shorter time to clinical stability and a shorter length of hospital stay.

levels.[117] suggesting that the calcium channel blocking activity of cortisol likely takes place on the cytoplasmic side of the calcium channels, since the cortisol receptors are located inside the cell. The antagonistic relationship between hydrocortisone and calcium is further defined by the fact that increased calcium exposure to adrenocortical cells (cells that secrete cortisol) provokes a prompt secretion of cortisol. This is consistent with the idea that a role of cortisol is to keep intracellular calcium levels down.[118] Essentially, cortisol lowers intracellular calcium, and the presence of excess calcium elicits the release of cortisol as a compensatory mechanism to keep the levels of cytoplasmic calcium under control.

The ability of cortisol to promote healing in general is also supported by a number of randomized studies that looked at the effects of short-term (one-time dose to 10 days of dosing) corticosteroid administration in the treatment of community-acquired pneumonia, an infection characterized by a strong inflammatory response. The ability of limited corticosteroid dosing to quell this inflammation, presumably via the mechanisms already discussed, resulted in a shorter time to clinical stability and a shorter length of hospital stay. Some of the studies suggested a mortality reduction effect as well. It was suggested that the studies collectively made a strong case for making corticosteroid administration part of the routine standard of care in the treatment of such patients.[119] Regardless of the other agents given, vitamin C always helps resolve infections more rapidly, and hydrocortisone helps get that vitamin C inside the affected cells.

Since hydrocortisone is a calcium channel blocker and works to keep intracellular calcium levels lower, it also serves as an antitoxin. That is true because all toxins effectively poison and/or kill affected cells by increasing calcium levels in the cell, which immediately translates to increased IOS.

Cyclosporin A is an immunosuppressive drug that

Essentially, cortisol lowers intracellular calcium, and the presence of excess calcium elicits the release of cortisol as a compensatory mechanism to keep the levels of cytoplasmic calcium under control.

consistently provokes toxic side effects in the heart, liver, and kidneys. This drug exerts its toxicity by increasing intracellular calcium levels and cellular oxidative stress. Cortisol has been shown to decrease the toxicity of cyclosporin A in therapeutic protocols. In animal cell studies, *in vivo* and *in vitro*, cortisol reduces the toxicity of this drug by decreasing intracellular calcium levels and dramatically reducing the calcium fluxes seen with the administration of this drug.[120,121]

Epinephrine in sufficient doses is also toxic, and it has been shown to increase myocardial calcium uptake when administered to dogs. The evidence of microscopic damage to the myocardium was significantly decreased when hydrocortisone was added to the epinephrine infusion.[122] This again shows that the ability of cortisol to prevent or significantly lower calcium uptake into any cell facing a toxic threat lessens or blocks that toxic effect. Of course, although not addressed in these studies, cortisol also works to block the threat of any toxin by increasing cellular vitamin C uptake. And vitamin C has been repeatedly shown to be the most impactful single agent in existence for its ability to neutralize toxins, to block their toxic impact, and to repair oxidized biomolecules already exposed directly to toxins.[123]

It is important to remember that hydrocortisone plays an important and direct role in lowering elevated IOS, at least *acutely*. Because of this, the clinician always needs to remember the following:

> **The many negative effects of long-term, high-dose hydrocortisone or corticosteroid therapy should <u>never</u> be used as a reason to deny the patient the incredibly beneficial benefits of short-term, lower-dose cortisol therapy.**

It turns outs that corticosteroid (dexamethasone) administration was shown to significantly enhance the cellular uptake of vitamin C. This was initially demonstrated in a mouse cell study.[124] Subsequently, in a human study on five volunteers, the uptake of orally-administered vitamin C into mononuclear white blood cells was greatly enhanced by intravenous hydrocortisone.[125] So, vitamin C keeps the intracellular hydrocortisone receptors in the reduced, active state, and hydrocortisone greatly facilitates the intracellular uptake of vitamin C. This is synergism at its best between the two most important anti-inflammatory agents in the body.

RECAP
Hydrocortisone properties that reduce or, cause to be reduced, increased IOS

1. Serves as a calcium channel blocker, decreasing intracellular concentrations of calcium

2. More calcium presence results in the reflex release of more hydrocortisone from adrenal cells

3. Serves as an antitoxin by decreasing intracellular concentrations of calcium

4. Increases the intracellular concentrations of vitamin C

5. Magnesium decreases the reflex need of hydrocortisone to lessen intracellular calcium levels

Thyroid hormone

Thyroid hormone (T3) appears to be the most important hormone in the body in terms of suppressing or minimizing body-wide oxidative stress when its levels are normal in the cells throughout the body. Both too much and too little thyroid hormone effect have been shown to be associated with increased oxidative stress.[126] Elevated levels of TSH (thyroid-stimulating hormone) that are generally seen in hypothyroid patients also correlate with increased systemic inflammation.[127]

In an animal study, it appeared that the initiation of the hypothyroid state directly increased oxidative stress in a cause-and-effect manner. Furthermore, the decline in thyroid function was promptly followed by microscopic evidence of inflammation in the heart tissue.[128] Effectively, it appears that loss of thyroid hormone effect in the cells assures the onset and maintenance of some degree of increased systemic inflammation. Therapeutically, this means that all otherwise effective treatment protocols for any disease will fall far short of their potential for success if any degree of decreased thyroid hormone function remains undiagnosed and/or untreated.

While many studies and trials have examined the clinical impact and treatment of any degree of hyperthyroidism or of marked degrees of hypothyroidism, it appears that there is literally an epidemic of minimal hypothyroidism ("subclinical hypothyroidism") that is often not detected on standard thyroid testing (typically significant elevations of TSH). However, even a subclinical deficiency can profoundly impact health in general and heart disease more specifically.[129-131]

The degree to which even minimal deficiencies of thyroid function negatively impact the redox balance in the body is supported strongly by the logical inferences from the clinical data of a clinician who specialized in the

Therapeutically, this means that all otherwise effective treatment protocols for any disease will fall far short of their potential for success if any degree of decreased thyroid hormone function remains undiagnosed and/or untreated.

treatment of hypothyroidism, Dr. Broda Barnes.[132] Dr. Barnes pioneered the concept of diagnosing low thyroid function by careful and repeated measurements of body temperature. He found many patients who demonstrated a good symptom and temperature response to dessicated thyroid therapy, yet who had normal conventional thyroid function tests. His observation was that a temperature consistently below 97.8 to 98.2 degrees Fahrenheit strongly suggested low thyroid function. And when any of the many symptoms of hypothyroidism was seen in the context of a lowered body temperature, thyroid therapy was initiated by Dr. Barnes. He also asserted that as long as basal temperature did not exceed 98.2 degrees Fahrenheit, there was "no risk of excessive thyroid dosage."

Over a 20-year period, Dr. Barnes conducted a study on 1,569 patients who he treated with dessicated thyroid utilizing his body temperature protocol and his clinical expertise on the resolution of hypothyroid symptoms. Some of the patients were not followed over a full 20 years. At the end of the study period, Dr. Barnes noted that there had occurred only _four_ heart attacks, all in men, ages ranging from 56 to 61. Retrospectively, Dr. Barnes suspected that these four individuals had been inadequately-dosed.

Based on a well-established prospective health study (Framingham study), the incidence of heart attacks in a comparable pool of adults over the same 20-year period should have been 22 for the women and 50 for the men. Of great additional significance, no patient in the study was directly asked to stop smoking, and the pool of patients studied logically had the same incidence of diabetes, high blood pressure, root canals and other infected teeth, and all of the other chronic degenerative diseases as those individuals followed in the Framingham study. Furthermore, Dr. Barnes also noted that at least 30 heart attacks occurred in patients who dropped out the study and stopped taking their thyroid replacement. A majority of these individuals were young (under 60), and 5 were seen under the age of 50.

Independent of his observation of the impact of low thyroid function in promoting coronary artery disease and heart attacks, Dr. Barnes also anecdotally noted that infectious diseases in general prospered when thyroid function was low, and was strikingly suppressed when the patient was in a normal (euthyroid) state of thyroid function. He also made the clinical observation that about 2 months of thyroid therapy was needed to clearly decrease the propensity towards contracting infectious diseases, and that the effect would wear off "in six months to a year if thyroid therapy is stopped."

Optimal Thyroid Status Provides Extra Protection Against the Systemic Spread of Dental Pathogens

It is now well-established in the medical and dental literature that the development and evolution of coronary artery disease leading to heart attacks is ***nearly always*** (>90%) caused by the chronic arterial inflammation fed by the continuous seeding of oral pathogens, especially from infected teeth (commonly root canal-treated) and chronic periodontal (gum) disease.[133,134]

Root canal-treated teeth, which are all chronically infected, appear to be especially important in seeding the pathogens that end up in the coronary arteries and lead to atherosclerosis and heart attack. Their very presence in the mouth is statistically linked to a significantly greater chance of heart attack.[135] Indeed, the oral pathogens characteristically seen in root canals and other sites of oral infection are the same as the ones seen in the linings of atherosclerotic coronary arteries. One investigator scraped out the obstructing plaques in coronary heart disease patients by a procedure called atherectomy and then analyzed them. He found bacterial DNA in these specimens in ***38 out of 38*** patients. Furthermore, over 50 different species of bacteria were found, and individual plaques typically had between 10 and 15 different bacterial DNAs.[136] Nearly all of the patients had fungal DNA as well.[137] Other investigators have also consistently found pathogens, especially of oral origin, in coronary artery plaques.[138-140] To be perfectly clear, pathogenic bacteria (and fungi as well) should **_NEVER_** be present in a normal coronary artery. The lining of the normal coronary artery should always be pathogen-free.

It is completely avoiding the obvious and logical conclusion to even suggest that these pathogens are not the primary reason for the evolution of atherosclerosis. Furthermore, the vast majority of acutely-formed platelet clots that are the immediate cause of complete coronary artery obstruction and heart attack have a very high concentration of these same pathogens.[141]

The clear conclusion would appear to be that:

> **Completely normal thyroid function protects strongly against both systemic infections as well as against the ability of chronic focal sites of infection to disseminate and to take hold at new sites.**

In other words, focal infections (teeth, gums, tonsils) strongly tend to **_STAY_** focal in persons with completely normal thyroid function. Effectively, thyroid normalcy allows individuals to **_coexist_** with their infections rather than have their general health eventually destroyed by their spread to distant, non-oral sites.

Dr. Barnes did an extraordinary job of clinically evaluating and effectively treating his minimal to mildly hypothyroid patients. While a doctor can certainly use the same approach as Dr. Barnes, it would appear that measuring free T3 levels and reverse T3 levels is also an effective way to discover minimally hypothyroid patients and then to document that they have been effectively returned to the normal thyroid state with dessicated thyroid administration. Reverse T3 is an inactive form of the thyroid hormone that binds and blocks the normal binding sites of T3, preventing active T3 from exerting its proper physiological effect. It also appears that following the reverse T3 level is a reliable way to monitor and quantify increased body-wide oxidative stress.

In diabetes, a prototypical disease featuring body-wide increased oxidative stress, T3 levels are consistently low and reverse T3 levels consistently elevated.[142] Consistent with this relationship with increased oxidative stress, reverse T3 has been shown *in vitro* to cause increased proliferation of breast cancer cells and glioblastoma cells.[143] However, even with the availability today of reverse T3 measurements, it would still be highly advisable for today's clinician to include Dr. Barnes' body temperature monitoring for the optimal identification, treatment, and long-term follow-up of minimally hypothyroid patients.

Monitoring free T3 and reverse T3 levels allows the physician to identify and treat the most common thyroid hormone malady: ***cellular hypothyroidism***, a condition typically not apparent on regular thyroid testing [TSH in normal range with normal thyroid hormone levels], but nevertheless very common, and very clinically significant (especially as a primary cause of atherosclerosis and heart attack).[144] Virtually all the cells in the body work to convert inactive T4 to active T3 with intracellular enzymes (deiodinases) that are subject to oxidation and inactivation as any other biomolecule.[145] Fully 80% of all the T3 in the body is generated in the cells of the body **_outside_** of the thyroid

It has also been shown that a severely low magnesium level not only increases the risk of hypothyroidism, it also is associated with an increased risk of autoimmune thyroid disease.

gland.[146] This means that a thyroid gland functionally normally enough to produce normal amounts of T4 can exist in a body with clinically significant hypothyroidism if enough oxidative stress is preventing its conversion to T3 in the peripheral tissues.[147,148]

As body-wide oxidative stress increases and more of the deiodinases become oxidized, reverse T3 levels reliably increase and T3 levels usually decrease. Optimally, there should be a ratio of T3 to reverse T3 of about 18/1 to 21/1. Slightly higher ratios should not be problematic as long as there is no clinical or other laboratory evidence of hyperthyroidism, and lower levels should always signal the need to begin some degree of thyroid therapy, while simultaneously looking to resolve sources of increased oxidative stress (e.g., infected teeth) to hopefully reactivate (reduce) the oxidized enzymes causing the abnormal T3 and reverse T3 levels. Many patients will need thyroid treatment for life, while others will just end up needing the identification and proper removal of focal infections to restore thyroid function normalcy after the reduction of increased systemic oxidative stress.

As magnesium and thyroid physiology is essential to the well-being of every cell in the body, it follows that magnesium and thyroid have been found to have some important interrelationships. One study showed that while significant exercise reduced thyroid hormone activity, magnesium supplementation was able to prevent this reduction.[149] In cell and animal studies, it appears that thyroid hormone plays a significant role in maintaining intracellular magnesium homeostasis. The administration of thyroid to hypothyroid or hypothyroid cell models restores the magnesium balance observed in animals or cells with a normal thyroid status.[150] When the thyroid gland is removed, magnesium levels often drop.[151] In an animal model of diabetes, magnesium administration appears to improve the thyroid dysfunction otherwise seen.[152] It has also been shown that a severely low magnesium level not only increases the risk of hypothyroidism, it also is associated with an increased risk of autoimmune thyroid disease.[153]

Thyroid hormone has also been shown to have largely opposite effects on calcium levels and calcium metabolism compared to its effects on magnesium. This is to be expected since calcium and magnesium have a reciprocal relationship throughout the body. Just as thyroid supplementation to hypothyroid animals restores intracellular magnesium levels in cardiac cells, thyroid hormone prevents intracellular calcium overload, a logical reciprocal effect.[154] Further consistent with these thyroid-magnesium-calcium relationship studies, it has been noted that in hypothyroid rats, myocardial calcium content is elevated while serum calcium is reduced.[155]

RECAP

Thyroid hormone properties and increased IOS

1. Thyroid hormone is a major, and probably the main, regulator of oxidative stress inside cells and throughout the body.
2. Thyroid hormone works to normalize intracellular magnesium levels in hypothyroid animals. Conversely, untreated hypothyroid animals have increased intracellular calcium and lower serum calcium. Thyroid hormone also acutely prevents intracellular calcium overload in animal heart cells.
3. Minimally decreased thyroid function facilitates the likelihood of contraction of systemic infectious diseases, and it facilitates the metastatic-like spread of focal infections such as are often found in the oral cavity. This decreased thyroid function likely also increases the aggressiveness and metastatic capacity of many cancers.
4. Minimally decreased thyroid function is extremely common, probably present in at least 50% of older individuals, especially those with significant chronic degenerative diseases.
5. Magnesium status strongly impacts the normalcy of thyroid status, and thyroid status significant impacts magnesium homeostasis.
6. Achieving an optimal impact from any clinical protocol must include the normalization of thyroid status.

Vitamin C Supplementation

An Essential Guide

The overall goal of any supplementation regimen should be to optimize the antioxidant status (stores) throughout as much of the body as possible. More specifically, as has been discussed at some length in this book, lowering or normalizing elevated intracellular oxidative stress (IOS) effectively treats all known diseases. When IOS can be reduced to normal physiological levels all disease-related symptoms should lessen or disappear. Furthermore, diseases that have not accumulated too extensive a degree of chronic oxidative damage in the body can actually be expected to resolve completely when this oxidative stress reduction goal is achieved and maintained.

As vitamin C is the most important antioxidant in the body and literally the fuel (electron source) required by every cell in body to function normally, the primary aim of all treatment protocols should center on optimizing the levels of this vitamin on a daily basis.

Other treatment protocols that lack this emphasis might still provide significant clinical benefits but those benefits will never be optimized if there is not a focus on keeping vitamin C levels normal in both the intracellular and extracellular spaces.

Unfortunately, being able to precisely define a problem does not necessarily make it a problem that is easy to correct. Restoring and maintain the levels of vitamin C and other important antioxidants to normal or near-normal levels is not as simple as one would hope. While popping a vitamin C pill of any size daily will help just about everyone, it will virtually always fall far short of the goal of reaching the state of optimized health that a normal antioxidant balance will bring in the body.

Many conditions, especially acute infections and acute toxin exposures, can readily be addressed and completely resolved with an aggressive administration of intravenous and/or oral multi-gram doses of vitamin C for several days.[1] However, optimizing vitamin C levels in various tissues and organs throughout the body to minimize the clinical impact and continued evolution of chronic diseases is a different story. This guide will first endeavor to outline the different ways in which vitamin C can be most effectively administered, along with important suggestions for both reaching and maintaining optimal tissue levels of vitamin C. Surprisingly, perhaps, getting vitamin C effectively into the body involves the interplay of many different administration factors.

Important Factors in the Effective Administration of Vitamin C

1. Dose
2. Route
3. Rate
4. Frequency
5. Duration of treatment period
6. Type of vitamin C
7. Adjunct therapies
8. Safety
9. Quality of overall protocol

1. Dose

While all of the factors of vitamin C administration to be discussed are important, inadequate dosing remains the single most important factor in preventing complete clinical success with the vitamin C treatment. This is especially for acute viral and bacterial infections. If enough vitamin C is not given to deal with the amount of increased oxidative stress involved with a significant infection, with an intoxication or poisoning, or with an ongoing medical condition, complete clinical success will never be realized. This is especially the case when an infection/poisoning/condition presents in a very acute and rapidly progressing fashion.

It is also important to emphasize that some success short of an optimal response can just about always be seen no matter how little vitamin C is given. In sick individuals, reduced, electron-replete vitamin C is always in short supply, and any amount will be of benefit. It's just a matter of whether the amount of vitamin C is able to help to the degree of being clinically apparent. Unlike many other clinical scenarios where more than the recommended dose of a clinically-indicated agent can cause toxicity or other clinical problems, more of vitamin C can expected to help even more.

Even with the ultra-high doses of vitamin C that have been administered over the previous decades, a toxic level has never been defined. As vitamin C is the main nutrient on which the body runs, expecting a toxic effect from vitamin C at some point of increased dosing is somewhat akin to expecting toxicity to result from assimilating too much nutrition from a quality diet.

In the treatment of acute infections and acute poisonings, optimal dosing is especially critical. If those conditions have been present for a long enough time before effective treatment is initiated, they can kill or cause long-term secondary organ damage. It is always important to give enough vitamin C to prevent new infection-induced oxidative damage while addressing repair of old oxidative damage. Lower dosing might eventually cure an infection, but achieving a cure as quickly as possible with higher vitamin C doses will always decrease the development of new oxidative damage while getting the infection under control before completely eradicating it.

Since vitamin C toxicity is not a significant concern, determining the initial dose requires only minimal clinical evaluation and expertise. This is especially so when considering the ramifications of an uncontrolled acute infection or the acute consequences of a highly toxic poisoning that is treated with an ineffective protocol for an extended time.

<u>ALWAYS</u>, when the patient is critically ill and in danger of imminent hemodynamic (blood pressure) collapse and death, be prepared to give additional dosing. Stabilizing the patient may even require direct injection over seconds to minutes by syringe. In an acutely poisoned or infected patient, *prompt administration of more vitamin C should always be given before any clinical evidence of deterioration develops.* When the patient is clinically stable and/or starting to show improvement, the clinician can then decide on the frequency and amount of future dosing from a less urgent perspective. It is always optimal to work with a clinician already familiar with vitamin C to monitor clinical progress and make dosing changes as indicated. But it is not necessary, and the lack of vitamin C toxicity always warrants an aggressive dosing approach in critically ill, clinically unstable patients.

While <u>not</u> an absolute rule, a reasonable guide for selecting the initial intravenous dose of vitamin C suggests between 1 to 1.5 grams per kilogram of body weight. Practically speaking, this would mean 25 grams for most children old enough to readily tolerate an IV line, 50 to 75 grams for a 100- to 120-pound person, and 75 to 150 grams for a 150- to 250-pound person. Larger children will benefit most by starting at 50 grams. Lower doses and higher doses can always be given as deemed appropriate clinically, depending on body size and the acuteness and clinical stability of the patient.

When determining long-term vitamin C dosing for general healthcare maintenance as well as the treatment of chronic disease, factors of affordability, convenience, symptom relief, and laboratory test results play significant roles in selecting both the type(s) and amounts of vitamin C to be taken daily.

Affordability. It is always optimal to include a quality preparation of liposome-encapsulated form of vitamin C if financially feasible, as these forms are generally more costly than regular, unencapsulated forms of vitamin C. While there is no absolute maximal dosage, most individuals will do very well on one to five grams of this form of vitamin C daily.

Be aware that there is a great deal of outright fraud among supplement manufacturers who claim they are selling a real liposome-encapsulated vitamin C. Also, note that all of the "homemade" formulations of "liposome-encapsulated" vitamin C tend to be emulsions and are not encapsulated at all. Although emulsions can somewhat improve initial uptake by the gut, they cannot provide the greatly-enhanced delivery of vitamin C into the cytoplasm and intracellular organelles (mitochondria, etc.) provided by quality liposomes of the right size and concentration. If this enhanced intracellular delivery is desired or needed, as in those with critical illness, a genuine liposome-encapsulated product is far better than other oral forms. But, a fraudulent product never makes sense from a health or economic standpoint.

Convenience. Oral vitamin C is best given several times a day, due to its rapid clearance through the kidneys. This is less of a concern with the liposome-encapsulated form of vitamin C, as its significantly enhanced intracellular uptake removes it from the blood where it would be subject to increased filtration by the kidneys with a more rapid and greater degree of excretion.

The best way to determine the appropriate daily dose of vitamin C the body needs is to administer a powdered form of sodium ascorbate or ascorbic acid in regular and increasing dosages to the point of diarrhea (bowel tolerance). Most reasonably healthy individuals will reach a daily bowel tolerance dose at somewhere between 5 and 15 grams. Some people have much more sensitive bowels, and cannot take more than one or two grams. If possible, such individuals should take more of the liposome-encapsulated vitamin C, as bowel tolerance is not an issue with that form of vitamin C. Other individuals have very high bowel tolerances of 20, 30, 40 grams or more of vitamin C, and even a handful of individuals cannot reliably reach a bowel tolerance level. Generally, these individuals have significant toxin levels in their bodies, often due-to dental infections, such as root canal-treated and other infected teeth.

Symptom Relief. Very few individuals have completely symptom-free lives. As all symptoms are mediated by increased oxidative stress in some area of the body, vitamin C can always be expected to lessen a symptom when dosed correctly, at the very least. Individuals who begin supplementing vitamin C quickly develop a sense for what amount of vitamin C makes them feel the best, and this is a good way to help determine long-term dosing. Other individuals who have no discernible symptoms will nevertheless begin to develop an increased "health awareness" the longer they supplement vitamin C. Such individuals often begin to feel even better than usual without having realized they were not feeling optimally before. Ultimately, as they sense just a slight impairment of wellness – even without clear-cut symptoms – they are able to discern that they are experiencing a toxic or infectious challenge. At that point, the vitamin C dose can be increased above maintenance levels for a few days to address the challenge and prevent an outright development of sickness.

Laboratory Testing. Only the rarest of individuals these days have complete normalcy when given a broad array of baseline laboratory tests. As such, many abnormal tests will significantly improve or even normalize as vitamin C is administered over time. An astute healthcare practitioner can readily see in routine laboratory testing whether the general antioxidant status of the body, lead by vitamin C, is having as much effect as possible by examining the interval changes in tests over time and relating those test results to the amount of vitamin C being taken at those times. Laboratory testing is an especially elegant way to fine-tune vitamin C dosing, as many individuals may still feel great while certain laboratory tests are worsening over time. Such testing can give a new meaning to preventive medicine by not just treating a patient based on symptomatology. It is also very important to realize that the "reference range" of very many laboratory tests do not represent a true "normal range." Such ranges are designed only to statistically group the tested population into subsets that are better considered to be "less abnormal" rather than actually normal. Some common blood tests actually have a "normal range" that doesn't even include a truly normal result, because some toxicities/conditions are shared by such a large percentage of the population (e.g., ferritin levels and iron toxicity).

2. Route

Vitamin C can be given in many different ways including:

- ✓ Intravenously
- ✓ Intramuscularly
- ✓ Orally
- ✓ Rectally
- ✓ Nasally via misting inhalers (nebulization)
- ✓ Topically on the eyes or in the ears, and both on the skin as well as through it (transdermally).

Most commonly, it is given orally and intravenously. The concept to keep in mind is that the success of any vitamin C treatment depends primarily on getting vitamin C molecules in direct contact with the pro-oxidant molecules at the site(s) of increased oxidative stress. When using vitamin C in the treatment of delicate areas, such as the eyes or the respiratory tract, it is important to always use pH-neutral solutions of vitamin C (sodium ascorbate or properly buffered ascorbic acid). Intramuscular injections, discussed further below, are great for babies and small children. Rectal administrations can also be an option if oral or intravenous routes are not feasible, or if a retention enema application is being used, as for a condition such as chronic ulcerative colitis. However, any inflammatory condition of the intestine or colon can also be very effectively treated by administering bowel tolerance doses of sodium ascorbate powder in water or juice, which also reaches the diseased areas quite effectively.

3. Rate

How fast a dose of vitamin C is given intravenously is a very important factor for maximizing the benefit of vitamin C therapy. Depending on the condition being treated and the effect that is desired, vitamin C can be given in seconds from a syringe as an IV push, or it can be infused rapidly, slowly, or even as a continuous infusion over 24 or more hours.

IV Push: When a patient is in shock or imminent danger of death (such as might be seen after an acute exposure to life-threatening amounts of venom or toxin that are still largely circulating in the bloodstream), multigram doses of vitamin C can be given IV push with sodium ascorbate or well-buffered ascorbic acid. The idea is to get as much vitamin C in direct contact with circulating toxins as rapidly as possible. The results can be dramatic. Dr. Klenner described how he treated a cyanotic patient who was acutely poisoned by the bite of a venomous Puss Caterpillar only 10 minutes earlier and complaining of severe chest pain, the inability to take a deep breath, and the feeling that he was dying:

"Twelve grams of vitamin C was quickly pulled into a 50 c.c. syringe and with a 20 gauge needle was given intravenously as fast as the plunger could be pushed. Even before the injection was completed, he exclaimed, 'Thank God.' The poison had been neutralized that rapidly." [2]

New variations on Dr. Klenner's approach described above include multi-gram vitamin C IV pushes augmented with magnesium, hydrocortisone, and insulin. These additions all enhance the ability to get vitamin C inside the cells of the body and rapidly decrease any elevated levels of IOS.

Rapid Infusion: Rapid infusion generally means an infusion rate that is as rapid as a wide-open IV line will permit. Practically speaking, this translates to 500 to 700 cc of vitamin C solution being administered between 40 and 60 minutes, typically containing between 50 and 100 grams of vitamin C.

Since the glucose and vitamin C molecules are very closely related chemically, when such an amount of vitamin C is infused this rapidly, the pancreas perceives the vitamin C load as a glucose load. As a result, the pancreas secretes substantial insulin into the blood to deal with what it considers an acute excess of glucose that needs to be metabolized. For most individuals, the insulin release is significant enough that a pronounced hypoglycemia, sometimes as low as 20 to 25 mg/dL, ensues and is maintained until the IV is completed or some oral or IV forms of glucose are supplied to increase the glucose level. This type of vitamin C infusion, then, can be viewed as an endogenously-induced form of insulin potentiation therapy (IPT).

IPT, involving the deliberate induction of substantial hypoglycemia with insulin injections, has been documented to be a very effective way to increase the cellular uptake of most nutrients and/or medications given at the same time.[3,4] The endogenously-induced IPT has the same effect, but also assuring a much larger uptake of vitamin C into the cells than would otherwise take place when it is infused at a slower rate and no significant release of insulin is stimulated. In cell studies, insulin has been documented to stimulate vitamin C accumulation.[5,6,7] Such studies, along with known effects of IPT, reliably indicate that similar mechanisms are in play for insulin promoting vitamin C uptake in all the metabolically active cells in the body

Slow Infusion: As noted rapid infusions can acutely push much more vitamin C inside the cells via the mechanism of reflex secretion of insulin by the pancreas. However, a much greater portion of the vitamin C also ends up being excreted through the kidneys in the process. Many chronic degenerative patients, including heart patients and cancer patients, will benefit optimally when their infusion takes place over two or more hours. Many such patients will benefit from both rapid and slow infusions during the course of their protocol administration, as vitamin C, somewhat like regular antibiotic therapy, can offer more benefit when given several times as a high-concentration, rapidly-infused "loading dose," to be followed over a more extended period of time with repeated slow infusions. This simply allows the underlying disease to be exposed to more vitamin C more of the time, often resulting in dramatic symptom lessening and even disease reversal.

Continuous Infusion: This is a form of administration that should be of great value, and trials are currently taking place (2019). Dr. Klenner first made the suggestion with regard to the possible treatment of cancer:

> "This is the reason we believe a dose range of 100 grams to 300 grams daily by continuous intravenous drip for a period of several months might prove surprisingly profitable." [8]

Perhaps the only flaw in Dr. Klenner's assertion is that it would seem unlikely that most cancers would require months to resolve with such an approach. Although intravenous vitamin C is finally making inroads (as of 2018) to being given more often in the hospitals of the United States, an administration such as suggested by Dr. Klenner is not yet being done. At the Riordan Clinic, the most prominent clinic in the world in terms of intravenous vitamin C (IVC) infusions and vitamin C-related clinical and basic science research, an elastic bladder form of administration containing vitamin C and other nutrients, such as magnesium, is now being utilized to allow an individual to get a controlled slow intravenous infusion of the bladder contents over a 24-hour period as an outpatient. And when the patients are in the clinic during operating hours, additional IV pushes (pulses) of vitamin C can also be given to further optimize the presence of vitamin C in the blood "24/7."

4. Frequency

The appropriate frequency of vitamin C dosing in any of its forms is completely based on the clinical response to the previous administration(s) of vitamin C. When treating an acute infectious disease or an acute intoxication/poisoning, the improvement of vital signs and the reported relief of any associated acute symptoms dictate how soon and how sizeable the next dose of vitamin C should be. When no significant improvement is seen, more vitamin C should be given immediately and generally infused more rapidly. IV push should generally be reserved for those circumstances when death or coma appear imminent.

If an appropriately-sized dose of vitamin C is administered the first time, a positive response should nearly always result, and the decision of when and how much the second dose of vitamin C should be will still be dictated by the clinical expertise of the treating healthcare practitioner, if intravenous administration is being utilized. An oral vitamin C regimen can also be pushed in a vigorous fashion by a caregiver at home if no healthcare provider is involved. The most important parameters to follow in the early stages of treatment include:

✓ Lowering of elevated temperatures
✓ Lessening of rapid heart rates and rapid breathing

✓ Normalization of elevated or depressed blood pressures
✓ Overall increased comfort level of the patient

It is also important to give sizeable doses of both regular vitamin C and liposome-encapsulated vitamin C orally regardless of whether the patient has also been receiving any intravenous administrations.

The value of the frequency of vitamin C administration was revealed in 2017 when a protocol for relatively small doses (1.5 grams) of vitamin C given every six hours (along with hydrocortisone and thiamine) resulted in the survival of most patients in septic shock treated in the intensive care unit (8.5% mortality versus a 40% mortality in an untreated group) .[9] Another similar study showed that a comparable dose of vitamin C by itself every six hours also produced the same impressive result in saving patients with advanced sepsis.[10]

Certainly, it remains clear that a large increase in toxin- or infection-induced oxidative stress requires a large amount of antioxidant administration to directly control and begin to resolve any clinical condition resulting from such stress. However, the studies cited above on vitamin C and sepsis (short of death, sepsis is the most advanced degree to which a systemic infection can evolve) appear to indicate that the frequency of vitamin C administration might be just as important as absolute dose. As it is known that vitamin C in the blood gets rapidly excreted via the urine, the takeaway lesson is that if 50 to 100 grams of vitamin C is going to be administered per day to an individual, it will probably have greater impact if given in divided doses every six to eight hours. This way, less will be excreted and more will be available to deal with the oxidative stress overload. Obviously, if the patient is not hospitalized but in a clinic, the one-time intravenous administration per day might be the only practical way to proceed.

5. Duration

Especially for significant acute infectious diseases, the duration of a vitamin C treatment regimen, by whatever route of administration, is important. Such a patient usually ~~does~~ responds very dramatically to a large initial dose of vitamin C. However, even when clinical normalcy appears to have been restored, it is very important to give sizeable doses of vitamin C for at least 48 hours after the patient "appears" completely cured. Acute infections, especially viral ones, can often rebound when vitamin C therapy is not extended for this length of time. Along the same line of thought, giving a large amount of vitamin C orally, IV, and/or IM every 4 to 6 hours around the clock will completely resolve an acute infectious syndrome much more rapidly than would be seen with much larger doses given 24 to 48 hours apart.

6. Types of Vitamin C

The essence of vitamin C is its ascorbate anion. The associated cations include the following:

✓ Hydrogen (ascorbic acid)
✓ Sodium
✓ Calcium
✓ Magnesium

✓ Transitional Metal (Manganese, Zinc, Molybdenum, Chromium)
✓ Ascorbyl Palmitate
✓ "Vitamin C Complex"

Ascorbic Acid is really the prototypical form of vitamin C. This is always a desirable form of vitamin C to take when there is no concern with stomach upset due to excess acid effect, or no concern of excess acidity causing pain at the catheter site when not sufficiently buffered and given intravenously. Sodium ascorbate is probably the optimal form of regular vitamin C that has not been encapsulated with liposomes. This is because very large amounts can be easily tolerated by the stomach, and it can be given up to the point of inducing a diarrhea-like effect when bowel tolerance is reached. If exceeding the bowel tolerance level is well-tolerated, this is also a very desirable effect as it neutralizes and eliminates a large amount of gut-generated toxins before they get absorbed, and the levels of bacterial pathogens are reduced as well. The amount of sodium ascorbate needed to exceed the bowel tolerance point can also be useful as a rough guide as to the degree of infection or toxicity that is present in the patient. Generally, the greater the infectious and/or toxic challenge, the more vitamin C gets absorbed earlier in the gut and the less of it reaches the colon to reach and exceed the bowel tolerance point.[11,12]

Calcium Ascorbate, which is commonly marketed as Ester C or buffered vitamin C, just adds another unnecessary source of calcium to the supplementing individual. While it is true that it is easy on the stomach, sodium ascorbate is tolerated just as easily and does not add to the pre-existing state of calcium excess already present in most older individuals. It should also be noted that large amounts of sodium ascorbate can be taken by most individuals, including those with high blood pressure and heart disease, without causing fluid retention or an increase in blood pressure. This is because it is sodium *chloride*, not sodium associated with another anion like ascorbate, citrate, or bicarbonate, that reliably causes fluid retention and aggravates high blood pressure in individuals sensitive to volume overload. The term "sodium-dependent" hypertension should forever be replaced with the term "sodium chloride-dependent" or "table salt-dependent" hypertension.[13,14] In any event, large doses of sodium ascorbate should not be avoided for fear of provoking elevated blood pressure.

Magnesium Ascorbate is an excellent form of vitamin C since it brings both magnesium and ascorbate into the body. The only practical limit to dosage with this form of vitamin C would the amount that starts to approach bowel tolerance and result in diarrhea. Probably the main reason against supplementing magnesium ascorbate on a regular basis is that it adds significant cost to what are two exceptionally inexpensive supplements when taken as separate supplements. It is also somewhat less well-tolerated by the stomach than sodium ascorbate, depending on the individual.

Potassium Ascorbate is also a good form of ascorbate for supplementation. The only problem is that it is relatively easy to overdose on potassium, which can cause fatal cardiac arrhythmias, especially if it is taken with the same abandon as so many other completely nontoxic supplements. Potassium should never really be taken on a regular basis unless advised by a healthcare practitioner who has done appropriate clinical and laboratory testing beforehand. For people who are in need of potassium supplementation, this can be an excellent supplement. It just needs some measure of regular monitoring to make sure blood levels of potassium do not get dangerously elevated.

Transitional Metal Forms of ascorbate are not really good forms of vitamin C to ingest in large amounts on a regular basis. While ascorbate has no real toxicity concerns, most of the transitional metal ascorbates, especially manganese, molybdenum, zinc, and chromium, can very easily be overdone. Also, as mentioned above, they are needlessly expensive and do not end up providing the amounts of vitamin C that most individuals should be taking on a regular basis. It is better to take a quality supplement with a wide range of bioavailable minerals along with multigram amounts of sodium ascorbate separately.

Ascorbyl Palmitate. Vitamin C, which is water-soluble in all the forms discussed above, also comes in a fat-soluble form known as ascorbyl palmitate. Including at least a gram or two of ascorbyl palmitate in a daily supplementation regimen can provide important additional antioxidant coverage in fat-rich tissues and areas not otherwise well-protected by the more common forms of vitamin C.[15,16,17] Ascorbyl palmitate has been demonstrated to protect the cell membrane of intact red blood cells[18] as well as to protect important anti-atherosclerotic lipoproteins in the body.[19] It has also been employed as an antioxidant to prevent skin aging.[20] Liposome delivery systems containing ascorbyl palmitate have been demonstrated to kill cancer cells *in vitro* as well as to slow tumor growth in mice more effectively than with free ascorbic acid.[21] All of these studies indicate the importance of including ascorbyl palmitate as part of an optimally effective vitamin C-centered protocol.

"Vitamin C Complex" There are also vitamin C supplements being marketed as "Vitamin C Complex," with the basic assertion that vitamin C must be present in a "food form" with multiple associated substances, such as antioxidant bioflavonoids like rutin and quercetin, in order to be of any benefit. Many of the sellers of a product like this even make the incredible assertion that pure vitamin C, as ascorbic acid or sodium ascorbate, is of little to no benefit and will not even reverse scurvy by itself. A few "vitamin C complex" voices even assert that ascorbic acid is bad for you and could cause cancer. In a nutshell, this is all marketing hyperbole (and outright fraud and deception) by companies trying to carve out a piece of the vitamin C sales pie. It seems that some "experts" feel that if something completely outlandish is asserted often enough with a straight face and the appearances of pseudoscientific "support" that the public will think they are "on to something." A deception or a lie remains just that no matter how many times it is repeated. Furthermore, all of these "experts" seem to have forgotten, or perhaps they never knew, that vitamin C-synthesizing animals make ascorbic acid and release it into the blood. They do not synthesize anything resembling a "vitamin C complex."

Certainly, vitamin C does function even better with as large a network of other antioxidants as can be assimilated. However, it is completely wrong and frankly ridiculous to assert that it will not reverse scurvy by itself, or that it is of very limited utility by itself. All the work of vitamin C pioneer Frederick Klenner, M.D. with infectious diseases and toxins demonstrated unequivocally the incredible and typically curative value of vitamin C utilized by itself in high doses in these conditions.[22] Just as crazy, some sellers of a vitamin C complex supplement actually claim ascorbic acid is not vitamin C, which is as dishonest as a statement can be. Presumably, this assertion is made in order to convince vitamin Consumers that their product is the only one that can deliver the many benefits of vitamin C ingestion. Not surprisingly, this form of vitamin C supplementation is substantially more expensive that regular supplemental forms of vitamin C. Although this is a product that will certainly provide benefits, more benefit is available for less money spent on just ascorbic acid or sodium ascorbate. Buyer, beware (or be aware).

7. Adjunct Therapies

Unless another therapy is inherently pro-oxidant or toxic in nature, vitamin C will only augment the desired effects. For example, if an individual is receiving chemotherapy for cancer, the vitamin C might neutralize the chemotherapy drug itself if it is circulating in the blood at the same time and enough vitamin C is circulating in the blood. The chemotherapy is a toxic, electron-seeking agent, and the vitamin C is an antioxidant, electron-donating agent. When any chemotherapy agent has received the electrons it is seeking, it ceases to be toxic and can no longer kill or help to kill a cancer cell. However, this effect is easily avoided by staggering the dosing of any inherently toxic drug and any administered vitamin C by a few hours or so. It should also be noted that when vitamin C is given after a cancer chemotherapy agent, it helps both to kill the cancer cell even more effectively while also repairing the damage that was done to normal cells by the chemotherapy. When the vitamin C is given before such chemotherapy, a greater cancer-killing effect is also seen, and many normal cells that would have been damaged are protected by the greater concentration of vitamin C present. The literature is now very clear that vitamin C substantially improves the anti-cancer effects of chemotherapy while dramatically lessening the side effects associated with chemotherapy.[23,24]

It is also important to note that vitamin C does not interfere with the antimicrobial effects of antibiotics. Quite the contrary, vitamin C enhances the effects of many antibiotics, and one should never avoid indicated antibiotic therapy if there is the possibility to take it along with the vitamin C. Vitamin C has many different supportive effects on the immune system,[25] including increasing the degree of antibody response to a pathogen. Even though vitamin C can often do the job on a bacterial infection by itself, there is no reason to avoid its synergistic effect with an appropriate antibiotic in resolving the infection.

8. Safety

An important factor in the administration of any therapy to treat a medical condition is how safe it is. Many traditional medical therapies can often have a desired clinical effect, but they can also have a significant side effect or toxicity some or even much of the time. "First, do no harm" continues to be the appropriate standard by which any therapeutic intervention should be measured, regardless of how effective it might be some of the time. Except in patients with significant chronic renal insufficiency or chronic renal failure, vitamin C has never exhibited toxicity at any level of administration. Of course, nearly all drugs have to be administered with caution in patients with kidney failure, and vitamin C is no exception. It should also be noted that many patients with deteriorating kidney function can benefit greatly from well-monitored vitamin C therapy, as inflammation, which is only another way of describing increased oxidative stress, is at the root of kidney disease evolution and eventual kidney failure.

Outside of the context of poor kidney function, vitamin C is enormously safe given in the highest of doses over extended periods of time in even the sickest of patients.[26] Also, vitamin C has no consistent relationship with the development of kidney stones, and vitamin C is not a risk factor for their development, even though there are continued efforts to assert other-wise.[27] In fact, vitamin C reliably **decreases** the chances of kidney stones, and the persons with the highest blood levels of vitamin C have the lowest inci-dence of kidney stone disease. The higher the blood level of vitamin C, the less chance there is of developing a kidney stone.[28] The real culprit for the development of kidney stones is excess dietary calcium and supple-mental calcium. For reasons that remain a mystery, the common calcium oxalate stone never seems to inspire investigation into the calcium intake of the stone-forming patient. Rather, the focus seems to target only foods and supplements that might increase urinary oxalate. Basically, if you eliminate calcium supple-ments, you eliminate any possibility of any oxalate source being a risk factor for stones. Excess dietary calcium, while a contributory factor, is probably less of a provocative stone-forming factor than just calcium supplementation.[29]

One very rare side effect of vitamin C can occur in patients with G6PD deficiency, an X-linked recessive hereditary disease. G6PD (glucose-6-phosphate dehy-drogenase) is an enzyme that is especially important in red blood cell metabolism. When is it severely deficient in the red blood cells, a hemolysis (rupture) of many of the red blood cells can be provoked by any of a number of agents, resulting in the acute development of anemia. A G6PD blood test is readily available and if possible, it is appropriate to conduct this test before initiating vitamin C therapy. However, even when this deficiency is present, it is still unlikely that the vitamin C will provoke any significant red blood cell hemolysis. If a test is positive and the need for vitamin C is urgent, treatment should proceed, but with closer clinical monitoring, slower infusion, lower doses, and a slower increase of the vitamin C dose over time. It should also be noted that the initial doses of vitamin C should decrease the susceptibility of the red blood cells to hemolysis as well, since vitamin C helps to bolster intracellular glutathione levels, which strongly protects them from hemolysis. When time permits, the administration of other agents that increase intracellular glutathione levels and lowered IOS inside the red blood cells (N-acetyl cysteine, whey protein, liposome-encapsulated glutathione, liposome-encapsulated magnesium) can also stabilize the red blood cells and increase their resistance to hemolysis before the initiation of vitamin C therapy.

9. Overall Protocol of Administration

This factor is much more important in dealing with the treatment of chronic degenerative diseases than when dealing with acute infectious diseases or acute toxin exposures. Toxins and infections will generally respond favorably and rapidly to the aggressive administration of vitamin C as discussed above. However, how-well-vitamin C impacts a chronic condition depends on how effectively multiple other factors that use up the antioxidant capacity of the body are minimized or eliminated. These factors include the following:

ENDOGENOUS Toxin Exposures. Such toxins result primarily from focal infections and areas of pathogen colonization. This includes endotoxins, exotoxins, aerobic and anaerobic metabolic byproducts. While there are many potential sites for focal infections to occur, well over 95% of significant focal infections originate in the oral cavity, in the form of root canal-treated and other symptom-free infected teeth, infected/inflamed gums, large sites of cavitational osteonecrosis, infected tonsils, infected sinuses, and infected lymph nodes draining oral cavity infections.

EXOGENOUS Toxin Exposures. This results from toxin exposure in air, food, water, and the environment in which one lives and/or works.

DIGESTIVE Toxin Exposures (technically an additional endogenous toxin exposure). Poor digestion and a sluggish, constipated gut permit a greater putrefaction of ingested foods that does not occur when bowel transit time is relatively brisk and normal. Highly toxic bacterial species such as *Clostridium* can proliferate, and the resulting toxicity can rival that of oral cavity infections. Chronically poor digestion is generally more toxic than generally poor food/nutrition choices. Less toxicity results from poor food optimally digested than perfect food choices poorly digested.

EXCESS IRON Exposure. This is strongly promoted by the persistent and completely unnecessary "enrichment" of food with iron, much of it in the form of metallic iron filings.

EXCESS CALCIUM Exposure. This is usually due to calcium supplementation, including from many antacid formulations. Excess dairy is statistically less important, but still a strong contributing factor to excessive calcium stores in many people. Low vitamin D levels further fuel the toxic contributions of excess calcium in the body.

GENETIC Contributions to the magnification of oxidative stress in the body. Generally, any given genetic disease/deficiency has biochemical pathways that are unable to function normally and ultimately amplify whatever oxidative stress is already present. This can be in the form of abnormal DNA sequences (genetic defect) or gene expression [transcription] deficiencies and errors (epigenetics).

HORMONE Deficiencies. Insufficient levels of testosterone, estrogen, thyroid hormone, and cortisol all independently serve to increase body-wide oxidative stress. All otherwise appropriate treatment protocols will never work optimally in the face of one or more of these hormone deficiencies.

SUPPLEMENTATION Status. In today's toxin-laden environment, a perfect diet perfectly digested will never give adequate, much less optimal, antioxidant support in the absence of adequate quality nutrient supplementation (vitamins, minerals, miscellaneous nutrient agents). Vitamin C is particularly important, since man should be synthesizing vitamin C from glucose in multi-gram amounts on a continual basis. However, the genetic expression of the enzyme necessary for this to occur in humans is missing. No diet could ever supply the amounts of vitamin C required for optimal health and metabolism.

Multi-C Protocol

As the ultimate goal of an optimally effective vitamin C protocol is to get as much of the active (reduced) vitamin C inside the cells of as many organs, tissues, and other sites in the body in the highest concentrations possible, the Multi-C Protocol utilizes multiple forms of vitamin C for supplementation. The basic outline of this protocol is as follows:

1. Oral Liposome-Encapsulated Vitamin C

This facilitates the optimal *intracellular* entry of vitamin C inside the cells as well as inside the intracellular structures (mitochondria, etc.). Although there is no absolute upper limit to the amount taken of this type of vitamin C, most health maintenance and health recovery programs will be well-served by a daily dose of one to five grams.

Additional Background/Considerations

Liposomes utilize a very unique biodelivery system, achieving a direct intracellular delivery of a substantial percentage of their payload,[30,31] **without the expenditure of energy in the process.** When that payload is vitamin C, the result is cells containing more vitamin C which reliably decreases IOS without an accompanying depletion of the energy resources in the body. All other forms of regular, unencapsulated vitamin C, administered either orally or intravenously, need to consume energy for cells to end up with an increased content of active, reduced vitamin C. While oxidized vitamin C circulating in the blood can be taken into cells passively without the immediate consumption of energy via the glucose transporter (GLUT), energy must still be spent inside the cells to reduce it back to its active antioxidant state. [32,33] Reduced vitamin C circulating in the blood, however, requires an active transport mechanism to get inside the cell, which means that energy must be consumed for the transport system to work. [34] Therefore, even when regular vitamin C is delivered straight into the blood by intravenous injection, significant energy consumption must take place to increase the levels of active, unoxidized vitamin C inside the cells. Liposome-encapsulated vitamin C, even though taken orally, does not deplete any of the energy stores in the body to deliver its payload to intracellular spaces.

In addition to their energy-sparing system of delivery, liposomes have an exceptionally rapid and enhanced form of absorption in the gastrointestinal tract, with very little remaining unabsorbed, unlike regular forms of vitamin C. [35] The payload encapsulation by lipids also prevents potential stomach upset by the liposome contents, as well as any premature breakdown or degradation of the liposome contents that might otherwise occur from enzyme and/or stomach acid exposure. In the case of liposome-encapsulated vitamin C, there is no issue of bowel tolerance and diarrhea as is seen with regular forms of vitamin C, although a very large dose of liposomes could potentially result in oily, greasy stools in some individuals.

In a nutshell, then, the unique intracellular delivery of vitamin C encapsulated in liposomes makes it an essential part of any protocol that strives to optimize support of intracellular vitamin C and antioxidant levels. An additional practical point is that it is very important to take a supplement with a high concentration of liposomes of an appropriately tiny size. Many commercial "liposome" formulations, incompetently or fraudulently, contain no liposome at all. The "homemade" formulations are actually only emulsions and also have zero liposome content, although advertised otherwise. An emulsion can contain two or more substances that do not normally go into solution, like fat and water, in what can be characterized as a smooth watery suspension containing small fat globules. However, these globules are as much larger than liposomes as a house is larger than a grain of sand. None of the unique **intracellular** biodelivery characteristics of incredibly tiny liposomes are shared by the much larger globules of fat. Nevertheless, the "homemade" preparations do improve vitamin C absorption from the gut and the general benefits of unencapsulated vitamin C can still be realized.

An emulsified supplement containing vitamin C and lecithin-derived phosphatidylcholine can certainly provide some clinical benefit since both substances are individually quality supplements. Phosphatidylcholine has been demonstrated to have multiple positive effects.[36-39] However, an emulsion does not have the ability to put anything directly inside cells without the consumption of energy like liposomes of the appropriately tiny size. Once again, buyer beware, as multiple manufacturers are trying to jump on the "liposome bandwagon" without going through the substantial expense and care involved in producing a consistently high-quality product. The benefits of vitamin C properly encapsulated in liposomes are literally exponentially better that the same amount of vitamin C delivered orally in an emulsion just containing phosphatidylcholine.

2. Sodium Ascorbate Powder

For most people a multigram dose of this form of vitamin C in divided doses, up to or even exceeding bowel tolerance ("C-flush") with large amounts of water (or juice) cleanses the gut of putrefying food, while neutralizing toxins that have been generated locally. This form of vitamin C supplementation also helps to optimize local **extracellular** ascorbate levels, especially supporting the many immune cells surrounding the gut. This should always be initiated before eating, and best if done on an empty stomach first thing in the morning. Ascorbic acid powder is perfectly acceptable as well if it does not cause stomach upset.

Additional Background/Considerations

The consumption of vitamin C on a regular (optimally daily) basis as sodium ascorbate powder facilitates the direct neutralization of toxins that are formed by the incomplete digestion, or putrefaction, of different foods. When the doses are pushed high enough and bowel tolerance is reached, further intake results in a watery diarrhea. This watery diarrhea, also known as a C-flush, further ensures that a substantial amount of toxins is directly eliminated without the need for neutralization as well. Inducing a C-flush at least once weekly is a great idea for general health support, as it allows for toxins to be eliminated, uneliminated toxins to be neutralized, and it helps keep the bowels regular even when the amounts of vitamin C being ingested are not up to bowel tolerance levels. If desired, inducing a C-flush even more frequently is fine.

Anything that induces bowel movements at least once a day, and preferably twice a day, will definitely promote good health. When ingested foodstuffs stay in the gut for more than 24 hours, significant putre-faction and anaerobic bacterial toxin formation will always result. Because of this, any degree of constipa-tion is a substantial additional challenge to maintaining a healthy level of vitamin C and other antioxidants in the body, as many of the most potent toxins generated in a sluggish gut are equal in toxicity to those seen in chronic dental infections, like root canals and other chronically (or acutely) infected teeth.

The regular ingestion of sodium ascorbate also assures a regular uptake of vitamin C into the extra-cellular fluids and spaces of the body. Just as the lipo-some-encapsulated vitamin C targets the intracellular spaces, the vitamin C powder continually supplies the extracellular areas while providing all of its other benefits in producing a healthy gut. Of course, some of the extracellular vitamin C also eventually makes its way inside the cells as well, just not with the efficiency of oral liposome-encapsulated vitamin C.

Finally, it is always best to proceed with a planned C-flush first thing in the morning before eating. It can be done at any time of the day, but when a large amount of undigested food is located midway in the gut and is not ready to be eliminated, a great deal of gas and uncomfortable abdominal distention can develop when the elimination of the upstream sodium ascorbate is effectively being blocked

3. Ascorbyl Palmitate.

Taking this form of vitamin C helps support vitamin C levels in areas requiring *fat-soluble access*, as regular vitamin C is water-soluble. One to three grams daily would be a good dose for most individuals.

Additional Background/Considerations

As noted above, ascorbyl palmitate is a unique form of vitamin C that is fat-soluble rather than water-soluble. As such, this allows the antioxidant effects of vitamin C to reach areas normally not as readily accessible to regular, water-soluble vitamin C. The cell membranes of the body are a particularly important site of oxidative stress in need of fat-soluble electron sources for repair. Vitamin E is also important in serving to repair oxidative stress in areas of high fat content.

4. Intravenous Vitamin C (IVC)

This form of vitamin C gets the blood levels of vitamin C vastly higher than any other form of administration, optimizing *extracellular* vitamin C levels throughout the body. Most IV vitamin C administrations will range between 25 and 150 grams at a time, depending on the condition being treated and the physical size of the patient. These high extracellular levels also result in a strong support of intracellular vitamin C levels, which also serves to support intracellular glutathione levels. Additional important ways to deliver vitamin C intravenously include low-dose, continuous infusions, with or without intermittent IV push vitamin C (pulsing protocols).

Additional Background/Considerations

IVC allows the administration of vastly higher doses of vitamin C than can be given by any other route. It results in very high concentrations in the blood and extracellular fluids. It also eventually increases intracellular vitamin C levels as well, even though energy consumption is required to achieve this, as noted above. Although all forms of vitamin C have been documented to have potent antitoxic and antimicrobial properties, a very large body of scientific evidence collected since the early 1940s has shown that properly-dosed IVC can result in a degree of toxin (poison) neutralization and infection resolution that simply has not been rivaled by any other agent up to now.[40] It is also important to emphasize that vitamin C need not be used instead of other traditional agents for combating toxins and infections, as it works well along with any other traditional measures used for these conditions. However, the evidence does clearly show that vitamin C works better as a monotherapy than any other single agent that contemporary medicine has to offer.

5. Intramuscular (IM) Vitamin C

Although much lower amounts of vitamin C can be injected into the muscles than can be delivered by intravenous infusion, this form of administration helps to maintain an increased blood level for a longer period of time than can be expected with intravenous infusions. Along with IV administration, IM injections serve to provide a longer-acting delivery of vitamin C before much of it is excreted in the urine.

Additional Background/Considerations

Another parenteral (non-oral) application of vitamin C that is little used today but that can be highly effective in certain situations is the intramuscular route. Frederick Klenner, MD, who singularly pioneered the field of the effective clinical applications of vitamin C, would often use intramuscular injections in young patients who were not optimal candidates for taking anything intravenously, or for ingesting sufficient quantities of anything orally. Regarding the intramuscular injection of vitamin C, Dr. Klenner had the following to say:

> "In small patients, where veins are at a premium, ascorbic acid can easily be given intramuscularly in amounts up to two grams at one site. Several areas can be used with each dose given. Ice held to the gluteal muscles until red, almost eliminates the pain. We always reapply the ice for a few minutes after the injection. Ascorbic acid is also given, by mouth, as followup treatment. Every emergency room should be stocked with vitamin C ampoules of sufficient strength so that time will never be counted—as a factor in saving a life. The 4 gram, 20 c.c. ampoule and 10 gram 50 c.c. ampoule must be made available to the physician." [4]

It should also be noted that the typical injection used by Dr. Klenner was sodium ascorbate or ascorbic acid buffered with sodium bicarbonate, not just straight ascorbic acid. As well, great care needs to be taken to ensure that the entire injection is intramuscular, with none of the injection being contained in the loose subcutaneous tissue. Whether by misguided intramuscular injection or by an infiltrated intravenous infusion of vitamin C, subcutaneous placement of any amount of vitamin C is enormously painful, often for up to an hour or so before resolving. While no damage is done by a subcutaneous infiltration, the pain is significant enough that the patient might not be so willing to permit future vitamin C infusions or injections, which would not be in the best interest of the patient.

6. Endogenous Vitamin C Production

Recent research has shown that a nutrient polyphenol exists which appears to "unblock" the genetic defect for producing vitamin C from the liver, long felt to be an irreversible genetic disease.[42] This can greatly expand the ability for optimally benefiting from the contributions that vitamin C can make to improving health and increasing longevity, as it has far more than a vitamin role, being the most important nutrient in the body.

Additional Background/Considerations

Nearly all mammals, reptiles, and amphibians have to ability to enzymatically synthesize vitamin C, with some animals far more capable than others in terms of amount per body size. Some synthesize vitamin C in their livers, others in their kidneys.[43,44] But they make it nevertheless. It has long been accepted that human beings, along with primates, guinea pigs, and fruit bats, cannot synthesize any vitamin C from glucose in their livers. However, the assertion is that the enzyme sequence needed for hepatic vitamin C synthesis functioned at some time in the past, but that the function of the last enzyme, L-gulonolactone oxidase (GLO), became non-functional for unclear reasons.

Just as importantly, animals that make their own vitamin C consistently make more vitamin C when increased oxidative stress (infection, toxin) appears in the blood stream. However, when humans face a large enough amount of oxidative stress, such as from a new viral exposure, they just get sick until their immune systems can gradually respond sufficiently to counter the infection and eventually resolve it. Also, humans frequently develop diabetes. Vitamin C-producing animals do not. This is probably due to the fact that the vitamin C-producing animals are continually converting their excess glucose into vitamin C while the human being just accumulates the glucose and either stores it or ends up sustaining damage from it when the glucose binds with different proteins in the body, causing a loss of their natural function (advanced glycation end-products).

As it turns out, there are human beings that can make vitamin C. The evidence has been "hiding in plain sight" for a long time. The actual GLO genome, or sequence of coding DNA, has been identified in humans, although it was felt to represent the "remnants" of the intact genome.[45] Although very many sailors died at sea of scurvy centuries ago, little attention is paid to the fact that a small percentage of sailors did survive, eating the same diet devoid of vitamin C as the others who succumbed.

It appears that a fetus developing in the womb not only makes vitamin C, it makes quite a lot, with levels in the brain running 400 to 1100% higher than the levels seen in adults. It has also been observed that umbilical cord blood had vitamin C levels 400% higher than seen in the maternal blood plasma.[46] Breastfed babies maintained a blood level of vitamin C roughly twice that of the vitamin C levels in the mothers, and it was noted that the maintenance of these vitamin C levels was "relatively independent" of the nutrition status of the mothers, or of the vitamin C concentration in the milk.[47] This at least suggests that the act of breastfeeding could be promoting by mechanisms unknown the transcription of the GLO gene with vitamin C production in the baby. Certainly, such an effect by itself would be a very significant reason why breastfeeding is vastly superior to bottle feeding for the support of good health and infectious disease prevention and resolution.

Even some children appear to be making their own vitamin C, as Bantu children subjected to what was termed "severe malnutrition" with estimated intakes of 3 to 8 mg of vitamin C daily did not develop overt scurvy.[48] A number of small studies looking at the conditions needed to induce severe vitamin C depletion found that a few individuals (adults) continued spilling substantial (saturation levels) of vitamin C in the urine after the other subjects had stopped such spillage. One young woman went 149 days without any dietary ascorbic acid and "never showed any symptoms," subsequently being taken out of the vitamin C-depletion study in which she was participating. Similar observations have been made with guinea pigs, as some of them appear likely to have the ability to make vitamin C as well. The most obvious conclusion is that some "genetically-deficient" humans and guinea pigs, two species supposedly incapable to making any vitamin C, are actually capable of such synthesis.[49-54] In a small but very compelling study, three guinea pigs were fed a vitamin C-free diet and manifested no symptoms of scurvy even after *4 to 8 months*. [It should be noted that guinea pigs deprived of vitamin C rapidly lose weight and start dying of scurvy by about the 30th day of deprivation.[55] Furthermore, these three animals had normal increases in body weight, and they excreted quantities of vitamin C in their urine far greater than the amount of the total body pool of vitamin C. Their healing response to experimental trauma was noted to be entirely normal. Finally, the vitamin C concentration in their livers after eight months of vitamin C abstinence was found to be more than twice that in guinea pigs given a daily intake of 10 mg of vitamin C. It was noted, however, that the frequency of finding such guinea pigs appeared to be "extremely small." [56]

The most logical takeaway point from the vitamin C depletion studies and observations discussed above is that the genetic deficiency of vitamin C possessed by most humans (and guinea pigs) is **NOT** a straightforward error or defect in genetic coding, with one or more nucleotide sequencing/substitution errors in the DNA coding for GLO. Rather, it would appear that the lack of GLO enzyme permitting the synthesis of vitamin C in the deficient human is due to problems with the transcription process by the ribosome that allows the normal "expression" of the nucleotide sequence into the GLO protein.

Such abnormal transcription falls in the realm of **epigenetics**, which basically refers to the variable genetic expression resulting from the impact of any of the modifiable factors that prevent or result in imperfect transcription of the DNA sequence. The DNA nucleotide sequence is normal, or normal enough, but the "machinery" needed to produce the protein coded from that sequencing is defective.

A sequence of three consecutive nucleotides in a chain of RNA, derived from the information in the DNA chain, and that provides the genetic information designating an amino acid to be transcribed into the protein being synthesized by the ribosome is known as a codon. There are 64 possible combinations of the four nucleotide bases, 61 of which code for amino acids, and 3 which do not code for amino acids. These 3 codons are known as stop, or termination codons, which normally serve to mark the end of a sequence of transcription, with the result of a normally-formed protein.

Scientific evidence supports the concept that many genetic "deficiencies" involve the presence of a **premature stop codon** being encountered too early in the transcription process to allow the formation/expression of a normal, or complete protein product. Why or how these stop codons appear in the RNA sequence prematurely is unclear, but there are now recognized various agents that promote the phenomenon of "premature termination codon readthrough." [57] This means that these stop codons are skipped or ignored, and the protein formation can proceed to completion, and the protein is functionally normal. It has been estimated that approximately one-third of genetic disorders are the result of mutations inserting premature termination codons in the genes that code for proteins.[58-61] Metaphorically, these premature stop codons are akin to a pieces of gum on a zipper, and there appear to be agents that effectively skip over the gum, allowing the unzipping (protein synthesis) to proceed to completion without interruption.

Different genetic conditions have been positively impacted, sometimes to apparent resolution, with agents that are felt to promote premature stop codon readthrough. Some aminoglycosides (a class of antibiotics) have been found to facilitate this readthrough.[62,63] In a mouse model of muscular dystrophy protein translation was restored by inducing the ribosome to bypass a premature stop codon.[64]

Resveratrol, a nutrient polyphenol found in grapes, red wine, some berries, and some plant extracts, has been found to induce the production of fetal hemoglobin in studies on cells from beta-thalassemia, who when left untreated end up needing repeated transfusions for life, as such patients have genetically impaired hemoglobin synthesis.[65] In one human study, resveratrol eliminated the need for transfusions in half of the thalassemia patients treated.[66] Other plant extracts in addition to resveratrol, as well as rapamycin (an antibiotic) have also been shown to be fetal hemoglobin inducers.[67]

All of the preceding information in this section should make it pretty clear that many genetic "diseases" are not conditions that have no hope of showing improvement, and in some cases, may have an actual clinical cure. Multiple agents, both prescription drugs along with plant- and food-sourced nutrients appear to have the ability to permit the protein expression of genes that otherwise appear to be completely blocked. With regard to the GLO expression in the liver that results in the synthesis of vitamin C in the liver, which is usually completely lacking in humans, there now appears to be another nutrient polyphenol along the lines of resveratrol that effectively unblocks this gene in humans. Found in olive oil and extracted from olive mill waste, this agent may prove to be one of the most incredible advances in the history of clinical medicine, when one realizes how valuable to longevity and overall good health having a steady production of vitamin C in the blood "24/7" would be. Preliminary unpublished research demonstrated an increase in vitamin C blood levels between 50 and 200% in five volunteers.

Perhaps just as exciting as the increased levels of vitamin C in the blood seen in response to this agent is the apparent response of the degree of vitamin C synthesis in the face of substantial oxidative stress. Most humans that make no vitamin C will rapidly metabolize whatever vitamin C they have in the blood as a new infectious or toxic oxidative challenge is faced. As such, the excretion of vitamin C in the urine rapidly drops to zero measurable amounts. However, another unpublished observation on one individual who was already demonstrating that the product kept vitamin C levels in the blood in the normal range without additional vitamin C supplementation was noted. Using urine dipstick testing for vitamin C, it appeared that the liver of this individual was already keeping the spillage of vitamin C in the urine in the low-normal range. However, when a large toxin load was relatively quickly ingested (Scotch whiskey), the urine vitamin C spillage rapidly shot up to the maximal dipstick level, and stayed at the maximal level for a full 24 hours before returning back down to the previously measured low-normal range. As a significant toxin capable of inducing substantial oxidative stress, it would appear that the whiskey load stimulated the liver to reflexively synthesize much more vitamin C to neutralize that acute stress load, and to **continue** that synthesis (24 hours) until that stress was fully negated. Remember that the "normal" human that cannot synthesize vitamin C will simply use up whatever vitamin C was circulating in the blood, and any large oxidative challenge would just quickly drop the urine levels of vitamin C to zero as no new vitamin C is being synthesized.

Practical IVC Considerations

In addition to how quickly vitamin C should be infused and how much should be given at a time, it is very important that the patient is completely comfortable and free of discomfort or pain in the process. Significant pain during the infusion of vitamin C, or anything else for that matter, is always an indication that the infusion is not being well-tolerated. Such pain virtually always leads to phlebitis, or inflammation of the vein, if not promptly addressed at the time of the infusion. And phlebitis leads to a thrombosis of the vein, sometimes leading to a permanent loss of the function of that vessel. No matter how good a vitamin C-centered protocol might be, it will do no little or no good if the patient becomes severely noncompliant in returning for continued IV infusions. Since it is clear that most patients will get their best clinical results with optimally-dosed vitamin C versus other traditional therapies, it is important not to let the patient get to the point of refusing further IVC treatment.

It should also be emphasized that most patients have no problem with vitamin C infusions, tolerating them without any symptomatology of any kind. However, when significant discomfort appears during an IV infusion, the following factors should all be considered in making the infusion as comfortable as possible:

✓ **Size of intravenous cannula, or infusion catheter.** A larger cannula inside a smaller vein can cause discomfort.

✓ **Placement of cannula.** Even though a cannula might be completely inside the vein, demonstrating venous backflow when tested, pain can ensue when the angle of the cannula abuts it directly against the side of the vein or when a venous valve is at the tip of the cannula. Oftentimes, nothing will stop the pain except cannula removal with reinsertion at another site in the vein, with greater care to insert the cannula in as *coaxial* an alignment as possible.

✓ **Size of the vein.** While some individuals can tolerate IV infusions in the tiniest of veins, many individuals cannot. The largest vein available should always be chosen, except when it is already known that smaller, more distal veins tolerate the infusion well, as in a larger man with substantially-sized veins on the back of the hand. If the patient is a smaller woman, or even a child, consideration should be given to having a central line placed if there appears to be no other way to get the amount of vitamin C infused at the rate desired, and the medical condition clearly warrants the therapy.

✓ **Rate of flow.** Many individuals tolerate a slower infusion perfectly well, while always noticing increasing discomfort the more rapid the infusion becomes. If this sensitivity is severe, consideration should again be given to the placement of a central line if deemed appropriate. Some patients will complain of discomfort and get relief when the infusion rate is slowed, and then later not feel any discomfort when the infusion rate is once again increased. Whatever the physiological reason for this is, it appears that the vein can show increased tolerance the longer it is exposed to the vitamin C infusion. Minimal discomfort can often be alleviated with cold (or even warm to hot) compresses gently applied and held over the infusion site as the infusion proceeds.

✓ **Concentration.** When a large enough vein cannot be found for infusion without significant discomfort, a more dilute infusion of vitamin C is warranted.

✓ **Temperature of the infusion solution.** Making sure the infusion solution is close to body temperature during the administration period can prevent a substantial amount of discomfort from ever developing in the first place.

Many offices are quite cold, and the IV
solutions often tend to be near to room
temperature, or less, as a refrigerated
vial of vitamin C is typically added to a
room temperature bag. To minimize any
degradation (oxidation) of the vitamin C
once it is mixed, place the IV bag in hot
water for 10 to 15 minutes before adding
the vitamin C. The vitamin C vial can
similarly be warmed immediately before
being added to the IV bag.

✓ **Presence of other solutes.** Generally,
it is best to infuse vitamin C and nothing
else. While other agents can be added, it is
important not to blame the vitamin C for
discomfort in the IV when something else
is at fault. Magnesium is usually very also
well-tolerated, and strong consideration
should always be given to adding this
mineral unless an extremely rapid infusion
is being planned.

✓ **pH of the infusion.** The more acidic
an infusion is, the more likely it will
hurt. A pH of 7.0 to 7.4 is ideal, and it is
characteristically reached when sodium
ascorbate powder is put into solution in
sterile water. When ascorbic acid is used, it
must be buffered with sodium bicarbonate.
Vials of ascorbic acid already buffered
with sodium bicarbonate are available,
but they are generally buffered only to be
somewhere in the range of pH 5.5 to 7.0.
For the exceptionally sensitive patient,
pH test paper should be utilized to make
sure pH is in the optimal range, and more

sodium bicarbonate should be added to the infusion if necessary to get into that pH range.

✓ **Nature of carrier solution.** Generally, it is best to infuse vitamin C mixed in sterile water. While normal saline, lactated Ringer's solution, or D5W (5% dextrose in water) can be used, it is best to stick with vitamin C in sterile water, buffered as close to a pH of 7.0 to 7.4 as possible. In general, D5W should still always be avoided, since the sugar (dextrose) directly competes with vitamin C for entry into the cells, and the uptake of vitamin C into the cells is the ultimate goal of the IV in the first place.

✓ **Presence of persistent or severe pain.** Any extravasation, or leakage, of vitamin C outside of the vein and into the subcutaneous tissue is severely painful, usually persisting for an hour or more before dissipation is complete and pain is resolved. Sometimes the cannula can move back out of the vein transiently, and a little leakage will take place. When the cannula is completely out of the vein, it is obvious to the experienced practitioner. Regardless of the reason, a severely painful infusion should always be promptly discontinued.

✓ **Vitamin C-induced hypoglycemia.** Rarely, some individuals are so sensitive to the infusion of multigram amounts of vitamin C that they will demonstrate some hypoglycemia secondary to increased insulin release from the pancreas at infusion rates well below what most other patients tolerate easily. When any inexplicable agitation, sweating, minimal disorientation, or unexplained increase in blood pressure occurs, be prepared to give some fruit juice orally or some glucose intravenously. Also, while very rare, an occasional individual, typically poorly nourished in general and appearing to be actively losing weight, can have a delayed hypoglycemia reaction hours later at home. All patients should be encouraged to promptly eat after an infusion session is complete.

✓ **Allergy-like reactions.** Technically, the ascorbate anion should never cause an allergic reaction in anyone, as it is an essential nutrient and a natural antioxidant molecule vital to health, as well as a substance that can be used to *treat* an allergic reaction. Nevertheless, rare individuals might demonstrate a rash and feel poorly. When this occurs shortly after the IV is started, an allergy-like reaction is likely, and the IV should be stopped. Consideration should then be given to obtaining vitamin C from a different source. Corn is commonly a source, but beet and casaba are also sources. When the reaction occurs late in the IV or shortly after its conclusion, a detoxification from the cells is more likely. This type of reaction and how to deal with it is addressed below in the "Mop-Up Vitamin C" section. If different types of vitamin C, mixed in different carrier solutions, continue to produce the same effect, premedication with an injection of 100 to 250 mg of hydrocortisone will usually blunt or prevent the reaction. This is a one-time dose, and further steroids would not generally be needed following the infusion.

✓ **No local anesthetics.** While used by some practitioners, I am not in favor of giving any types of anesthetic agents that would prevent the perception of pain in the vein. If pain is reported by the patient, and pain relief through anesthesia is obtained, the pain-causing inflammation in the vein can still result in enough of a reaction that vein thrombosis and subsequent sclerosis, or scarring of the vein, can occur. Relieving infusion pain with anesthesia is not a good idea for the long-term health of the veins. However, this does not refer to the use of a small amount of lidocaine in the subcutaneous tissue to lessen or block the pain of the initial needle stick for placement of the intravenous cannula, if felt to be indicated.

Mop-Up IVC

Many individuals, especially sicker ones with acute and chronic infections, as well as substantial toxin accumulations in their bodies, will feel anywhere from minimally to substantially ill late during an infusion of vitamin C or directly following it. These symptoms flare-ups have been called Herxheimer, or Herxheimer-like reactions. The first described Herxheimer reaction occurred when syphilis patients with a high pathogen load took their first injection of penicillin. The kill-off of the pathogens was so extensive that massive amounts of pro-oxidant, dead pathogen-related debris was released into the blood as a result. The clinical result was a much sicker patient, at least in the short term, while the body processed and eliminated the toxic debris. Following an infusion of vitamin C, these Herxheimer-like reactions can occur because of one or more of the following reasons:

✓ **Whenever an acute or chronic infection responds dramatically enough to the antimicrobial effect of vitamin C.** This results in the release of toxic debris into the blood and lymphatics, similar to the syphilis example above, as viruses, bacteria, and other pathogens are broken down and metabolized.

✓ **Whenever a legitimate detoxification occurs.** When some individuals with longstanding and substantial accumulations of toxins inside the cells receives a high enough dose of vitamin C quickly enough, toxins are then mobilized out of the cells and flood the blood and lymphatics. Generally, this occurs only when IOS levels are so high that many of the natural enzymatic chelators and toxin mobilizers are themselves in an oxidized and relatively or completely nonfunctional state. The massive vitamin C administration then causes a big intracellular rise in vitamin C, the enzymes are repaired by reduction (electron donation) from the vitamin C, and the toxins are released in large quantities as the enzymes again begin to function normally. It is very important to realize that detoxification is also retoxification, and many newly mobilized toxins are just as free to be redeposited anew somewhere else in the body as to be excreted in the urine or feces. Detoxification should never be deliberately done vigorously without the ability to promote neutralization and excretion of those toxins after they are released from the cells.

✓ **Whenever a substantial quantity of cancer cells are rapidly killed via necrosis:** When dosed and administered correctly, many different cancers will begin to resolve, often eventually to the point of complete resolution. When a patient has a relatively large physical mass of cancer cells in their body, this type of reaction is more likely to occur than when the collective cancer mass is small. This reaction can be very dramatic in some patients, and several days may be needed for the patient to properly neutralize, process, and excrete the pro-oxidant debris. Of note as well, both cancer cells and most infectious agents have very large concentrations of unbound, reactive iron inside them, and the rupture of cancer cells *and pathogens* via vitamin C-fed mechanisms can release quite abruptly large amounts of reactive iron into the blood and lymphatics. Iron is highly toxic (pro-oxidant) when concentrated in its unbound, reactive form. It is high amounts of iron that facilitate

the proliferation of many cancer cells and
pathogens in the first place.

The Mop-Up vitamin C infusion, at first, might
seem paradoxical. That is to say, the very same agent
(vitamin C) that caused the flood of pro-oxidant debris
into the blood and lymphatics is also the very same
agent best suited to deal with that situation. The trick
is in the *amount* of vitamin C infused and the *rate* at
which it is infused. All three of the types of pro-oxidant reactions noted above share one thing in common.
Namely, they needed large amounts of vitamin C given
quickly to become manifest. However, at the termination of such an infusion, a "Low & Slow" follow-up
infusion of vitamin C at 25% or less of the initial
amount infused, infused over two hours or more, will
readily "mop-up" much or all of the pro-oxidant debris
released by the larger rapid infusion. The mop-up
infusion does not significantly worsen the pro-oxidant
release because its lower concentration and slower rate
of infusion does not result in the same rapid increase
in intracellular vitamin C uptake. However, it does
very effectively neutralize the toxins already released
while they are circulating in the blood and lymphatics.
While the figures are not precise, this would mean
that someone who was feeling well at the outset of a
50-gram infusion of vitamin C but began feeling poorly
after the completion of the infusion in about one hour,
should then receive about 12.5 grams of vitamin C
infused over another two hours. However, be aware
that this is very approximate, and the clinician must
make adjustment to the individual needs of the patient.
At the Riordan Clinic, a modified "Mop-Up" approach
was developed, when some patients receiving the first

half of their infusion quite rapidly, followed simply by a much slower infusion of the second half. Such an approach also appears to prevent many significant detoxification reactions from occurring in the first place.

While most pro-oxidant debris release scenarios occur when acutely stimulated, as with a vitamin C infusion, it also important to appreciate what is going on in a patient with an extended, chronic detoxification process. For example, when an older patient has an exceptionally large amount of stored toxins in the body, the stage is set for a chronic release of toxins when enough other circumstances come to bear. The relatively abrupt initiation of a quality supplement regimen, especially when accompanied or preceded by a removal of ongoing sources of toxin exposure, as seen in root canal-treated teeth, can result in enough of a reactivation of natural detoxification enzymes inside the cells that a chronic detoxification results. As such, the patient can begin to feel poorly a greater percentage of the time the less effectively the antioxidant capacity of the body is supported.

Just as with the acute pro-oxidant debris release scenario, this chronic one is readily dealt with by the same "Low & Slow" vitamin C infusions, with a good clinical response typically realized. However, many chronic detoxifications can take months or sometimes years before the individual truly feels well, so experimentation must take place with finding the best amounts of vitamin C to also take orally that will neutralize the pro-oxidant products of detoxification without significantly further stimulating their release from the cells.

Another especially important consideration about the Mop-Up vitamin C infusion is that is allows the healthcare practitioners to push vitamin C doses higher than might have been possible otherwise. **As long as a patient feels good by the time they leave the office, they will generally come back for more treatment**. Mop-Up vitamin C, then, is a tool that allows a large group of patients that could otherwise only tolerate substantially lower doses of vitamin C to push their doses into a range that will produce even more positive clinical outcomes that were not otherwise attainable, while optimizing patient compliance with a treatment regimen.

RECAP

All infections, all toxin exposures, and all chronic degenerative diseases will benefit some and often greatly from vitamin C that is properly-dosed and administered in an appropriate manner. The different forms of vitamin C and the various ways to give it offer a wide range of treatment possibilities, capable of being appropriately individualized for optimal clinical response. The new concept of Mop-Up vitamin C now allows the vitamin C practitioner to push the therapeutic envelope to previously unattainable levels. Utilized properly, vitamin C-centered protocols have already gone and will continue to go where no medicines have gone before or can ever expect to go.

Companion Supplements

Importance and Considerations

Supplementation should actually be a highly-individualized process, and most definitely "one size does **not** fit all." With all of the vitamins, minerals, herbs, plants and plant extracts, and other nutrient or nutrient-based formulations available, the number of potential supplementation regimens is virtually limitless. That is not to say, however, that supplementation along with vitamin C is not extremely important. Vitamin C just remains singularly important since the amounts of vitamin C present in any dietary regimen will not remotely approach the amount needed to support optimal health.

Certain supplements are extremely important for literally everyone. The only time any of these should not be supplemented is when you are being treated by a highly-informed healthcare provider who advises you not to, or to at least modify dosage, for whatever reason. However, these are so important that you should definitely consider having a second opinion if you are advised to avoid any or all of them. Bear in mind that nearly all quality-produced dietary supplements available today have some beneficial impact on health. So, if your favorite supplement is not listed below, and you feel it is serving you well, do not feel that its absence on this recommended listing means you should no longer take it.

AVOID calcium, iron, and copper supplementation.

IMPORTANT SUPPLEMENTATION NOTE

Any dosages mentioned herein are very general in nature only and should not be considered as a direct recommendation to any individual; as with prescription medicine, an optimal supplementation regimen should be achieved in conjunction with your physician or other healthcare provider.

Vital and Essential Supplements

1. Vitamin C
2. Magnesium
3. Vitamin D
4. Vitamin K

All four of these supplements have been documented to decrease the chances of death from any medical condition (all-cause mortality). They all play integral roles in normalizing calcium metabolism while antagonizing the pro-oxidant effects of calcium in the intracellular space. All disease is both directly caused by, as well as directly related to, increased intracellular oxidative stress secondary to increased intracellular calcium. No supplement regimen should fail to include these "top 4" supplements.

Vitamin C

Already discussed with regard to dosing and administration, vitamin C has been shown to decrease all-cause mortality. The higher the blood levels, the lower the mortality.[1-5]

Magnesium

Higher magnesium intake and higher plasma levels have been correlated with lower all-cause mortality.[6] In general, regular oral forms of magnesium cannot be overdosed before diarrhea is induced. A prominent exception to this is the extended retention of magnesium cathartics in the gut with chronically constipated older individuals. Enough magnesium can be absorbed to result in severe toxicity under these circumstances when the bowels do not promptly evacuate after its administration. Many different forms are available and can be chosen based on pocketbook and preference. Transdermal application is an additional option. The liposome-encapsulated magnesium is another oral form that can also be overdone due to its advanced bioavailability with deep intracellular access. Too much of this form can result in lowered blood pressures to the point of feeling sleepy and tired.

Vitamin D

A deficiency in vitamin D also increases all-cause mortality, and individuals with higher vitamin D levels clearly live longer than those with the lowest vitamin D levels.[7-15] When evaluating optimal vitamin D levels by looking at reduction in fracture risk, it would appear that maintaining a blood level above 50 ng/cc would be optimal.[16] Defining a maximal level is less clear-cut, although vitamin D can definitely be overdone to the point of toxicity. As a rough guide, it would probably be best to maintain a vitamin D level between 50 and 80 ng/cc. Many individuals will get into this range with about 5,000 units of vitamin D3 daily, but long-term supplementation should be supported by blood testing verifying that circulating levels are in this range.

<u>Vitamin K</u>

The intake of vitamin K, especially vitamin K2 (menaquinone), also appears to reduce all-cause mortality.[17,18] While supplements with less than one milligram of K2 are common, it is probably best to take more than this amount daily, although benefits are still seen with daily doses of K2 less than one milligram.

Highly Important Supplements

These 4 additional supplements (along with the top 4) are relatively inexpensive, and an argument could be made for considering them to be essential as well.

5. Omega-3 fatty acids
6. Vitamin E
7. B vitamins
8. Iodine

<u>Omega-3 Fatty Acids</u>

Essential fatty acids of the omega-3 form also have calcium channel blocking properties, further elevating the importance of this supplement. Omega-3 fatty acid supplementation has also been shown to be associated with decreased all-cause mortality, which is likely largely secondary to its calcium antagonist effects. It has also been shown that individuals with the highest blood levels of these fatty acids have a decreased all-cause mortality relative to those with the lowest levels.[19-21] While fish oil is a common source of these fatty acids, any supplements with EPA (eicosapentaenoic acid) and DHA (docosahexaenoic acid) can be taken. However, the supplement with the highest concentrations of EPA and DHA is a quality fish oil supplement, and is the least costly way to go.

Vitamin E

There are eight substances in nature known to have "vitamin E" activity. These are alpha-, beta-, gamma-, and delta-tocopherol, along with alpha-, beta-, gamma-, and delta-tocotrienols.[22] All of the different forms of vitamin E are fat-soluble, and their antioxidant function is especially important in protecting the fatty cell membranes from oxidation.[23] There are many variations of vitamin E supplements. In general, taking as broad a spectrum of the eight forms mentioned above will offer the most benefit. Also, unlike the more rapidly excreted water-soluble vitamins and nutrients, vitamin E can be overdosed, and it is advisable to follow the directions supplied on the supplement bottle.

B Vitamins

The B vitamins are water-soluble, and they all play important roles in cellular metabolism. They are all also quite chemically distinct, in spite of being grouped together.

Most of the time, the B vitamins are supplemented in the form of a vitamin B complex, combining the eight different known B vitamins. They are:

✓ B_1 – thiamine (also thiamin): helps to generate cellular energy, promote fatty acid synthesis, and support normal membrane and nerve conduction

✓ B_2 – riboflavin: important for energy-transfer reactions in the cell

✓ B_3 – niacin (also nicotinic acid): important in the function of many enzymes, the synthesis of hormones, and the function of the brain and nervous system

✓ B_5 – pantothenic acid: a precursor for the synthesis of coenzyme A; very important in energy generation

✓ B_6 – pyridoxine (also pyridoxal or pyridoxamine): important in amino acid metabolism

✓ B_7 – biotin—important in energy metabolism

✓ B_9 – folate (also folic acid): important in DNA synthesis

✓ B_{12} – cobalamin (different forms: hydroxo-, methyl-, cyano-): important for blood synthesis and the maintenance of proper nerve function

A relatively large number of compounds have been labeled as B vitamins in the past, but ended up losing this designation, as they were shown not to be essential to humans. Many of them can still be considered good supplements, but they no longer qualify as being members of the B vitamin family.

Iodine

Iodine is essential for the normal functioning of the thyroid gland, and normal thyroid function is absolutely vital not only to general good health, but also for preventing body-wide elevations of oxidative stress. It also plays an important role in preventing the spread of both focal infections and localized cancers to other places in the body. While very many, possibly most, adults who do not supplement iodine are deficient in it, supplementation with iodine is best done with the help of your doctor or chosen healthcare provider. Iodized salt has helped decrease the presence of iodine deficiency statistically, but the amount of iodine delivered in this fashion falls short of what very many people need.

Important Supplements

9. Lysine
10. Vitamin A
11. Alpha lipoic acid
12. Acetyl L-carnitine
13. Zinc
14. Carnosine
15. Coenzyme Q10
16. Methylsulfonylmethane (MSM)
17. Pantethine (vitamin B_5 source)
18. N-acetylcysteine and glutathione
19. Chondroitin and glucosamine
20. Amino acids, especially essential
21. Resveratrol
22. Olive leaf extract
23. Curcumin
24. Multivitamin, multimineral formulations, WITHOUT copper and iron, and very minimal to no calcium
25. Lutein, zeaxanthin, and astaxanthin (eye antioxidant support)

Lysine

Lysine is an amino acid that has been shown to be especially effective in helping to prevent the evolution of atherosclerosis, as well as to probably even reverse it. This has been to shown to be true especially when combined with vitamin C and other nutrients.[24-26]

Vitamin A

Vitamin A is a fat-soluble vitamin that is essential for good vision and a strong immune system. It is also an antioxidant. It is probably best supplemented as beta-carotene, which converts to vitamin A and minimizes the chances of taking too much vitamin A. Due to its fat-soluble nature, it can accumulate to undesirable levels since it is not rapidly excreted as with water-soluble supplements.

Alpha Lipoic Acid (ALA)

ALA is an organosulfur compound that has both water-soluble and fat-soluble characteristics. It is essential for aerobic metabolism, serving as a cofactor for at least five enzyme systems, two in the ATP-generating Krebs cycle. It is a strong antioxidant, which accounts for most of its positive biological effects. It also serves to regenerate active, reduced vitamin C, vitamin E, and glutathione after they donate electrons and are in an oxidized state. ALA can also increase insulin sensitivity and possibly have a hypoglycemic effect in some individuals.

Acetyl L-Carnitine

Acetyl L-carnitine is another supplement that helps the body to produce energy. It is often taken by individuals hoping to improve memory, as with Alzheimer's disease and other dementias, and also to lessen easy fatiguability.

Zinc

Zinc is an important mineral for optimizing immune function, recovery from infection, and healing in general. Accumulation can occur over time and result in varying degrees of toxicity. Generally, staying below 40 mg daily will prevent this from occurring. However, there is nothing wrong with just adding zinc to a supplementation regimen when facing the need to overcome an infection or improve healing after an injury.

Carnosine

Carnosine is a dipeptide made up of two amino acids, alanine and histidine, linked together. It is highly concentrated in the brain and in muscle tissue. It is known to be a powerful antioxidant, and there is evidence that it can slow the processes that worsen both Alzheimer's disease and the body-wide impact of uncontrolled blood sugar levels.

Coenzyme Q10 (CoQ10)

Present in every cell of the body, CoQ10 plays an important role in the synthesis of ATP inside the mitochondria. Consistent with this role, the highest concentrations of CoQ10 are found in the organs that consume the most energy, such as the heart, kidneys, lungs, and liver. There is some evidence that supplementation with CoQ10 is useful for heart failure, fertility, healthy skin, headaches, exercise endurance, diabetes, and brain function.

Methylsulfonylmethane (MSM)

As a sulfur-containing agent, MSM supplementation provides a source of added sulfur to the body. It has anti-inflammatory properties and helps to boost glutathione levels. It can decrease joint pain and promote a quicker recovery of muscle damage (soreness) after exercise. It also offers strong support to the immune system.

Pantethine (Vitamin B₅ Source)

Pantethine is noted here separately since the most common supplemental form of pantothenic acid is calcium pantothenate. Whenever possible, added sources of calcium should be avoided. Panthethine is actually two derivative molecules of pantothenic acid hooked together by a sulfur bond, with no calcium involved. It is also a better biologically available form of pantothenic acid. Pantethine is the substrate needed to synthesize coenzyme A. Coenzyme A is needed to initiate the sequence of chemical reactions needed to generate ATP in the Krebs cycle. It is also a pivotal nutrient in at least 70 metabolic pathways. While available in the diet, most people generate energy much more readily with its supplementation. Its deficiency in the body results in an array of wide-ranging effects.

N-Acetylcysteine and Glutathione

As the most important and highly concentrated intracellular antioxidant, it is always a good goal to support intracellular glutathione levels as much as possible.

While benefits do result from taking unaltered glutathione as a supplement, it is a highly inefficiency way to take this tripeptide antioxidant. Even when it is administered in an intravenous infusion, glutathione is quickly broken down into its three constituent amino acids in the blood, and each amino acid requires energy consumption to get inside the cell, and once in the cell, two more steps consuming energy are needed to reconstitute active, reduced glutathione inside the cell. As amazing as it may seem, the best way to boost glutathione levels inside the cell, without utilizing energy in the process (5 steps of consumption when given intravenously), is to take orally a quality liposome-encapsulated form of glutathione.

N-acetylcysteine is an inexpensive supplement that supports intracellular glutathione levels in a much more economic fashion than either taking it by vein or by an oral liposome-encapsulated supplement.

Chondroitin and Glucosamine

Many people, regardless of whatever else might be bothering them, suffer from degenerative joint disease, with chronic joint (arthritic) pain. Although they can be taken apart from one another, chondroitin and glucosamine make a good supplement combination for helping to alleviate osteoarthritis pain, while providing elements needed to keep joints fluid and to help them repair, at least to a limited degree.

Amino Acids, Especially Essential

Amino acids are literally the building blocks that link together and make up all proteins. Proteins and peptides perform countless important functions throughout the body, in both the intracellular and extracellular spaces. If economically feasible, a quality broad-spectrum amino acid supplement is a good idea, although a supplement limited to the amino acids that the body cannot synthesize (essential amino acids) is good as well.

Resveratrol

Resveratrol is a nutrient polyphenol, present in many different plants, fruits, and vegetables. Along with other naturally-occurring polyphenols, it actually serves to protect its host against pathogens, parasites, and predators. Especially significant sources of resveratrol are red wine, red grapes, blueberries, bilberries, cranberries, and peanuts. It has a wide spectrum of positive health benefits, exerting antidiabetic, anti-inflammatory, and antioxidant effects throughout the body.[27]

Olive Leaf Extract

Olive leaf extract has been demonstrated in very many studies to have a wide array of important health benefits including, but not limited to, improved blood pressure control, better cardiovascular health, better regulation of blood sugar, improved brain function, strengthened immune function, and even some protection against cancer. A nutrient polyphenol in olive leaf extract appears to help the body support/ produce endogenous vitamin C from the liver.[28] Such an effect could single-handedly account for all of the known positive effects of olive leaf extract supplementation. However, this product also has many other compounds that positively impact good health and health maintenance.

Curcumin

Curcumin is the most important active ingredient in turmeric, a plant root which provides the spice that gives curry its yellow color and has been ingested in India for thousands of years as both a spice and a medicinal herb. As a fat-soluble agent that is not especially well-absorbed into the blood, curcumin is probably better assimilated if taken with a fatty meal.

Curcumin is a strong antioxidant and has powerful anti-inflammatory effects. As such, it is also promoted as having anti-aging, pain-reducing, and detoxifying properties.

Multivitamin, Multimineral Formulations –
WITHOUT copper and iron, and very minimal to no calcium

This is only being recommended since it is an economical way to get a wide variety of supplements that positively impact health. Few formulations are optimal, as less costly (and less desirable) forms of the different compounds are often included in these products. Nevertheless, as long as no iron or copper is in the supplement, and little to no calcium is contained in it as well, the various different formulations are certainly better than no supplementation at all. However, iron, copper, and calcium can largely negate the otherwise positive impact of such supplements.

Lutein, Zeaxanthin, and Astaxanthin –
(eye antioxidant support)

These three agents are classified as carotenoids, making them akin to beta-carotene, which metabolizes to vitamin A. Zeaxanthin is concentrated in the center of the retina of the eye (macula), and in concert with lutein, it affords protection against the oxidative damage that can be inflicted by certain wavelengths of light. One study showed that a high dietary intake of zeaxanthin and lutein appeared to result in a significantly decreased risk of cataracts.[29] Another study reached the same result related to the ingestion of these two agents along with vitamin E.[30] Astaxanthin is another powerful antioxidant that would be expected to augment the protection of the eye against oxidative damage.

Summary

An optimal supplementation regimen for one individual may bear little resemblance to an optimal supplementation regimen for another individual. Economics, gastrointestinal tolerance, the presence of certain prominent symptoms, the presence of one or more diseases unique to an individual, and the unique reaction (positive or negative) that any one individual has to a given combination of supplements are all important factors in determining what serves that individual best.

It is always important to remember that the "bottom line" for any supplementation and overall treatment protocol is to alleviate as much intracellular oxidative stress as possible, while aiming to avoid as many new oxidative challenges as possible. Nutrient supplement intake is only really half of the equation. As important, or more important, is the identification and elimination/attenuation of new daily toxin exposures in order that cellular damage can be prevented as well as healed. No treatment protocol is complete unless PREVENTION of new oxidative damage gets as much attention as REPAIR of old oxidative damage.

Magnesium Supplementation

An Essential Guide

Forms and Applications

There are many different forms and routes of magnesium supplementation. Depending on the needs of the patient, along with considerations of expense and convenience, any of a number of different forms of magnesium can be taken by an individual. Magnesium has many different chemical forms, and it has been administered intravenously, intramuscularly, orally, transdermally, via enema, and via inhalation by nebulization. Also, while magnesium in all of its forms and all of its applications remains greatly underutilized today, it must nevertheless be acknowledged that progress, however slow, is being made in seeing its use become more common and widespread. A study looking at the use of intravenous magnesium in the hospitalized setting (a Canadian tertiary care center) between 2003 and 2013 was conducted. A 2.86 fold (almost 300%) increase in the use of infused magnesium in patients was seen during this period. Note was also made by the authors that the increase "cannot be explained for

by medical indications." Some areas (wards) of the
hospital actually saw a 1000% increase.[1] At the very
least, it would appear that the awareness of the benefits
of magnesium for many different indications is on the
rise.

Oral Forms

Traditional Oral Forms

There are a large number of different magnesium supplements that can be taken orally. While
they all can deliver beneficial amounts of magnesium
depending on the doses taken, the efficiency of absorption, the unique contributions of the associated anion
that is hooked to the magnesium (cation), and the
degree of side effects, like loosened stools or diarrhea,
can vary widely. Because of all these factors, the costs
of different magnesium supplements can also vary
widely. The most common forms are inexpensive, as
supplements go in general. These common oral forms
include the following:

1. **Magnesium Citrate**
   This is an especially common and inexpensive form of magnesium. It is often used in
   large doses to deliberately induce a cleansing,
   watery diarrhea in order to prepare an individual for a major surgery or colonoscopy.[2,3]

2. **Magnesium Sulfate**
   This form of magnesium is also known as
   Epsom salt. While it can be taken orally, it
   readily results in a diarrhea or loosening
   of the stools as is seen with magnesium

citrate. Although not the optimal form for oral supplementation, magnesium sulfate is the most common form of magnesium given intravenously for many different medical conditions.[4-6] Taking Epsom salt baths appears to offer much of the known benefits of magnesium administration, as significant amounts of magnesium can be assimilated transdermally from this practice.

3. **Magnesium Taurate**
   This is a very bioavailable form of magnesium that is complexed with taurine, an important sulfur-containing amino acid.[7] Taurine is known to have antioxidant and anti-inflammatory properties. It is the most plentiful amino acid in the body, and it plays an important role in supporting normal physiology, especially beneficial in supporting good cardiac, brain, and eye health. Relative to other forms of magnesium, it does not readily result in diarrhea at lower doses.

4. **Magnesium Gluconate**
   The gluconate form of magnesium is an organic salt that is noteworthy for having a high degree of absorption. In a study on magnesium-depleted rats, this form of magnesium was absorbed and retained better than 9 other forms of magnesium that were studied (oxide, chloride, sulfate, carbonate, acetate, pidolate, citrate, lactate, and aspartate).[8] Sodium gluconate is also known for its ability to chelate heavy metals, including calcium, iron, copper,

and aluminum. This likely provides a substantial additional benefit for taking the gluconate form of magnesium.

5. **Magnesium Chloride**

   This form of magnesium has been shown to have impressive anti-viral properties,[9,10] and it would appear to be an especially good form of magnesium to take whenever any symptoms of an acute infectious disease appear, viral or otherwise (see Chapter 11). It should be part of any infection or infectious disease protocol, and it should prove to have at least additive and probably synergistic effects with other anti-pathogen agents, including vitamin C, ozone, and even antibiotics. It is very inexpensive, and it is absorbed very well relative to the other oral forms of magnesium. And while any form of magnesium should be expected to be a good adjunct therapy to add to a treatment protocol for infection, it appears that the chloride anion is also an important factor in the ability of magnesium chloride to deal with infection.[11]

6. **Magnesium Glycinate**

   This form of magnesium is bound to an amino acid, glycine. This magnesium supplement is more bioavailable and absorbable than many of the other forms of oral magnesium, and less likely to cause the diarrhea effect. While not one of the essential amino acids that must be supplied by diet or supplementation, glycine is one of the three amino acids needed for the body to synthesize glutathione, an antioxidant especially critical for maintaining a normal intracellular level of oxidative stress. Glycine is also essential for the synthesis of creatine and collagen in the body. Additional sources of glycine in supplementation and the diet are always good practices.

7. **Magnesium Oxide**
   This form of magnesium is especially inexpensive, and it is probably the most common form of magnesium supplementation sold in pharmacies and supplement stores. While it has one of the poorest absorption rates, the literature has nevertheless documented many clear-cut benefits from its administration, often in doses of 500 mg daily.

8. **Magnesium Aspartate and Magnesium Glutamate**
   While aspartate and glutamate are not toxic *per se,* they are probably both best avoided for relatively high dosing on a regular basis, especially in light of the many other forms of magnesium with clearly beneficial anions that can be supplemented.

9. **Magnesium Carbonate**
   This form of magnesium effectively becomes magnesium chloride after mixing with the acid in the stomach (and also forming carbon dioxide and water). Additionally, it has significant antacid properties.

✓ **Magnesium Threonate**
This is a form of magnesium that was
developed to better cross the blood-
brain barrier and positively impact brain
function and neurological conditions.[12]

Liposome-Encapsulated Oral Form

Vitamins, minerals, and other nutrient agents are
becoming increasingly available in oral liposome-encapsulated forms. When the liposome formulation
is a quality product, the encapsulated agents generally get inside the cells more readily than when those
agents are given intravenously, and typically without
the consumption of energy, amazingly enough. This
certainly appears to be particularly true for liposome-encapsulated vitamin C. It must be pointed out,
however, that there is a great deal of fraud among
supplements that are now labeled as being encapsulated in liposomes. The Suggested Resources section of
this book recommends sources for liposome products
and some other selected supplements. More detailed
information on this liposome form of supplementation
is available elsewhere.[13]

Liposome-encapsulated magnesium (as threonate) has only recently become available (early 2019),
and undoubtedly many other companies will start
selling fraudulent "liposome-encapsulated" versions
of this product as they have with vitamin C and other
nutrients. Currently, LivOn Laboratories is the only
company producing this form of magnesium encapsulated in liposomes. Early anecdotal feedback is indicating that a quality liposome-encapsulated form of

magnesium appears to have a high degree of intracellular bioavailability, capable of getting significant amounts of magnesium into the cytoplasm without the consumption of energy, as would be seen when utilizing active transport mechanisms into the cell. Many agents not liposome-encapsulated yet given intravenously still need to consume energy via active transport to end up inside the cells. While the mechanisms for magnesium cellular uptake remain to be fully elucidated, the normally extremely high intracellular magnesium concentrations relative to extracellular concentrations logically demands that an energy-consuming active transport process must be involved to further concentrate magnesium inside cells.[14-17]

The capability of this orally-administered liposome product to deliver magnesium into the cells appears to be so effective that taking too much of this product seems to have the ability to induce some of the early signs of magnesium excess, as discussed below. It also appears that the absorption initially into the blood is nearly 100%, without resulting in any of the loose stools or diarrhea characteristic of the incomplete absorption of other oral magnesium preparations. One of the best ways to track magnesium status clinically is by following blood pressures. When blood pressures begin to be consistently lowered significantly by liposome-encapsulated magnesium (or any other form of magnesium), greater care must then be exerted with regard to long-term dosing and frequency of supplementation. However, even though monitoring must be more vigilant, a lowering of blood pressure is a very clear indication that body-wide magnesium stores are being normalized, which is the ultimate goal of any magnesium supplementation regimen. It is also a goal that is not routinely achieved with other forms of oral magnesium supplementation, regardless of the dosing schedule.

Intravenous and Intramuscular Magnesium

Intravenous

The intravenous administration of magnesium is the most common form given in the hospital and clinic setting. While the circumstances of magnesium toxicity are discussed further below, it needs to be emphasized that intravenous magnesium is a safe way to administer magnesium, and it has a wide margin of safety. However, unlike many other nutrient supplements, magnesium can be overdone and cannot be given with the abandon of something like the virtually nontoxic vitamin C. A partial listing of the many situations in which intravenous magnesium has been safely given, including in many subsets of very critically ill patients, include the following:

✓ A large number of different drug intoxications and overdoses (see Chapter 10)
✓ Following cardiothoracic surgery[18]
✓ Pain management in routine post-cesarean delivery care[19,20]
✓ Treatment of migraine[21]
✓ Treatment of children with acute asthma in the emergency room[22]
✓ Pain reduction after abdominal hysterectomy[23]

✓ Treatment of reversible cerebral vasoconstriction syndrome: case series[24]

✓ Treatment of sickle cell crises in children[25]

✓ In prevention of contrast-induced nephropathy[26]

✓ Treatment of pregnant women for fetal/neonatal neuroprotection[27]

✓ Treatment of exacerbations of chronic obstructive pulmonary disease[28,29]

✓ Acute treatment of headaches in pediatric patients[30]

✓ Treatment of laryngospasm in children post-adenotonsillectomy[31]

✓ As an adjuvant to morphine for postoperative analgesia[32,33]

✓ Treatment of aneurysmal subarachnoid hemorrhage[34]

✓ Treatment of eclampsia[35,36]

✓ Treatment of stroke[37]

✓ Treatment of severe tetanus[38]

✓ Treatment of fetal arrhythmia[39]

✓ Treatment of neuropathic pain[40]

✓ Treatment of severe mania[41]

✓ Treatment of neonates[42,43]

✓ Treatment of AIDS patients[44]

✓ Infants of mothers given long-term magnesium sulfate during pregnancy[45]

✓ Treatment of cluster headaches[46]

✓ Treatment of hydrofluoric acid burns[47]

✓ Preanesthetic administration for better hemodynamic stabilization[48]

✓ Treatment of suspected acute myocardial infarction[49]

✓ Treatment of supraventricular
   arrhythmias[50]
✓ Treatment of diastolic dysfunction[51]
✓ Treatment for acute respiratory failure
   (from asthma)[52]
✓ Treatment of preeclampsia[53]
✓ Treatment of acute digitalis poisoning[54]

It would also appear that a substantial amount of intravenous magnesium is ultimately retained inside the cells of the body. Studies on patients with acute myocardial infarction or suspected acute myocardial infarction who received high doses of magnesium sulfate intravenously demonstrated a profoundly positive longevity effect after the one-time hospital dosing. The patients in one study received 22 grams of magnesium over 48 hours. All-cause mortality was significantly decreased over as long as 5 years post-infusion.[55-57]

Because of these well-established effects of intravenous magnesium on longevity, along with the established benefits of optimized magnesium concentrations in all the cells of the body, anyone receiving an IV for any reason should not miss the opportunity to have magnesium added to the solution. The only reasons to avoid adding magnesium would be the rare situations of preexisting magnesium toxicity or advanced kidney disease, or when it is desired to give an IV or an infusion extremely rapidly (say, over 15 to 30 minutes) as might be desired at times when giving vitamin C intravenously rapidly to induce an endogenous release of insulin.

Intramuscular

Intramuscular magnesium is another effective way to deliver magnesium. In one study, intramuscular magnesium sulfate has proven to be equally effective for the control and prevention of seizures in eclampsia patients compared to an IV regimen.[58] Another study reached a similar conclusion with preeclampsia patients given either intramuscular or intravenous magnesium.[59] It also appears that the intramuscular administration of magnesium disseminates throughout the body well, as eclampsia patients given IM injections showed good uptake of magnesium into the brain.[60]

Other Routes of Administration

Transdermal

Transdermal delivery of an agent simply means a form of administration that goes into and ultimately through the skin. Depending on the nature of the components being used in the transdermal application or delivery system (e.g., patch), substantial amounts of the agent being dosed can enter the systemic circulation and treat conditions remote from the application site.[61,62] Transdermal preparations of various agents are also used to treat skin conditions and wounds more effectively by improved delivery of those agents.[63,64]

Magnesium can be reliably introduced into the body via transdermal delivery. However, the degree to which that delivery delivers magnesium and the consistency with which it is delivered from one application to the next remains in doubt.[65] One study showed that the application of magnesium cream resulted in a rise in both serum and urinary magnesium markers.[66] Another study found that the application of a magne-

sium chloride solution on the limbs appeared to alleviate symptoms of fibromyalgia.[67]

Transdermal magnesium avoids the gastrointestinal side effects seen with regular oral forms of
magnesium supplementation. This form of magnesium
is a good adjunct in helping to support the magnesium
levels resulting from its other more common forms of
administration. Its regular use is also one good way to
support good skin health. The typical forms of magnesium for transdermal use are as an oil, a gel, a lotion, or
as bath salts. Magnesium oil is a concentrated solution
of magnesium chloride and water. A gel or lotion is
less concentrated and mixed with any of a number of
different agents commonly used for skin or cosmetic
applications. The bath salts are generally magnesium
chloride flakes or granular magnesium sulfate (Epsom
salt).

An additional "form" of transdermal magnesium
application comes in the form of a magnesium-containing enema. The mucosal lining throughout the
gastrointestinal tract is very effective in absorbing just
about any agent with which it comes in contact for a
long enough period of time. Applications of magnesium via enema are especially useful when oral intake
is impaired or limited, and when intravenous infusions are not readily available or economically feasible.
However, the amount of rectal absorption of magnesium can be difficult to predict and toxicity can occur
even in the face of normal renal function.

Nebulization

Nebulization is the process that effectively
converts a medicament from a liquid form into a fine
mist that can be readily inhaled into the upper respi-

ratory tract and the lungs.[68] The administration of a drug or nutrient agent via such a route of inhalation has an extensive history, actually dating back more than 3,500 years ago to ancient Egypt.[69] Except for the direct treatment of pulmonary and upper airway conditions, the delivery of therapeutic agents via inhalation remains greatly underutilized, in spite of its ease of usage and lack of expense. To be fair, many clinicians simply rarely think in terms of inhalation as an effective means of systemic deliverance of a drug or nutrient. However, while it can sometimes be effective as a primary means of drug administration, it is virtually always of value in the adjunctive administration of a therapeutic agent. Nebulization offers multiple benefits, including the following:

- ✓ Moistens the inhaled air, helping to thin secretions and mucus and allowing them to be mobilized and expelled
- ✓ Lessens the need to cough as more secretions and mucus end up getting eliminated
- ✓ Allows the direct inhalation of bronchodilating therapeutic agents
- ✓ Allows the direct inhalation of agents that can combat pathogens colonizing and/or grossly infecting the upper respiratory tract and lungs
- ✓ Permits the use of lower amounts of therapeutic agents that would be more prone to toxicity when given systemically in much higher doses, either orally or intravenously

✓ Permits some systemic assimilation of the
nebulized agent throughout the body

Magnesium has been administered via nebulization for infections, a number of pulmonary conditions,
and as an adjunctive agent in lessening the bronchospasm of an asthmatic attack.[70-72] One study showed
that the preoperative administration of nebulized
magnesium sulfate significantly reduced the incidence
of postoperative sore throat following tracheal intubation and the administration of general anesthesia.[73]

While there is some question of the benefits of
inhaled magnesium in adults with stable asthma, it
appears to be especially effective in alleviating bronchospasm in asthmatic children, even when compared
to intravenous magnesium.[74-77] Also, while there is still
a relative scarcity of studies on nebulizing medicines
in general, and on nebulizing magnesium more specifically, many unlabeled uses of nebulized medicaments
are now emerging, including antibiotics, antifungals,
and narcotics such as opioids.[78] Nebulized magnesium can be used as a primary or an adjunctive therapy
for pneumona, lung cancer, pulmonary and systemic
intoxications, and to a limited degree for just about
any condition for which magnesium is given orally or
intravenously.

Magnesium, along with many other nutrients and anti-pathogen agents, can also be administered via nebulization for acute upper respiratory
tract infections, lung infections, and sinus infections.
Furthermore, many people who do not have an acute
flu, cold, or other respiratory tract infection have
chronic pathogen colonization. Such pathogens, while
not having the negative clinical impact of an advanced

case of influenza, for example, are capable of a substantial chronic negative health impact that could significantly limit the degree of positive response that could otherwise be achieved in the optimal treatment of many medical conditions. Pathogens always produce prooxidant metabolic byproducts (toxins), and when growing in the upper airway, they are chronically swallowed "24/7." It is probable that this constant state of pathogen colonization is a strong contributor to most of the chronic gastrointestinal disorders, including ulcer disease, leaky gut syndrome, and even gastrointestinal malignancy. States of chronic pathogen colonization often have biofilms (an extracellular envelope of proteins, lipids, and polysaccharides) lessening or blocking the access of traditional anti-pathogen agents to the pathogens.[79] A number of different agents that can be nebulized appear to be able to break through such biofilms (e.g., hydrogen peroxide or DMSO).[80,81]

While no studies were found addressing the issue of chronic pathogen colonization and its consequences, it would make good sense to always help resolve any acute respiratory syndrome with nebulized magnesium chloride (probably the best form of magnesium for nebulization for anti-pathogen effects — see Chapter 11) and any of a number of other nebulized anti-pathogen agents. Any persistent post-infection symptoms (residual cough, yellow and/or green sputum production, however minimal) would likely benefit significantly from such a protocol of nebulization.

It would probably be a good practice to periodically nebulize magnesium and/or other agents to re-establish and/or maintain a more normal throat and respiratory tract flora as well. Other anti-pathogen agents that can be nebulized include hydrogen peroxide, N-acetyl cysteine, sodium bicarbonate, DMSO, nascent iodine, colloidal silver, and vitamin C as sodium ascorbate. Dosing and administration protocols should be worked out with a physician or other chosen health care provider. Generally, any nebulization should be comfortable and any odor should not be overly pungent or off-putting. However, it should be discontinued if any coughing or even minimal compromise of breathing results. Often, when not well-tolerated, it can be continued subsequent to greater dilution of the nebulized agents. Most agents can be nebulized together, although hydrogen peroxide is best nebulized by itself.

Magnesium Toxicity

Traditionally, there has only been concern with magnesium toxicity when giving magnesium intravenously, or when giving enough of any form of magnesium to an individual with diminished kidney function. Oral magnesium has been typically been felt to be a "protected" form of magnesium intake, resulting in abdominal cramping and/or a diarrhea response before enough magnesium can be absorbed to ever approach systemic magnesium toxicity. And for patients with normal kidney function who take any of the traditional forms of oral magnesium supplementation, this is a good working rule of thumb.

Constipated elderly individuals comprise a subset of patients especially susceptible to significant magnesium toxicity, even from oral sources. Such patients, often but not necessarily in the setting of a nursing home, can receive sizeable amounts of magnesium-based cathartics (such as magnesium citrate) as a therapy for their constipation. When a large enough amount of magnesium, even a relatively poorly-absorbed form, is taken orally and remains in the gut for a long enough time, toxic amounts of magnesium can eventually be assimilated. This is especially true if any compromise of kidney function is present as well. Furthermore, this magnesium toxicity can even be fatal if bowel function does not sufficiently respond quickly enough.[82-84] Severe hypermagnesemia with clinical magnesium toxicity from repeated administration of magnesium citrate as a cathartic in overdose patients has also been reported.[85,86] A 14-year-old girl who received magnesium hydroxide for a week for constipation eventually presented with hypotension and lethargy, but survived.[87] In a patient with megacolon, a condition in which the colon is dilated and the contractile nature of the bowel is severely diminished or even paralyzed, an enema with magnesium sulfate resulted in fatal magnesium poisoning.[88]

Intravenous magnesium can be administered very safely, but attention must be paid to dose, rate of administration, and the condition of the patient being treated. Toxicity, to the point of being fatal, will reliably occur if too much is given too rapidly, especially in the setting of a severely ill patient, as in an acute drug overdose, or in the setting of significantly decreased kidney function. Magnesium overdoses have often been noted to be due to erroneous overdosing.[89] Early clinical signs of magnesium toxicity when giving intravenous magnesium include nausea and vomiting, feeling warm and flushed, slowed heart rate and/or new cardiac arrhythmias, sleepiness, double vision, slurred speech, and weakness. Of note, visual disturbances during intravenous magnesium administration are common, including blurred and double vision. These findings were not necessarily associated with any other symptoms and the visual changes resolved upon discontinuation of the magnesium infusion.[90] Generally, many of these symptoms of early magnesium excess appear after the blood pressure drops, either to levels low for the patient's history, or to levels of frank hypotension, due to excessive calcium channel blocking effect on the arteries and excessive vasodilation. A similar profile of signs and symptoms is seen with a prescription calcium channel blocker overdose. At the highest of plasma magnesium levels muscular paralysis, with respiratory or cardiac arrest, can occur. Because of their mutual antagonism, calcium administration serves as an acute and effective antidote for advanced magnesium toxicity or overdose.[91]

However, it is also important to realize that the lowering of blood pressure in some clinical settings is the desired outcome of intravenous magnesium administration. In some types of surgery intraoperative blood loss can be substantial and often requires blood transfusion. An infusion of magnesium while such surgery is performed is an accepted approach for maintaining lowered blood pressure in what is known as "controlled" or "deliberate" hypotension. Not surprisingly, such uses of magnesium require very careful and continued monitoring, since a state of intentionally-inflicted hypotension is getting very close to frank magnesium toxicity with multiple undesired side effects. Depending on the surgery and the preferences of the operating team, mean arterial blood pressures between 50 and 65 mm Hg are maintained, while the normal range is considered to be between 70 and 110 mm Hg.[92-97]

Magnesium Supplementation Guidelines

As with the dosing of any agent that has great benefits yet potentially substantial toxicity, these guidelines can only be considered approximate. A perfect dose for one person might be toxic for another, and vice-versa. Nevertheless, as stated above, magnesium has a very large safety margin in all its forms of administration, but aggressive and reckless regimens, especially when there is compromised kidney function, can completely nullify this safety cushion, especially in its intravenous application.[98] Furthermore, as has been pointed out repeatedly throughout this book, very many people, likely a substantial majority, are magnesium-deficient, and this deficiency still must be addressed, as it has a wide-ranging negative impact on the public health. Some degree of supplementation is in order for just about everyone, especially older individuals who have magnesium-deficient diets, diseases that decrease magnesium stores, and/or medications that further lower magnesium levels. It has been estimated that under "typical physiological conditions," a daily intake of 3.6 mg/kg of body weight is indicated (elemental magnesium). This ends up being an average daily intake (ADI) of 320 to 420 mg/day (13 to 17 mmol/day).[99]

The most common test for assessing the magnesium status in the body is the serum total magnesium concentration. However, as discussed before, magnesium levels that fall into the established reference range (0.75 to 0.95 mmol/L, or 1.82 mg/dL to

2.30 mg/dL) can be present when the magnesium levels in the tissues of the body are still significantly depleted.[100] A reference range level of magnesium indicates a better magnesium status in the body than a level that is clearly low, but little more can be definitively concluded from it. In other words, a chronically low serum magnesium level clearly indicates body-wide depletion, but a reference range, or "normal" serum magnesium level is in no way an assurance of normal magnesium levels in the cells and tissues. Less than 1% of magnesium in the body is in the blood. Greater than 99% is outside the blood, nearly all of which is inside the cells of the body, predominantly the bones and the muscles.[101] Clinically speaking, then:

> **A low serum magnesium is an unequivocal indication FOR magnesium supplementation, but a normal serum magnesium level by itself is NOT an argument against supplementation.**

An elevated serum magnesium can be present even when a body-wide deficiency exists. However, such an elevated level does indicate that further magnesium should not be given acutely, and the elevated serum magnesium, along with the circumstances provoking it, should be resolved prior to considering any schedule of supplementation. Other tests, as noted below, should be considered to establish whether body-wide magnesium stores are at all deficient before proceeding with supplementation after the elevated serum magnesium has normalized.

Key indicators of magnesium status include the serum magnesium levels, urinary magnesium excretion, and dietary/supplemental intake. This information must then be correlated with the clinical and laboratory status of an individual, particularly with regard to the parameters measuring cardiovascular (lipid panel), renal, and sugar metabolism (diabetes) status.[102]

Other laboratory tests that help in establishing the magnesium status in the body include the following:

1. **Red Blood Cell (RBC) Magnesium Level**
   RBC magnesium levels give a better idea of the magnesium status in the body than serum magnesium levels, but they can still be misleading. An RBC has cytoplasm, but it has no nucleus and it does not have any mitochondria, which is where the vast majority of the body-wide content of magnesium is stored. When both the RBC magnesium levels and the serum magnesium levels are in the reference ("normal") ranges, the magnesium status in the body is certainly better than if these levels were low. However, it is not a guarantee that the body magnesium stores are normal, or that magnesium supplementation is still not warranted. Generally, normal RBC magnesium levels will not be seen when serum magnesium levels have been chronically low. Unfortunately, the limitations of RBC magnesium levels remain unappreciated by many researchers and clinicians who continue to regard the RBC magnesium content as being a clear-cut measure of intracellular magnesium content in all the other cells of the body.[103]

2. **Platelet Magnesium Level**
   Platelet magnesium levels are primarily
   available for research and not general laboratory testing, like RBC magnesium levels.
   However, they suffer from largely the same
   shortcomings as noted above for the RBC
   measurements. Like an RBC, a platelet lacks
   mitochondria and a nucleus, along with most
   known intracellular organelles. Platelets are
   essentially fragments of cytoplasm derived
   from megakaryocytes (large bone marrow
   cells). Platelets probably more accurately
   reflect recent changes in magnesium availability compared to RBCs, as their life span
   is only 8 to 9 days compared to the RBC life
   span of 100 to 120 days.

3. **Mononuclear Cell Magnesium Level**
   Mononuclear cell magnesium levels are also
   primarily for research purposes. However,
   they better reflect body-wide magnesium
   levels than RBCs, platelets, or serum.[104-106]
   Mononuclear cells are complete cells, with
   nuclei, subcellular organelles, and cytoplasm, and the measured levels directly
   reflect the large stores of magnesium found
   in the mitochondria. However, mononuclear cells are largely circulating cells that
   will assimilate new magnesium intake
   better than a cell that is non-mobile and
   part of a tissue or organ, as with a skeletal
   muscle cell. Presumably, this would make
   the monocyte less reflective of long-term
   magnesium assimilation than would the

skeletal muscle cells.

Quite literally, the magnesium level measurement sites in the body are much like the layers of an onion. The serum is the outermost layer, the fragmented cells are the next layer, the intact but mobile cells are the next layer, and the "fixed" cells in the tissues and organs are the innermost layer. Normal tissue cell magnesium levels mean normal magnesium levels everywhere, but normal "outer layer" magnesium levels do not assure that the innermost layers are yet optimized in magnesium content.

4. **Intravenous Magnesium Load Test**

   The intravenous magnesium load test is a practical way to infer that the body is depleted of magnesium. After taking a given intravenous dose of magnesium, a later analysis of the urine directly reflects how well your body retained the magnesium. The less that magnesium appears in the urine, the greater the presumption that there exists a significant need for the magnesium, and the greater the degree of overall magnesium deficiency is inferred.[107]

5. **Magnesium Content in Muscle Biopsies**

   Magnesium content measurements in muscle biopsies are quite accurate, and they probably represent the best way to clearly assess the normalcy of magnesium content in the body.[108,109] However, they are invasive, expensive, and largely limited to research settings.

6. **Sublingual Epithelial Cell Magnesium Assay**
The sublingual epithelial cell magnesium assay has been reported in the literature for many years now, but it is only relatively recently being utilized as an optimal way to assess the magnesium content in the body. It needs to be emphasized that this test measures total cellular magnesium content (not just cytoplasmic), which makes it a good reflection of the stores of magnesium in the body, as 95% of the magnesium in the cell is in the mitochondria. The literature addressing this test, although limited, indicates that it is a reliable assessment of the body-wide magnesium stores, as it measures both bound and unbound magnesium inside the cells tested (sublingual epithelial cells from the mouth), and that the magnesium content of these cells correlates well with the magnesium content in tissues remote from them (atrial tissue and muscle biopsies). These cells are readily accessible and easily sampled. Currently, the test is available at www.exatest.com.[110-112]

Basically, then, the best and probably most economic approach to knowing your body-wide magnesium status would be to first measure your serum magnesium. If it is low, you are low everywhere else in the body. If it is normal or even high-normal, then proceed to the sublingual epithelial assay test to see if the normal serum level has completely made its way to the magnesium stores in the intact tissue cell, the "innermost" layer of the onion. Of course, undergoing magnesium supplementation does not require such testing as a guideline. Positive interval changes in blood tests, like the blood glucose and the lipid panel, are clear indicators that your body was magnesium deficient and is improving with magnesium administration. It later becomes a judgment call with your physician whether you are reaching a level of magnesium in your body that permits a cutting back or stopping of magnesium supplementation. However, the daily excretion of magnesium (further aggravated by various medications) along with the chronic depletion of magnesium in so many foods and the excessive utilization of magnesium in so many chronic diseases makes it enormously unlikely that magnesium supplementation would ever need to be completely stopped, especially in the presence of normal kidney function.

Suggested Resources

Biological Dentistry
http://www.hugginsappliedhealing.com
http://www.iaomt.org
http://www.iabdm.org
http://www.biologicaldent.com
http://www.biodentist.com

Integrative/Complementary Medicine
http://www.riordanclinic.org/
http://www.acam.org
http://acam.site-ym.com/search/custom.asp?id=1758
http://orthomolecular.org/
http://www.a4m.com/directory.html
http://www.icimed.com/
http://www.acimconnect.com/
http://www.grossmanwellness.com

Supplement sources
http://www.livonlabs.com
http://www.altrient-europe.com

http://www.lef.org
http://www.mcguff.com
http://www.meritpharm.com

For further information

http://www.peakenergy.com
http://www.medfoxpub.com
http://www.doctoryourself.com
http://www.riordanclinic.org
http://www.vitamincfoundation.org
http://www.naturalhealth365.com

These websites are for general reference only, and any information, treatments, or products derived from them cannot be guaranteed to be beneficial or to be in agreement with the information in this book.

References

Chapter 1

1. de Baaji J, Hoenderop J, Bindels R (2015) Magnesium in man: implications for health and disease. *Physiological Reviews* 95:1-46. PMID: 25540137

2. Workinger J, Doyle R, Bortz J (2018) Challenges in the diagnosis of magnesium status. *Nutrients* 10:1202. PMID: 30200431

3. Grober U, Schmidt J, Kisters K (2015) Magnesium in prevention and therapy. *Nutrients* 7:8199-8226. PMID: 26404370

4. Hsu J, Rubenstein B, Paleker A (1982) Role of magnesium in glutathione metabolism of rat erythrocytes. *The Journal of Nutrition* 112:488-496. PMID: 7062145

5. Mills B, Lindeman R, Lang C (1986) Magnesium deficiency inhibits biosynthesis of blood glutathione and tumor growth in the rat. *Proceedings of the Society for Experimental Biology and Medicine* 181:326-332. PMID: 3945642

6. Barbagallo M, Dominguez L, Tagliamonte M et al. (1999) Effects of glutathione on red blood cell intracellular magnesium: relation to glucose metabolism. *Hypertension* 34:76-82. PMID: 10406827

7. Regan R, Guo Y (2001) Magnesium deprivation decreases cellular reduced glutathione and causes oxidative neuronal death in murine cortical cultures. *Brain Research* 890:177-183. PMID: 11164781

8. DiNicolantonio J, O'Keefe J, Wilson W (2018) Subclinical magnesium deficiency: a principal driver of cardiovascular disease and a public health crisis. *Open Heart* 5:e000668. PMID: 29387426

9. Ahmed F, Mohammed A (2019) Magnesium: the forgotten electrolyte—a review on hypomagnesemia. *Medical Sciences* 7:56. PMID: 30987399

10. Eftekhari M, Rostami Z, Emami M, Tabatabaee H (2014) Effects of "vitex agnus castus" extract and magnesium supplementation, along and in combination, on osteogenic and angiogenic factors and fracture healing in women with long bone fracture. *Journal of Research in Medical Sciences* 19:1-7. PMID: 24672557

11. Zhang Y, Xu J, Ruan Y et al. (2016) Implant-derived magnesium induces local neuronal production of CGRP to improve bone-fracture healing in rats. *Nature Medicine* 22:1160-1169. PMID: 27571347

12. Galli S, Stocchero M, Andersson M et al. (2017) The effect of magnesium on early osseointegration in osteoporotic bone: a histological and gene expression investigation. *Osteoporosis International* 28:2195-2205. PMID: 28349251

13. Schaller B, Saulacic N, Beck S et al. (2017) Osteosynthesis of partial rib osteotomy in a miniature pig model using human standard-sized magnesium plate/screw systems: effect of cyclic deformation on implant integrity and bone healing. *Journal of Cranio-Maxillo-Facial Surgery* 45:862-871. PMID: 28457825

14. Akhtar M, Ullah H, Hamid M (2011) Magnesium, a drug of diverse use. *The Journal of the Pakistan Medical Association* 61:1220-1225. PMID: 22355971

15. Altura BM, Altura BT (1984) Microcirculatory actions and uses of naturally-occurring (magnesium) and novel synthetic calcium channel blockers. *Microcirculation, Endothelium, and Lymphatics* 1:185-220. PMID: 6400430

16. Iseri L, French J (1984) Magnesium: nature's physiologic calcium blocker. *American Heart Journal* 108:188-193. PMID: 6375330

17. Yago M, Manas M, Singh J (2000) Intracellular magnesium: transport and regulation in epithelial secretary cells. *Frontiers in Bioscience* 5:D602-D618. PMID: 10877998

18. Lin C, Tsai P, Hung Y, Huang C (2010) L-type calcium channels are involved in mediating the anti-inflammatory effects of magnesium sulphate. *British Journal of Anaesthesia* 104:44-51. PMID: 19933511

19. Libako P, Nowacki W, Castiglioni S et al. (2016) Extracellular magnesium and calcium blockers modulate macrophage activity. *Magnesium Research* 29:11-21. PMID: 27160489

20. Razzaghi R, Pidar F, Momen-Heravi M et al. (2018) Magnesium supplementation and the effects on wound healing and metabolic status in patients with diabetic foot ulcer: a randomized, double-blind, placebo-controlled trial. *Biological Trace Element Research* 181:207-215. PMID: 28540570

21. Afzali H, Jafari Kashi A, Momen-Heravi M et al. (2019) The effects of magnesium and vitamin E co-supplementation on wound healing and metabolic status in patients with diabetic foot ulcer: a randomized, double-blind, placebo-controlled trial. *Wound Repair and Regeneration* Jan 28 [Epub ahead of print]. PMID: 30693609

22. De Oliveira G, Bialek J, Fitzgerald P et al. (2013) Systemic magnesium to improve quality of post-surgical recovery in outpatient segmental mastectomy: a randomized, double-blind, placebo-controlled trial. *Magnesium Research* 26:156-164. PMID: 24491463

23. Afshari D, Moradian N, Rezaei M (2013) Evaluation of the intravenous magnesium sulfate effect in clinical improvement of patients with acute ischemic stroke. *Clinical Neurology and Neurosurgery* 115:400-404. PMID: 22749947

24. Cox R, Osgood K (1994) Evaluation of intravenous magnesium sulfate for the treatment of hydrofluoric acid burns. *Journal of Toxicology. Clinical Toxicology* 32:123-136. PMID: 8145352

25. Lin D, Hung F, Yeh M, Lui T (2015) Microstructure-modified biodegradable magnesium alloy for promoting cytocompatibility and wound healing *in vitro*. *Journal of Materials Science. Materials in Medicine* 26:248. PMID: 26411444

26. Sasaki Y, Sathi G, Yamamoto O (2017) Wound healing effect of bioactive ion released from Mg-smectite. *Materials Science & Engineering. C, Materials for Biological Applications* 77:52-57. PMID: 28532061

27. Grzesiak J, Pierschbacher M (1995) Shifts in the concentrations of magnesium and calcium in early porcine and rat wound fluids activate the cell migratory response. *The Journal of Clinical Investigation* 95:227-233. PMID: 7814620

28. Bravi M, Armiento A, Laurenti O et al. (2006) Insulin decreases intracellular oxidative stress in patients with type 2 diabetes mellitus. *Metabolism* 55:691-695. PMID: 16631447

29. Barbagallo M, Dominguez L, Tagliamonte M et al. (1999) Effects of glutathione on red blood cell intracellular magnesium: relation to glucose metabolism. *Hypertension* 34:76-82. PMID: 10406827

30. Barbagallo M, Dominguez L, Tagliamonte M et al. (1999a) Effects of vitamin E and glutathione on glucose metabolism: role of magnesium. *Hypertension* 34:1002-1006. PMID: 10523398

31. De Mattia G, Bravi M, Laurenti O et al., (1998) Influence of reduced glutathione infusion on glucose metabolism in patients with non-insulin-dependent diabetes mellitus. *Metabolism* 47:993-997. PMID: 9711998 glucose metabolism: role of magnesium. *Hypertension* 34:1002-1006. PMID: 10523398

32. Cheung B, Li C (2012) Diabetes and hypertension: is there a common metabolic pathway? *Current Atherosclerosis Reports* 14:160-166. PMID: 22281657

33. Resnick L, Gupta R, Gruenspan H, Laragh J (1988) Intracellular free magnesium in hypertension: relation to peripheral insulin resistance. *Journal of Hypertension. Supplement* 6:S199-S201. PMID: 3241201

34. Resnick L, Gupta R, Laragh J (1984) Intracellular free magnesium in erythrocytes of essential hypertension: relation to blood pressure and serum divalent cations. *Proceedings of the National Academy of Sciences of the United States of America* 81:6511-6515. PMID: 6593713

35. Barbagallo M, Dominguez L, Bardicef O, Resnick L (2001) Altered cellular magnesium responsiveness to hyperglycemia in hypertensive subjects. *Hypertension* 38:612-615. PMID: 11566941

36. Altura B (1994) Introduction: importance of Mg in physiology and medicine and the need for ion selective electrodes. *Scandinavian Journal of Clinical and Laboratory Investigation. Supplementum* 217:5-9. PMID: 7939385

37. Worthington V (2001) Nutritional quality of organic versus conventional fruits, vegetables, and grains. *Journal of Alternative and Complementary Medicine* 7:161-173. PMID: 11327522

38. Davies B (2015) The UK geochemical environment and cardiovascular diseases: magnesium in food and water. *Environmental Geochemistry and Health* 37:411-427. PMID: 25528218

39. Maraver F, Vitoria I, Ferreira-Pego C et al. (2015) Magnesium in tap and bottled mineral water in Spain and its contribution to nutritional recommendations. *Nutricion Hospitalaria* 31:2297-2312. PMID: 25929407

40. Jiang L, He P, Chen J et al. (2016) Magnesium levels in drinking water and coronary heart disease mortality risk: a meta-analysis. *Nutrients* 8:5. PMID: 26729158

41. Yang C, Chiu H (1999) Calcium and magnesium in drinking water and the risk of death from hypertension. *American Journal of Hypertension* 12:894-899. PMID: 10509547

42. Chiu H, Chang C, Yang C (2004) Magnesium and calcium in drinking water and risk of death from ovarian cancer. *Magnesium Research* 17:28-34. PMID: 15083566

Chapter 2

1. Bolland M, Avenell A, Baron J et al. (2010) Effect of calcium supplements on risk of myocardial infarction and cardiovascular events: meta-analysis. *BMJ* 341:c3691. PMID: 20671013

2. Bolland M, Grey A, Avenell A et al. (2011) Calcium supplements with or without vitamin D and risk of cardiovascular events: reanalysis of the Women's Health Initiative limited access dataset and meta-analysis. *BMJ* 342:d2040. PMID: 21505219

3. Reid I, Bolland M, Avenell A, Grey A (2011) Cardiovascular effects of calcium supplementation. *Osteoporosis International* 22:1649-1658. PMID: 21409434

4. Michaelsson K, Melhus H, Warensjo Lemming E et al. (2013) Long term calcium intake and rates of all cause and cardiovascular mortality: commonly based prospective longitudinal cohort study. *BMJ* 346:f228. PMID: 23403980

5. Rodriguez A, Scott D, Khan B et al. (2018) High calcium intake in men not women is associated with all-cause mortality risk: Melbourne Collaborative Cohort Study. *Archives of Osteoporosis* 13:101. PMID: 30242518

6. Graham G, Blaha M, Budoff M et al. (2012) Impact of coronary artery calcification on all-cause mortality in individuals with and without hypertension. *Atherosclerosis* 225:432-437. PMID: 23078882

7. Jacobs P, Gondrie M, van der Graaf Y et al. (2012) Coronary artery calcium can predict all-cause mortality and cardiovascular events on low-dose CT screening for lung cancer. *American Journal of Roentgenology* 198:505-511. PMID: 22357989

8. Kiramijyan S, Ahmadi N, Isma'eel H et al. (2013) Impact of coronary artery calcium progression and statin therapy on clinical outcome in subjects with and without diabetes mellitus. *The American Journal of Cardiology* 111:356-361. PMID: 23206921

9. Nakanishi R, Li D, Blaha M et al. (2016) All-cause mortality by age and gender based on coronary artery calcium scores. *European Heart Journal Cardiovascular Imaging* 17:1305-1314. PMID: 26705490

10. Budoff M, Lutz S, Kinney G et al. (2018) Coronary artery calcium on noncontrast thoracic computerized tomography scans and all-cause mortality. *Circulation* 138:2437-2438. PMID: 30571584

11. Orimoloye O, Budoff M, Dardari Z et al. (2018) Race/ethnicity and the prognostic implications of coronary artery calcium for all-cause and cardiovascular disease mortality: The Coronary Artery Calcium Consortium. *Journal of the American Heart Association* 7:e010471

12. Iseri L, French J (1984) Magnesium: nature's physiologic calcium blocker. *American Heart Journal* 108:188-193. PMID: 6375330

13. Anghileri L (1999) Magnesium, calcium and cancer. *Magnesium Research* 22:247-255. PMID: 20228002

14. Sasaki Y, Sathi G, Yamamoto O (2017) Wound healing effect of bioactive ion released from Mg-smectite. *Materials Science & Engineering. C, Materials for Biological Applications* 77:52-57. PMID: 28532061

15. De Oliveira G, Bialek J, Fitzgerald P et al. (2013) Systemic magnesium to improve quality of post-surgical recovery in outpatient segmental mastectomy: a randomized, double-blind, placebo-controlled trial. *Magnesium Research* 26:156-164. PMID: 24491463

16. Afzali H, Jafari Kashi A, Momen-Heravi M et al. (2019) The effects of magnesium and vitamin E co-supplementation on wound healing and metabolic status in patients with diabetic foot ulcer: a randomized, double-blind, placebo-controlled trial. *Wound Repair and Regeneration* 27:277-284. PMID: 30693609

17. Razzaghi R, Pidar F, Momen-Heravi M et al. (2018) Magnesium supplementation and the effects on wound healing and metabolic status in patients with diabetic foot ulcer: a randomized, double-blind, placebo-controlled trial. *Biological Trace Element Research* 181:207-215. PMID: 28540570

18. Zhang Z, Zhou Y, Li W et al. (2019) Local administration of magnesium promotes meniscal healing through homing of endogenous stem cells: a proof-of-concept study. *The American Journal of Sports Medicine* 47:954-967. PMID: 30786213

19. Gillman M, Ross-Degnan D, McLaughlin T et al. (1999) Effects of long-acting versus short-acting calcium channel blockers among older survivors of acute myocardial infarction. *Journal of The American Geriatrics Society* 47:512-517. PMID: 10323641

20. Gibson R, Hansen J, Messerli F et al. (2000) Long-term effects of diltiazem and verapamil on mortality and cardiac events in non-Q-wave acute myocardial infarction without pulmonary congestion: post hoc subset analysis of the multicenter diltiazem postinfarction trial and the second Danish verapamil infarction trial studies. *The American Journal of Cardiology* 86:275-279. PMID: 10922432

21. Lubsen J, Wagener G, Kirwan B et al. (2005) Effect of long-acting nifedipine on mortality and cardiovascular morbidity in patients with symptomatic stable angina and hypertension: the ACTION trial. *Journal of Hypertension* 23:641-648. PMID: 15716708

22. Constanzo P, Perrone-Filardi P, Petretta M et al. (2009) Calcium channel blockers and cardiovascular outcomes: a meta-analysis of 175,634 patients. *Journal of Hypertension* 27:1136-1151. PMID: 19451836

23. Deshmukh H, Barker E, Anbarasan T et al. (2018) Calcium channel blockers are associated with improved survival and lower cardiovascular mortality in patients with renovascular disease. *Cardiovascular Therapeutics* 36:e12474. PMID: 30372589

24. Mittal S, Mathur A, Prasad N (1993) Effect of calcium channel blockers on serum levels of thyroid hormones. *International Journal of Cardiology* 38:131-132. PMID: 8454374

25. Morad F, Elsayed E, Mahmoud S (1997) Inhibition of steroid sex hormones release in rats by two Ca2+ channel blockers. *Pharmacological Research* 35:177-180. PMID: 9229405

26. Verhoeven F, Moerings E, Lamers J et al. (2001) Inhibitory effects of calcium channel blockers on thyroid hormone uptake in neonatal rat cardiomyocytes. *American Journal of Physiology. Heart and Circulatory Physiology* 281:H1985-H1991. PMID: 11668059

27. Reffelmann T, Ittermann T, Dorr M et al. (2011) Low serum magnesium concentrations predict cardiovascular and all-cause mortality. *Atherosclerosis* 219:280-284. PMID: 21703623

28. Ferre S, Li X, Adams-Huet B et al. (2018) Association of serum magnesium with all-cause mortality in patients with and without chronic kidney disease in the Dallas Heart Study. *Nephrology, Dialysis, Transplantation* 33:1389-1396. PMID: 29077944

29. Zhang X, Xia J, Del Gobbo L et al. (2018) Serum magnesium concentrations and all-cause, cardiovascular, and cancer mortality among U.S. adults: results from the NHANES I epidemiologic follow-up study. *Clinical Nutrition* 37:1541-1549. PMID: 28890274

30. Weisinger J, Bellorin-Font E (1998) Magnesium and phosphorus. *Lancet* 352:391-396. PMID: 9717944

31. Elin R (2010) Assessment of magnesium status for diagnosis and therapy. *Magnesium Research* 23:S194-S198. PMID: 20736141

32. Munoz-Castaneda J, Pendon-Ruiz de Mier M, Rodriguez M, Rodriguez-Ortiz M (2018) Magnesium replacement to protect cardiovascular and kidney damage? Lack of prospective clinical trials. *International Journal of Molecular Sciences* Feb 27; 19(3). PMID: 29495444

33. Woods K, Fletcher S (1994) Long-term outcome after intravenous magnesium sulphate in suspected acute myocardial infarction: the second Leicester Intravenous Magnesium Intervention Trial (LIMIT-2). *Lancet* 343:816-819. PMID: 7908076

34. Shechter M, Hod H, Rabinowitz B et al. (2003) Long-term outcome of intravenous magnesium therapy in thrombolysis-ineligible acute myocardial infarction patients. *Cardiology* 99:205-210. PMID: 12845247

35. Steidl L, Ditmar R (1990) Soft tissue calcification treated with local and oral magnesium therapy. *Magnesium Research* 3:113-119. PMID: 2133625

36. Ter Braake A, Shanahan C, de Baaij J (2017) Magnesium counteracts vascular calcification: passive interference or active modulation? *Arteriosclerosis, Thrombosis, and Vascular Biology* 37:1431-1445. PMID: 28663256

37. Ter Braake A, Tinnemans P, Shanahan C et al. (2018) Magnesium prevents vascular calcification *in vitro* by inhibition of hydroxyapatite crystal formation. *Scientific Reports* 8:2069. PMID: 29391410

38. Hisamatsu T, Miura K, Fujiyoshi A et al. (2018) Serum magnesium, phosphorus, and calcium levels and subclinical calcific aortic valve disease: a population-based study. *Atherosclerosis* 273:145-152. PMID: 29655832

39. Ishimura E, Okuno S, Kitatani K et al. (2007) Significant association between the presence of peripheral vascular calcification and lower serum magnesium in hemodialysis patients. *Clinical Nephrology* 68:222-227. PMID: 17969489

40. Sato H, Takeuchi Y, Matsuda K et al. (2018) Evaluation of the predictive value of the serum calcium-magnesium ratio for all-cause and cardiovascular mortality in incident dialysis patients. *CardioRenal Medicine* 8:50-60. PMID: 29344026

41. Razzaque M (2018) Magnesium: are we consuming enough? *Nutrients* 10:1863. PMID: 30513803

42. Kass G, Orrenius S (1999) Calcium signaling and cytotoxicity. *Environmental Health Perspectives* 107 (Suppl 1):25-35. PMID: 10229704

43. Vormann J (2016) Magnesium: nutrition and homoeostasis. *AIMS Public Health* 3:329-340. PMID: 29546166

44. D'Agostino A (1963) An electron microscopic study of skeletal and cardiac muscle of the rat poisoned by plasmocid. *Laboratory Investigations* 12:1060-1071. PMID: 14083316

45. Caulfield J, Schrag P (1964) Electron microscopic study of renal calcification. *The American Journal of Pathology* 44:365-381. PMID: 14126660

46. D'Agostino A (1964) An electron microscopic study of cardiac necrosis produced by 9 alpha-fluorocortisol and sodium phosphate. *The American Journal of Pathology* 45:633-644. PMID: 14217676

47. Giacomelli F, Spiro D, Wiener J (1964) A study of metastatic renal calcification at the cellular level. *The Journal of Cell Biology* 22:189-206. PMID: 14195609

48. Montes de Oca A, Guerrero F, Martinez-Moreno J et al. (2014) Magnesium inhibits Wnt/β-catenin activity and reverses the osteogenic transformation of vascular smooth muscle cells. *PLoS One* 9:e89525. PMID: 24586847

49. Bressendorff I, Hansen D, Schou M et al. (2016) Oral magnesium supplementation in chronic kidney disease stages 3 and 4: efficacy, safety, and effect on serum calcification propensity—a prospective randomized double-blinded placebo-controlled clinical trial. *Kidney International Reports* 2:380-389. PMID: 29142966

50. Yue J, Jin S, Li Y et al. (2016) Magnesium inhibits the calcification of the extracellular matrix in tendon-derived stem cells via the ATP-P2R and mitochondrial pathways. *Biochemical and Biophysical Research Communications* 478:314-322. PMID: 27402270

51. Bressendorff I, Hansen D, Shou M et al. (2018) The effect of increasing dialysate magnesium on serum calcification propensity in subjects with end stage kidney disease: a randomized, controlled clinical trial. *Clinical Journal of the American Society of Nephrology* 13:1373-1380. PMID: 30131425

52. Henaut L, Massy Z (2018) Magnesium as a calcification inhibitor. *Advances in Chronic Kidney Disease* 25:281-290. PMID: 29793668

53. Kaesler N, Goettsch C, Weis D et al. (2019) Magnesium but not nicotinamide prevents vascular calcification in experimental uraemia. *Nephrology, Dialysis, Transplantation* [Epub ahead of print]. PMID: 30715488

54. Roos D, Seeger R, Puntel R, Vargas Barbosa N (2012) Role of calcium and mitochondria in MeHg-mediated cytotoxicity. *Journal of Biomedicine & Biotechnology* 2012:248764. PMID: 22927718

55. Chi Y, Zhang X, Cai J et al. (2012) Formaldehyde increases intracellular calcium concentration in primary cultured hippocampal neurons partly through NMDA receptors and T-type calcium channels. *Neuroscience Bulletin* 28:715-722. PMID: 23160928

56. Gao F, Ding B, Zhou L et al. (2013) Magnesium sulfate provides neuroprotection in lipopolysaccharide-activated primary microglia by inhibiting NF-κB pathway. *The Journal of Surgical Research* 184:944-950. PMID: 23628437

57. Li J, Wang P, Yu S et al. (2012) Calcium entry mediates hyperglycemia-induced apoptosis through Ca(2+)/calmodulin-dependent kinase II in retinal capillary endothelial cells. *Molecular Vision* 18:2371-2379. PMID: 23049237

58. Kawamata H, Manfredi G (2010) Mitochondrial dysfunction and intracellular calcium dysregulation in ALS. *Mechanisms of Ageing and Development* 131:517-526. PMID: 20493207

59. Corona C, Pensalfini A, Frazzini V, Sensi S (2011) New therapeutic targets in Alzheimer's disease: brain deregulation of calcium and zinc. *Cell Death & Disease* 2:e176. PMID: 21697951

60. Surmeier D, Guzman J, Sanchez-Padilla J, Schumacker P (2011) The role of calcium and mitochondrial oxidant stress in the loss of substantia nigra pars compacta dopaminergic neurons in Parkinson's disease. *Neuroscience* 198:221-231. PMID: 21884755

61. Surmeier D, Halliday G, Simuni T (2017) Calcium, mitochondrial dysfunction and slowing the progression of Parkinson's disease. *Experimental Neurology* 298:202-209. PMID: 28780195

62. Levy T (2011) *Curing the Incurable: Vitamin C, Infectious Diseases, and Toxins.* Henderson, NV: MedFox Publishing

63. Chang Y, Kao M, Lin J et al. (2018) Effects of $MgSO_4$ on inhibiting Nod-like receptor protein 3 inflammasome involve decreasing intracellular calcium. *The Journal of Surgical Research* 221:257-265. PMID: 29229137

64. Brvar M, Chan M, Dawson A et al. (2018) Magnesium sulfate and calcium channel blocking drugs as antidotes for acute organophosphorus insecticide poisoning—a systematic review and meta-analysis. *Clinical Toxicology* 56:725-736. PMID: 29557685

65. Guzel A, Dogan E, Turkcu G et al. (2018) Dexmedetomidine and magnesium sulfate: a good combination treatment for acute lung injury? *Journal of Investigative Surgery* Jan 23:1-12 [Epub ahead of print]. PMID: 29359990

66. Chen N, Xu R, Wang L et al. (2018) Protective effects of magnesium sulfate on radiation induced brain injury in rats. *Current Drug Delivery* 15:1159-1166. PMID: 29366417

67. Khalilzadeh M, Abdollahi A, Abdolahi F et al. (2018) Protective effects of magnesium sulfate against doxorubicin induced cardio-toxicity in rats. *Life Sciences* 207:436-441. PMID: 29940240

68. Altura BM, Zhang A, Cheng T, Altura BT (1995) Alcohols induce rapid depletion of intracellular free Mg2+ in cerebral vascular muscle cells: relation to chain length and partition coefficient. *Alcohol* 12:247-250. PMID: 7639959

69. Zhang A, Cheng T, Altura BT, Altura BM (1997) Chronic treatment of cultured cerebral vascular smooth cells with low concentration of ethanol elevates intracellular calcium and potentiates prostanoid-induced rises in [Ca2+]i: relation to etiology of alcohol-induced stroke. *Alcohol* 14:367-371. PMID: 9209552

70. Zhang A, Cheng T, Altura BT, Altura BM (1996) Acute cocaine results in rapid rises in intracellular free calcium concentration in canine cerebral vascular smooth muscle cells: possible relation to etiology of stroke. *Neuroscience Letters* 215:57-59. PMID: 8880753

71. Zhang A, Altura BT, Altura BM (1997) Elevation of extracellular magnesium rapidly raises intracellular free Mg2+ in human aortic endothelial cells: is extracellular Mg2+ a regulatory cation? *Frontiers in Bioscience* 2:a13-a17. PMID: 9206991

72. Altura BM, Zhang A, Cheng T, Altura BT (2001) Extracellular magnesium regulates nuclear and perinuclear free ionized calcium in cerebral vascular smooth muscle cells: possible relation to alcohol and central nervous system injury. *Alcohol* 23:83-90. PMID: 11331105

73. Saito Y, Okamoto K, Kobayashi M et al. (2017) Magnesium co-administration decreases cisplatin-induced nephrotoxicity in the multiple cisplatin administration. *Life Sciences* 189:18-22. PMID: 28864226

74. Simental-Mendia L, Sahebkar A, Rodriguez-Moran M et al. (2017) Effect of magnesium supplementation on plasma C-reactive protein concentrations: a systematic review and meta-analysis of randomized controlled trials. *Current Pharmaceutical Design* 23:4678-4686. PMID: 28545353

75. Afshar Ebrahimi F, Foroozanfard F, Aghadavod E et al. (2018) The effects of magnesium and zinc co-supplementation on biomarkers of inflammation and oxidative stress, and gene expression related to inflammation in polycystic ovary syndrome: a randomized controlled clinical trial. *Biological Trace Element Research* 184:300-307. PMID: 29127547

76. Mazidi M, Rezaie P, Banach M (2018) Effect of magnesium supplements on serum C-reactive protein: a systematic review and meta-analysis. *Archives of Medical Science* 14:707-716. PMID: 30002686

77. Mojtahedzadeh M, Chelkeba L, Ranjvar-Shahrivar M et al. (2016) Randomized trial of the effect of magnesium sulfate continuous infusion on IL-6 and CRP serum levels following abdominal aortic aneurysm surgery. *Iranian Journal of Pharmaceutical Research* 15:951-956. PMID: 28243294

78. Nielsen F (2018) Magnesium deficiency and increased inflammation: current perspectives. *Journal of Inflammation Research* 11:25-34. PMID: 29403302

79. Touyz R, Milne F (1995) Alterations in intracellular cations and cell membrane ATPase activity in patients with malignant hypertension. *Journal of Hypertension* 13:867-874. PMID: 8557964

80. Touyz R, Schiffrin E (1997) Role of calcium influx and intracellular calcium stores in angiotensin II-mediated calcium hyper-responsiveness in smooth muscle from spontaneously hypertensive rats. *Journal of Hypertension* 15:1431-1439. PMID: 9431849

81. Touyz R, Mercure C, Reudelhuber T (2001) Angiotensin II type I receptor modulates intracellular free Mg2+ in renally derived cells via Na+-dependent Ca2+-independent mechanisms. *The Journal of Biological Chemistry* 276:13657-13663. PMID: 11278387

82. Touyz R, Schiffrin E (2001) Measurement of intracellular free calcium ion concentration in vascular smooth muscle cells: fluorescence imaging of cytosolic calcium. *Methods in Molecular Medicine* 51:341-354. PMID: 21331728

83. Touyz R, Schiffrin E (1993) The effect of angiotensin II on platelet intracellular free magnesium and calcium ionic concentrations in essential hypertension. *Journal of Hypertension* 11:551-558. PMID: 8390527

84. Touyz R, Milne F, Reinach S (1992) Intracellular Mg2+, Ca2+, Na2+ and K+ in platelets and erythrocytes of essential hypertension patients: relation to blood pressure. *Clinical and Experimental Hypertension. Part A, Theory and Practice* 14:1189-1209. PMID: 1424233

85. Adachi M, Nara Y, Mano M et al. (1993) Intralymphocytic free calcium and magnesium in stroke-prone spontaneously hypertensive rats and effects of blood pressure and various antihypertensive agents. *Clinical and Experimental Pharmacology & Physiology* 20:587-593. PMID: 8222339

86. Adachi M, Nara Y, Mano M, Yamori Y (1994) Effect of dietary magnesium supplementation on intralymphocytic free calcium and magnesium in stroke-prone spontaneously hypertensive rats. *Clinical and Experimental Hypertension* 16:317-326. PMID: 8038757

Chapter 3

1. Kolte D, Vijayaraghavan K, Khera S et al. (2014) Role of magnesium in cardiovascular diseases. *Cardiology in Review* 22:182-192. PMID: 24896250

2. DiNicolantonio J, O'Keefe J, Wilson W (2018) Subclinical magnesium deficiency: a principal driver of cardiovascular disease and a public health crisis. *Open Heart* 5:e000668. PMID: 29387426

3. Mottillo S, Filion K, Genest J et al. (2010) The metabolic syndrome and cardiovascular risk: a systematic review and meta-analysis. *Journal of the American College of Cardiology* 56:1113-1132. PMID: 20863953

4. Dibaba D, Xun P, Fly A et al. (2014) Dietary magnesium intake and risk of metabolic syndrome: a meta-analysis. *Diabetic Medicine* 31:1301-1309. PMID: 24975384

5. Guerrero-Romero F, Jaquez-Chairez F, Rodriguez-Moran (2016) Magnesium in metabolic syndrome: a review based on randomized, double-blind clinical trials. *Magnesium Research* 29:146-153. PMID: 27834189

6. Liao F, Folsom A, Brancati F (1998) Is low magnesium concentration a risk factor for coronary heart disease? The Atherosclerosis Risk in Communities (ARIC) Study. *American Heart Journal* 136:480-490. PMID: 9736141

7. Kieboom B, Niemeijer M, Leening M et al. (2016) Serum magnesium and the risk of death from coronary heart disease and sudden cardiac death. *Journal of the American Heart Association* 5. PMID: 26802105

8. Zhang W, Iso H, Ohira T et al. (2012) Associations of dietary magnesium intake with mortality from cardiovascular disease: the JACC study. *Atherosclerosis* 221:587-595. PMID: 22341866

9. Abbott R, Ando F, Masaki K et al. (2003) Dietary magnesium intake and the future risk of coronary heart disease (the Honolulu Heart Program). *The American Journal of Cardiology* 92:665-669. PMID: 12972103

10. Park B, Kim M, Cha C et al. (2017) High calcium-magnesium ratio in hair is associated with coronary artery calcification in middle-aged and elderly individuals. *Biological Trace Element Research* 179:52-58. PMID: 28168532

11. Chakraborty P, Hoque M, Paul U, Husain F (2014) Serum magnesium status among acute myocardial infarction patients in Bangladesh. *Mymensingh Medical Journal* 23:41-45. PMID: 24584371

12. Woods K, Fletcher S (1994) Long-term outcome after intravenous magnesium sulphate in suspected acute myocardial infarction: the second Leicester Intravenous Magnesium Intervention Trial (LIMIT-2). *Lancet* 343:816-819. PMID: 7908076

13. Shechter M, Hod H, Rabinowitz B et al. (2003) Long-term outcome of intravenous magnesium therapy in thrombolysis-ineligible acute myocardial infarction patients. *Cardiology* 99:205-210. PMID: 12845247

14. ISIS-4: a randomized factorial trial assessing early oral captopril, oral mononitrate, and intravenous magnesium sulphate in 58,050 patients with suspected acute myocardial infarction. ISIS-4 (Fourth International Study of Infarct Survival) Collaborative Group. *Lancet* 345:669-685. PMID: 7661937

15. Seelig M, Elin R, Antman E (1998) Magnesium in acute myocardial infarction: still an open question. *The Canadian Journal of Cardiology* 14:745-749. PMID: 9627532

16. MAGIC trial (2002) Early administration of intravenous magnesium to high-risk patients with acute myocardial infarction in the Magnesium in Coronaries (MAGIC) Trial: a randomized controlled trial. *Lancet* 360:1189-1196. PMID: 12401244

17. Ganga H, Noyes A, White C, Kluger J (2013) Magnesium adjunctive therapy in atrial arrhythmias. *Pacing and Clinical Electrophysiology* 36:1308-1318. PMID: 23731344

18. Baker W (2017) Treating arrhythmias with adjunctive magnesium: identifying future research directions. *European Heart Journal. Cardiovascular Pharmacotherapy* 3:108-117. PMID: 27634841

19. Falco C, Grupi C, Sosa E et al. (2012) Successful improvement of frequency and symptoms of premature complexes after oral magnesium administration. *Arquivos Brasileiros de Cardiologia* 98:480-487. PMID: 22584491

20. Shiga T, Wajima Z, Inoue T, Ogawa R (2004) Magnesium prophylaxis for arrhythmias after cardiac surgery: a meta-analysis of randomized controlled trials. *The American Journal of Medicine* 117:325-333. PMID: 15336582

21. Lee H, Ghimire S, Kim E (2013) Magnesium supplementation reduces postoperative arrhythmias after cardiopulmonary bypass in pediatrics: a meta-analysis of randomized controlled trials. *Pediatric Cardiology* 34:1396-1403. PMID: 23443885

22. Salaminia S, Sayemiri F, Angha P et al. (2018) Evaluating the effect of magnesium supplementation and cardiac arrhythmias after acute coronary syndrome: a systematic review and meta-analysis. *BMC Cardiovascular Disorders* 18:129. PMID: 29954320

23. Fairley J, Zhang L, Glassford N, Bellomo R (2017) Magnesium status and magnesium therapy in cardiac surgery: a systematic review and meta-analysis focusing on arrhythmia prevention. *Journal of Critical Care* 42:69-77. PMID: 28688240

24. Jannati M, Shahbazi S, Eshaghi L (2018) Comparison of the efficacy of oral versus intravascular magnesium in the prevention of hypomagnesemia and arrhythmia after CABG. *Brazilian Journal of Cardiovascular Surgery* 33:448-453. PMID: 30517252

25. Narang A, Ozcan C (2016) Severe torsades de pointes with acquired QT prolongation. *European Heart Journal. Acute Cardiovascular Care* May 6 [Epub ahead of print]. PMID: 27154527

26. Coppola C, Rienzo A, Piscopo G et al. (2018) Management of QT prolongation induced by anti-cancer drugs: target therapy and old agents. Different algorithms for different drugs. *Cancer Treatment Reviews* 63:135-143. PMID: 29304463

27. Ceremuzynski L, Gebalska J, Wolk R, Makowska E (2000) Hypomagnesemia in heart failure with ventricular arrhythmias. Beneficial effects of magnesium supplementation. *Journal of Internal Medicine* 247:78-86. PMID: 10672134

28. Lutsey P, Alonso A, Michos E et al. (2014) Serum magnesium, phosphorus, and calcium are associated with risk of incident heart failure: the Atherosclerosis Risk in Communities (ARIC) Study. *The American Journal of Clinical Nutrition* 100:756-764. PMID: 25030784

29. Angkananard T, Anothaisintawee T, Eursiriwan S et al. (2016) The association of serum magnesium and mortality outcomes in heart failure patients: a systematic review and meta-analysis. *Medicine* 95:e5406. PMID: 27977579

30. Kunutsor S, Khan H, Laukkanen J (2016) Serum magnesium and risk of new onset heart failure in men: the Kuopio Ischemic Heart Disease Study. *European Journal of Epidemiology* 31:1035-1043. PMID: 27220323

31. Wannamethee S, Papacosta O, Lennon L, Whincup P (2018) Serum magnesium and risk of incident heart failure in older men: the British Regional Heart Study. *European Journal of Epidemiology* 33:873-882. PMID: 29663176

32. Liu M, Jeong E, Liu H et al. (2019) Magnesium supplementation improves diabetic mitochondrial and cardiac diastolic function. *JCI Insight* Jan 10; 4. [Epub ahead of print]. PMID: 30626750

33. Witte K, Nikitin N, Parker A et al. (2005) The effect of micronutrient supplementation on quality-of-life and left ventricular function in elderly patients with chronic heart failure. *European Heart Journal* 26:2238-2244. PMID: 16081469

34. Alon I, Gorelik O, Berman S et al. (2006) Intracellular magnesium in elderly patients with heart failure: effects of diabetes and renal dysfunction. *Journal of Trace Elements in Medicine and Biology* 20:221-226. PMID: 17098580

35. Almoznino-Sarafian D, Sarafian G, Berman S et al. (2009) Magnesium administration may improve heart rate variability in patients with heart failure. *Nutrition, Metabolism, and Cardiovascular Diseases* 19:641-645. PMID: 19201586

36. Fang X, Wang K, Han D et al. (2016) Dietary magnesium intake and the risk of cardiovascular disease, type 2 diabetes, and all-cause mortality: a dose-response meta-analysis of prospective cohort studies. *BMC Medicine* 14:210. PMID: 27927203

37. Dyckner T, Wester P (1984) Intracellular magnesium loss after diuretic administration. *Drugs* 28 Suppl 1:161-166. PMID: 6499698

38. Dorup I, Skajaa K, Thybo N (1994) [Oral magnesium supplementation to patients receiving diuretics—normalization of magnesium, potassium and sodium, and potassium pumps in the skeletal muscles]. Article in Danish. *Ugeskr Laeger* 156:4007-4010. PMID: 8066894

39. Cohen N, Alon I, Almoznino-Sarafian D et al. (2000) Metabolic and clinical effects of oral magnesium supplementation in furosemide-treated patients with severe congestive heart failure. *Clinical Cardiology* 23:433-436. PMID: 10875034

40. Iezhitsa I (2005) Potassium and magnesium depletions in congestive heart failure—pathophysiology, consequences and replenishment. *Clinical Calcium* 15:123-133. PMID: 16272623

41. Kusama Y, Kodani E, Nakagomi A et al. (2011) Variant angina and coronary artery spasm: the clinical spectrum, pathophysiology, and management. *Journal of the Nippon Medical School* 78:4-12. PMID: 21389642

42. Minato N, Katayama Y, Sakaguchi M, Itoh M (2006) Perioperative coronary artery spasm in off-pump coronary artery bypass grafting and its possible relation with perioperative hypomagnesemia. *Annals of Thoracic and Cardiovascular Surgery* 12:32-36. PMID: 16572072

43. Teragawa H, Kato M, Yamagata T et al. (2000) The preventive effect of magnesium on coronary artery spasm in patients with vasospastic angina. *Chest* 118:1690-1695. PMID: 11115460

44. Cohen L, Kitzes R (1984) Magnesium sulfate in the treatment of variant angina. *Magnesium* 3:46-49. PMID: 6541279

45. Ryzen E, Elkayam U, Rude R (1986) Low blood mononuclear cell magnesium in intensive cardiac care unit patients. *American Heart Journal* 111:475-480. PMID: 3953355

46. Tanabe K, Noda K, Mikawa T et al. (1991) Magnesium content of erythrocytes in patients with vasospastic angina. *Cardiovascular Drugs and Therapy* 5:677-680. PMID: 1888691

47. Tanabe K, Noda K, Kamegai M et al. (1990) Variant angina due to deficiency of intracellular magnesium. *Clinical Cardiology* 13:663-665. PMID: 2208825

48. Ducros A (2012) Reversible cerebral vasoconstriction syndrome. *The Lancet. Neurology* 11:906-917. PMID: 22995694

49. Hokkoku K, Furukawa Y, Yamamoto J et al. (2018) Reversible cerebral vasoconstriction syndrome accompanied by hypomagnesemia. *Neurological Sciences* 39:1141-1142. PMID: 29455396

50. Mijalski C, Dakay K, Miller-Patterson C et al. (2016) Magnesium for treatment of reversible cerebral vasoconstriction syndrome: case series. *The Neurohospitalist* 6:111-113. PMID: 27366294

51. Romani A (2018) Beneficial role of Mg^{2+} in prevention and treatment of hypertension. *International Journal of Hypertension* 2018:9013721. PMID: 29992053

52. Kass L, Weekes J, Carpenter L (2012) Effect of magnesium supplementation on blood pressure: a meta-analysis. *European Journal of Clinical Nutrition* 66:411-418. PMID: 22318649

53. Laragh J, Resnick L (1988) Recognizing and treating two types of long-term vasoconstriction in hypertension. *Kidney International. Supplement* 25:S162-S174. PMID: 3054233

54. Han H, Fang X, Wei X et al. (2017) Dose-response relationship between dietary magnesium intake, serum magnesium concentration and risk of hypertension: a systematic review and meta-analysis of prospective cohort studies. *Nutrition Journal* 16:26. PMID: 28476161

55. Wu L, Zhu X, Fan L et al. (2017) Magnesium intake and mortality due to liver diseases: results from the Third National Health and Nutrition Examination Survey Cohort. *Scientific Reports* 7:17913. PMID: 29263344

56. Kostov K, Halacheva L (2018) Role of magnesium deficiency in promoting atherosclerosis, endothelial dysfunction, and arterial stiffening as risk factors for hypertension. *International Journal of Molecular Sciences* 19(6). PMID: 29891771

57. Durlach J, Lebrun R (1959) [Magnesium and pathogenesis of idiopathic constitutional spasmophilia]. Article in French. *C R Seances Soc Biol Fil* 153:1973-1975. PMID: 13818852

58. Durlach J (1962) [Tetany caused by magnesium deficiency: Constitutional idiopathic spasmophilia]. Article in German. *Munch Med Wochenschr* 104:57-60. PMID: 13888681

59. James M, Wright G (1986) Tetany and myocardial arrhythmia due to hypomagnesaemia. A case report. *South Africa Medical Journal* 69:48-49. PMID: 3941943

60. Koppel H, Gasser R, Spichiger U (2000) [Free intracellular magnesium in myocardium—measurement and physiological role—state of the art]. Article in German. *Wiener Medizinische Wochenschrift* 150:321-324. PMID: 11105326

61. Kisters K, Tokmak F, Kosch M et al. (1999) Lowered total intra-cellular magnesium status in a subgroup of hypertensives. *The International Journal of Angiology* 8:154-156. PMID: 10387123

62. Huijgen H, Soesan M, Sanders R et al. (2000) Magnesium levels in critically ill patients. What should we measure? *American Journal of Clinical Pathology* 114:688-695. PMID: 11068541

63. Lajer H, Bundgaard H, Secher N et al. (2003) Severe intracel-lular magnesium and potassium depletion in patients after treat-ment with cisplatin. *British Journal of Cancer* 89:1633-1637. PMID: 14583761

64. Kubota T, Shindo Y, Tokuno K et al. (2005) Mitochondria are intracellular magnesium stores: investigation by simultaneous fluorescent imagings in PC12 cells. *Biochimica et Biophysica Acta* 1744:19-28. PMID: 15878394

65. Belfort M, Anthony J, Saade G et al. (2003) A comparison of magnesium sulfate and nimodipine for the prevention of eclampsia. *The New England Journal of Medicine* 348:304-311. PMID: 12540643

66. Douglas W, Rubin R (1963) The mechanism of catecholamine release from the adrenal medulla and the role of calcium in stim-ulus-secretion coupling. *The Journal of Physiology* 167:288-310. PMID: 16992152

67. Seelig M (1994) Consequences of magnesium deficiency on the enhancement of stress reactions: preventive and thera-peutic implications (a review). *Journal of the American College of Nutrition* 13:429-446. PMID: 7836621

68. Gromova O, Torshin I, Kobalava Z et al. (2018) Deficit of magnesium and states of hypercoagulation: intellectual analysis of data obtained from a sample of patients aged 18-50 years from medical and preventive facilities in Russia. *Kardiologiia* 58:22-35. PMID: 30704380

69. An G, Du Z, Meng X et al. (2014) Association between low serum magnesium level and major adverse cardiac events in patients treated with drug-eluting stents for acute myocardial infarction. *PLoS One* 9:e98971. PMID: 24901943

70. Cicek G, Acikgoz S, Yayla C et al. (2016) Magnesium as a predictor of acute stent thrombosis in patients with ST-segment eleva-tion myocardial infarction who underwent primary angioplasty. *Coronary Artery Disease* 27:47-51. PMID: 26513291

71. Hansi C, Arab A, Rzany A et al. (2009) Differences of platelet adhesion and thrombus activation on amorphous silicon carbide, magnesium alloy, stainless steel, and cobalt chromium stent surfaces. *Catheterization and Cardiovascular Interventions* 73:488-496. PMID: 19235237

72. Mazur A, Maier J, Rock E et al. (2007) Magnesium and the inflammatory response: potential physiopathological implica-tions. *Archives of Biochemistry and Biophysics* 458:48-56. PMID: 16712775

73. Maier J, Malpuech-Brugere C, Zimowska W et al. (2004) Low magnesium promotes endothelial cell dysfunction: implications for atherosclerosis, inflammation and thrombosis. *Biochimica et Biophysica Acta* 1689:13-21. PMID: 15158909

74. Maier J, Bernardini D, Rayssiguier Y, Mazur A (2004a) High concentrations of magnesium modulate vascular endothelial cell behaviour *in vitro*. *Biochimica et Biophysica Acta* 1689:6-12. PMID: 15158908

75. Emami Z, Mesbah Namin A, Kojuri J et al. (2019) Expression and activity of platelet endothelial nitric oxide synthase are decreased in patients with coronary thrombosis and stenosis. *Avicenna Journal of Medical Biotechnology* 11:88-93. PMID: 30800248

76. Sheu J, Hsiao G, Shen M et al. (2003) Antithrombotic effects of magnesium sulfate in *in vivo* experiments. *International Journal of Hematology* 77:414-419. PMID: 12774935

77. Ravn H, Kristensen S, Hjortdal V et al. (1997) Early administration of intravenous magnesium inhibits arterial thrombus formation. *Arteriosclerosis, Thrombosis, and Vascular Biology* 17:3620-3625. PMID: 9437213

78. Toft G, Ravn H, Hjortdal V (2000) Intravenously and topically applied magnesium in the prevention of arterial thrombosis. *Thrombosis Research* 99:61-69. PMID: 10904104

79. Shechter M (1999) Oral magnesium supplementation inhibits platelet-dependent thrombosis in patients with coronary artery disease. *The American Journal of Cardiology* 84:152-156. PMID: 10426331

80. Shechter M (2000) The role of magnesium as antithrombotic therapy. *Wiener Medizinische Wochenschrift* 150:343-347. PMID: 11105330

81. Shechter M, Merz C, Rude R et al. (2000) Low intracellular magnesium levels promote platelet-dependent thrombosis in patients with coronary artery disease. *American Heart Journal* 140:212-218. PMID: 10925332

Chapter 4

1. Ferrannini E, Cushman W (2012) Diabetes and hypertension: the bad companions. *Lancet* 380:601-610. PMID: 22883509

2. Tatsumi Y, Ohkubo T (2017) Hypertension with diabetes mellitus: significance from an epidemiological perspective for Japanese. *Hypertension Research* 40:795-806. PMID: 28701739

3. Petrie J, Guzik T, Touyz R (2018) Diabetes, hypertension, and cardiovascular disease: clinical insights and vascular mechanisms. *The Canadian Journal of Cardiology* 34:575-584. PMID: 29459239

4. Lima Mde L, Cruz T, Rodrigues L et al. (2009) Serum and intra-cellular magnesium deficiency in patients with metabolic syndrome—evidences for its relation to insulin resistance. *Diabetes Research and Clinical Practice* 83:257-262. PMID: 19124169

5. Wang Y, Wei J, Zeng C et al. (2018) Association between serum magnesium concentration and metabolic syndrome, diabetes, hypertension and hyperuricaemia in knee osteoarthritis: a cross-sectional study in Hunan Province, China. *BMJ Open* 8:e019159

6. Rodriguez-Moran M, Simental-Mendia L, Gamboa-Gomez C, Guerrero-Romero F (2018) Oral magnesium supplementation and metabolic syndrome: a randomized double-blind placebo-controlled clinical trial. 25:261-266. PMID: 29793665

7. Schutten J, Gomes-Neto A, Navis G et al. (2019) Lower plasma magnesium, measured by nuclear magnetic resonance spectroscopy, is associated with increased risk of developing type 2 diabetes mellitus in women: results from a Dutch Prospective Cohort Study. *Journal of Clinical Medicine* 8. 30717286

8. Zhang X, Xia J, Del Gobbo L et al. (2018) Serum magnesium concentrations and all-cause, cardiovascular, and cancer mortality among U.S. adults: results from the NHANES I epidemiologic follow-up study. *Clinical Nutrition* 37:1541-1549. PMID: 28890274

9. Paolisso G, Barbagallo M (1997) Hypertension, diabetes mellitus, and insulin resistance: the role of intracellular magnesium. *American Journal of Hypertension* 10:346-355. PMID: 9056694

10. Moctezuma-Velazquez C, Gomez-Samano M, Cajas-Sanchez M et al. (2017) High dietary magnesium intake is significantly and independently associated with higher insulin sensitivity in a Mexican-Mestizo population: a brief cross-sectional report. *Revista de Investigation Clinica* 69:40-46. PMID: 28239181

11. Shahbah D, Hassan T, Morsy S et al. (2017) Oral magnesium supplementation improves glycemic control and lipid profile in children with type 1 diabetes and hypomagnesaemia. *Medicine* 96:e6352. PMID: 28296769

12. Verma H, Garg R (2017) Effect of magnesium supplementation on type 2 diabetes associated cardiovascular risk factors: a systematic review and meta-analysis. *Journal of Human Nutrition and Dietetics* 30:621-633. PMID: 28150351

13. Konishi K, Wada K, Tamura T et al. (2017) Dietary magnesium intake and the risk of diabetes in the Japanese community: results for the Takayama study. *European Journal of Nutrition* 56:767-774. PMID: 26689794

14. Hruby A, Guasch-Ferre M, Bhupathiraju S et al. (2017) Magnesium intake, quality of carbohydrates, and risk of type 2 diabetes: results from three U.S. cohorts. *Diabetes Care* 40:1695-1702. PMID: 28978672

15. Gant C, Soedamah-Muthu S, Binnenmars S et al. (2018) Higher dietary magnesium intake and higher magnesium status are associated with lower prevalence of coronary artery disease in patients with type 2 diabetes. *Nutrients* 10. PMID: 29510564

16. Richter E, Hargreaves M (2013) Exercise, GLUT4, and skeletal muscle glucose uptake. *Physiological Reviews* 93:993-1017. PMID: 23899560

17. ELDerawi W, Naser I, Taleb M, Abutair A (2018) The effects of oral magnesium supplementation on glycemic response among type 2 diabetes patients. *Nutrients* 11. PMID: 30587761

18. Morakinyo A, Samuel T, Adekunbi D (2018) Magnesium upregulates insulin receptor and glucose transporter-4 in strepto-zotocin-nicotinamide-induced type-2 diabetic rats. *Endocrine Regulators* 52:6-16. PMID: 29453923

19. Takaya J, Higashino H, Kobayashi Y (2004) Intracellular magnesium and insulin resistance. *Magnesium Research* 17:126-136. PMID: 15319146

20. Kostov K (2019) Effects of magnesium deficiency on mechanisms of insulin resistance in type 2 diabetes: focusing on the processes of insulin secretion and signaling. *International Journal of Molecular Sciences* 20. PMID: 30889804

21. Ozcaliskan Ilkay H, Sahin H, Tanriverdi F, Samur G (2019) Association between magnesium status, dietary magnesium intake, and metabolic control in patients with type 2 diabetes mellitus. *Journal of the American College of Nutrition* 38:31-39. PMID: 30160617

22. Takaya J, Higashino, Kotera F, Kobayashi Y (2003) Intracellular magnesium of platelets in children with diabetes and obesity. *Metabolism* 52:468-471. PMID: 12701060

23. Takaya J, Yamato F, Kuroyanagi Y et al. (2010) Intracellular magnesium of obese and type 2 diabetes mellitus children. *Diabetes Therapy* 1:25-31. PMID: 22127671

24. Zghoul N, Alam-Eldin N, Mak I et al. (2018) Hypomagnesemia in diabetes patients: comparison of serum and intracellular measurement of responses to magnesium supplementation and its role in inflammation. *Diabetes, Metabolic Syndrome and Obesity* 11:389-400. PMID: 30122966

25. Delva P, Degan M, Trettene M, Lechi A (2006) Insulin and glucose mediate opposite intracellular ionized magnesium variations in human lymphocytes. *The Journal of Endocrinology* 190:711-718. PMID: 17003272

26. Bardicef M, Bardicef O, Sorokin Y et al. (1995) Extracellular and intracellular magnesium depletion in pregnancy and gestational diabetes. *American Journal of Obstetrics and Gynecology* 172:1009-1013. PMID: 7892840

27. Maktabi M, Jamilian M, Amirani E et al. (2018) The effects of magnesium and vitamin E co-supplementation on parameters of glucose homeostasis and lipid profiles in patients with gestational diabetes. *Lipids in Health and Disease* 17:163. PMID: 30025522

28. de Valk H (1999) Magnesium in diabetes mellitus. *The Netherlands Journal of Medicine* 54:139-146. PMID: 10218382

29. Kostov K (2019) Effects of magnesium deficiency on mechanisms of insulin resistance in type 2 diabetes: focusing on the processes of insulin secretion and signaling. *International Journal of Molecular Sciences* 20. PMID: 30889804

30. Guerrero-Romero F, Rodriguez-Moran M (2011) Magnesium improves the beta-cell function to compensate variation of insulin sensitivity: double-blind, randomized clinical trial. *European Journal of Clinical Investigation* 41:405-410. PMID: 21241290

31. Rodriguez-Moran M, Guerrero-Romero F (2011) Insulin secretion is decreased in non-diabetic individuals with hypomagnesaemia. *Diabetes/Metabolism Research and Reviews* 27:590-596. PMID: 21488144

32. Gommers L, Hoenderop J, Bindels R, de Baaij J (2016) Hypomagnesemia in type 2 diabetes: a vicious circle? *Diabetes* 65:3-13. PMID: 26696633

Chapter 5

1. Kirkland A, Sarlo G, Holton K (2018) The role of magnesium in neurological disorders. *Nutrients* 10. PMID: 29882776

2. Vink R, Nechifor M (2011) *Magnesium in the Central Nervous System.* Adelaide, Australia: University of Adelaide Press

3. Uteva A, Pimenov L (2012) [Magnesium deficiency and anxiety-depressive syndrome in elderly patients with chronic heart failure]. Article in Russian. *Advances in Gerontology* 25:427-432. PMID: 23289218

4. Jacka F, Overland S, Stewart R et al. (2009) Association between magnesium intake and depression and anxiety in community-dwelling adults: the Hordaland Health Study. *The Australian and New Zealand Journal of Psychiatry* 43:45-52. PMID: 19085527

5. Sartori S, Whittle N, Hetzenauer A, Singewald N (2012) Magnesium deficiency induces anxiety and HPA axis dysregulation: modulation by therapeutic drug treatment. *Neuropharmacology* 62:304-312. PMID: 21835188

6. Tarleton E, Littenberg B (2015) Magnesium intake and depression in adults. *Journal of the American Board of Family Medicine* 28:249-256. PMID: 25748766

7. Serefko A, Szopa A, Poleszak E (2016) Magnesium and depression. *Magnesium Research* 29:112-119. PMID: 27910808

8. Li B, Lv J, Wang W, Zhang D (2017) Dietary magnesium and calcium intake and risk of depression in the general population: a meta-analysis. *The Australian and New Zealand Journal of Psychiatry* 51:219-229. PMID: 27807012

9. Anjom-Shoae J, Sadeghi O, Hassanzadeh Keshteli A et al. (2018) The association between dietary intake of magnesium and psychiatric disorders among Iranian adults: a cross-sectional study. *The British Journal of Nutrition* 120:693-702. PMID: 30068404

10. You H, Cho S, Kang S et al. (2018) Decreased serum magnesium levels in depression: a systematic review and meta-analysis. *Nordic Journal of Psychiatry* 72:534-541. PMID: 30444158

11. Sun C, Wang R, Li Z, Zhang D (2019) Dietary magnesium intake and risk of depression. *Journal of Affective Disorders* 246:627-632. PMID: 30611059

12. Tarleton E, Littenbers B, MacLean C et al. (2017) Role of magnesium supplementation in the treatment of depression: a randomized clinical trial. *PLoS One* 12:e0180067. PMID: 28654669

13. Rajizadeh A, Mozaffari-Khosravi H, Yassini-Ardakani M, Dehghani A (2017) Effect of magnesium supplementation on depression status in depressed patients with magnesium deficiency: a randomized double-blind, placebo-controlled trial. *Nutrition* 35:56-60. PMID: 28241991

14. Mehdi S, Atlas S, Qadir S et al. (2017) Double-blind, randomized crossover study of intravenous infusion of magnesium sulfate versus 5% dextrose on depressive symptoms in adults with treatment-resistant depression. *Psychiatric and Clinical Neurosciences* 71:204-211. PMID: 27862658

15. Petrovic J, Stanic D, Bulat Z et al. (2018) ACTH-induced model of depression resistant to tricyclic antidepressants: neuroendocrine and behavioral changes and influence of long-term magnesium administration. *Hormones and Behavior* 105:1-10. PMID: 30025718

16. Gorska N, Cubala W, Slupski J, Galuszko-Wegielnik M (2018) Ketamine and magnesium common pathology of antidepressant action. *Magnesium Research* 31:33-38. PMID: 30398153

17. Ryszewska-Pokrasniewicz B, Mach A, Skalski M et al. (2018) Effects of magnesium supplementation on unipolar depression: a placebo-controlled study and review of the importance of dosing and magnesium status in the therapeutic response. *Nutrients* 10. PMID: 30081500

18. Pouteau E, Kabir-Ahmadi M, Noah L et al. (2018) Superiority of magnesium and vitamin B6 over magnesium alone on severe stress in healthy adults with low magnesemia: a randomized, single-blind clinical trial. *PLoS One* 13:e0208454. PMID: 30562392

19. Szewczyk B, Szopa A, Serefko A et al. (2018) The role of magnesium and zinc in depression: similarities and differences. *Magnesium Research* 31:78-89. PMID: 30714573

20. Kovacevic G, Stevanovic D, Bogicevic D et al. (2017) A 6-month follow-up of disability, quality of life, and depressive and anxiety symptoms in pediatric migraine with magnesium prophylaxis. *Magnesium Research* 30:133-141. PMID: 29637898

21. Gu Y, Zhao K, Luan X et al. (2016) Association between serum magnesium levels and depression in stroke patients. *Aging and Disease* 7:687-690. PMID: 28053818

22. Strapasson M, Ferreira C, Ramos J (2018) Associations between postpartum depression and hypertensive disorders of pregnancy. *International Journal of Gynaecology and Obstetrics* 143:367-373. PMID: 30194695

23. Nechifor M (2018) Magnesium in addiction—a general view. *Magnesium Research* 31:90-98. PMID: 30714574

24. Li L, Wu C, Gan Y et al. (2016) Insomnia and the risk of depression: a meta-analysis of prospective cohort studies. *BMC Psychiatry* 16:375. PMID: 27816065

25. Manber R, Buysse D, Edinger J et al. (2016) Efficacy of cognitive-behavioral therapy for insomnia combined with antidepressant pharmacotherapy in patients with comorbid depression and insomnia: a randomized controlled trial. *The Journal of Clinical Psychiatry* 77:e1316-e1323. PMID: 27788313

26. Gebara M, Siripong N, DiNapoli E et al. (2018) Effect of insomnia treatments on depression: a systematic review and meta-analysis. *Depression and Anxiety* 35:717-731. PMID: 29782076

27. Mason E, Harvey A (2014) Insomnia before and after treatment for anxiety and depression. *Journal of Affective Disorders* 168:415-421. PMID: 25108278

28. Abbasi B, Kimiagar M, Sadeghniiat K et al. (2012) The effect of magnesium supplementation on primary insomnia in elderly: a double-blind, placebo-controlled clinical trial. *Journal of Research in Medical Sciences* 17:1161-1169. PMID: 23853635

29. Rondanelli M, Opizzi A, Monteferrario F et al. (2011) The effect of melatonin, magnesium, and zinc on primary insomnia in long-term care facility residents in Italy: a double-blind, placebo-controlled clinical trial. *Journal of the American Geriatrics Society* 21226679

30. Hornyak M, Haas P, Veit J et al. (2004) Magnesium treatment of primary alcohol-dependent patients during subacute withdrawal: an open pilot study with polysomnography. *Alcoholism, Clinical and Experimental Research* 28:1702-1709. PMID: 15547457

31. Hornyak M, Voderholzer U, Hohagen F et al., (1998) Magnesium therapy for periodic leg movements-related insomnia and restless legs syndrome: an open pilot study. *Sleep* 21:501-505. PMID: 9703590

32. Naziroglu M, Ovey I (2015) Involvement of apoptosis and calcium accumulation through TRPV1 channels in neurobiology of epilepsy. *Neuroscience* 293:55-66. PMID: 25743251

33. Pal S, Sun D, Limbrick D et al. (2001) Epileptogenesis induces long-term alterations in intracellular calcium release and sequestration mechanisms in the hippocampal neuronal culture model of epilepsy. *Cell Calcium* 30:285-296. PMID: 11587552

34. Delorenzo R, Sun D, Deshpande L (2005) Cellular mechanisms underlying acquired epilepsy: the calcium hypothesis of the induction and maintenance of epilepsy. *Pharmacology & Therapeutics* 105:229-266. PMID: 15737406

35. Pisani A, Bonsi P, Martella G et al. (2004) Intracellular calcium increase in epileptiform activity: modulation by levetiracetam and lamotrigine. *Epilepsia* 45:719-728. PMID: 15230693

36. Nagarkatti N, Deshpande L, DeLorenzo R (2009) Development of the calcium plateau following status epilepticus: role of calcium in epileptogenesis. *Expert Review of Neurotherapeutics* 9:813-824. PMID: 19496685

37. Meldrum B (1986) Cell damage in epilepsy and the role of calcium in cytotoxicity. *Advances in Neurology* 44:849-855. PMID: 3706026

38. Cain S, Snutch T (2011) Voltage-gated calcium channels and disease. *BioFactors* 37:197-205. PMID: 21698699

39. Walden J, Grunze H, Bingmann D et al. (1992) Calcium antagonistic effects of carbamazepine as a mechanism of action in neuropsychiatric disorders: studies in calcium dependent model epilepsies. *European Neuropsychopharmacology* 1490097

40. Igelstrom K, Shirley C, Heyward P (2011) Low-magnesium medium induces epileptiform activity in mouse olfactory bulb slices. *Journal of Neurophysiology* 106:2593-2605. PMID: 21832029

41. Xu J, Tang F (2018) Voltage-dependent calcium channels, calcium binding proteins, and their interaction in the pathological process of epilepsy. *International Journal of Molecular Sciences* 19. PMID: 30213136

42. Wiemann M, Jones D, Straub H et al. (1996) Simultaneous blockade of intracellular calcium increases and of neuronal epileptiform depolarizations by verapamil. *Brain Research* 734:49-54. PMID: 8896807

43. Yuen A, Sander J (2012) Can magnesium supplementation reduce seizures in people with epilepsy? A hypothesis. *Epilepsy Research* 100:152-156. PMID: 22406257

44. Osborn K, Shytle R, Frontera A et al. (2018) Addressing potential role of magnesium dyshomeostasis to improve treatment efficacy for epilepsy: a reexamination of the literature. *Journal of Clinical Pharmacology* 56:260-265. PMID: 26313363

45. Dhande P, Ranade R, Ghongane B (2009) Effect of magnesium oxide on the activity of standard anti-epileptic drugs against experimental seizures in rats. *Indian Journal of Pharmacology* 41:268-272. PMID: 20407558

46. Safar M, Abdallah D, Arafa N, Abdel-Aziz M (2010) Magnesium supplementation enhances the anticonvulsant potential of valproate in pentylenetetrazol-treated rats. *Brain Research* 1334:58-64. PMID: 20353763

47. Abdelmalik P, Politzer N, Carlen P (2012) Magnesium as an effective adjunct therapy for drug resistant seizures. *The Canadian Journal of Neurological Sciences* 39:323-327. PMID: 22547512

48. Visser N, Braun K, Leijten F et al. (2011) Magnesium treatment for patients with refractory status epilepticus due to POLG1-mutations. *Journal of Neurology* 258:218-222. PMID: 20803213

49. Oladipo O, Ajala M, Okubadejo N et al. (2003) Plasma magnesium in adult Nigerian patients with epilepsy. *The Nigerian Postgraduate Medical Journal* 10:234-237. PMID: 15045017

50. Baek S, Byeon J, Eun S et al. (2018) Risk of low serum levels of ionized magnesium in children with febrile seizure. *BMC Pediatrics* 18:297. PMID: 30193581

51. Yary T, Kauhanen J (2019) Dietary intake of magnesium and the risk of epilepsy in middle-aged and older Finnish men: a 22-year follow-up study in a general population. *Nutrition* 58:36-39. PMID: 30273823

52. Toffa D, Magnerou M, Kassab A et al. (2019) Can magnesium reduce central neurodegeneration in Alzheimer's disease? Basic evidences and research needs. *Neurochemistry International* Mar 21. [Epub ahead of print]. PMID: 30905744

53. Durlach J (1990) Magnesium depletion and pathogenesis of Alzheimer's disease. *Magnesium Research* 3:217-218. PMID: 2132752

54. Glick J (1990) Dementias: the role of magnesium deficiency and an hypothesis concerning the pathogenesis of Alzheimer's disease. *Medical Hypotheses* 31:211-225. PMID: 2092675

55. Perl D, Brody A (1980) Alzheimer's disease: X-ray spectrometric evidence of aluminum accumulation in neurofibrillary tangle-bearing neurons. *Science* 208:297-299. PMID: 7367858

56. Perl D (1985) Relationship of aluminum to Alzheimer's disease. *Environmental Health Perspectives* 63:149-153. PMID: 4076080

57. Hashimoto T, Nishi K, Nagasao J et al. (2008) Magnesium exerts both preventive and ameliorating effects in an in vitro rat Parkinson disease model involving 1-methyl-4-phenylpyridinium (MPP+) toxicity in dopaminergic neurons. *Brain Research* 1197:143-151. PMID: 18242592

58. Shindo Y, Yamanaka R, Suzuki K et al. (2015) Intracellular magnesium level determines cell viability in the MPP(+) model of Parkinson's disease. *Biochimica et Biophysica Acta* 1853:3182-3191. PMID: 26319097

59. Li W, Yu J, Liu Y et al. (2014) Elevation of brain magnesium prevents synaptic loss and reverses cognitive deficits in Alzheimer's disease mouse model. *Molecular Brain* 7:65. PMID: 25213836

60. Sadir S, Tabassum S, Emad S et al. (2019) Neurobehavioral and biochemical effects of magnesium chloride (MgCl2), magnesium sulphate (MgSO4) and magnesium-L-threonate (MgT) supplementation in rats: a dose dependent comparative study. *Pakistan Journal of Pharmaceutical Sciences* 32:277-283. PMID: 30829204

61. Xu Z, Li L, Bao J et al. (2014) Magnesium protects cognitive functions and synaptic plasticity in streptozotocin-induced sporadic Alzheimer's model. *PLoS One* 9:e108645. PMID: 25268773

62. Cilliler A, Ozturk S, Ozbakir S (2007) Serum magnesium level and clinical deterioration in Alzheimer's disease. *Gerontology* 53:419-422. PMID: 17992016

63. Volpe S (2013) Magnesium in disease prevention and overall health. *Advances in Nutrition* 4:378S-383S. PMID: 23674807

64. Kieboom B, Licher S, Wolters F et al. (2017) Serum magnesium is associated with the risk of dementia. *Neurology* 89:1716-1722. PMID: 28931641

65. Jin X, Liu M, Zhang D et al. (2018) Elevated circulating magnesium levels in patients with Parkinson's disease: a meta-analysis. *Neuropsychiatric Disease and Treatment* 14:3159-3168. PMID: 30510425

66. Shindo Y, Yamanaka R, Suzuki K et al. (2015) Intracellular magnesium level determines cell viability in the MPP(+) model of Parkinson's disease. *Biochimica et Biophysica Acta* 1853:3182-3191. PMID: 26319097

67. Vink R (2016) Magnesium in the CNS: recent advances and developments. *Magnesium Research* 29:95-101. PMID: 27829572

68. Iotti S, Malucelli E (2008) *In vivo* assessment of Mg2+ in human brain and skeletal muscle by 31P-MRS. *Magnesium Research* 21:157-162. PMID: 19009818

69. Veronese N, Zurlo A, Solmi M et al. (2016) Magnesium status in Alzheimer's disease: a systematic review. *American Journal of Alzheimer's Disease and other Dementias* 31:208-213. PMID: 26351088

70. Barbagallo M, Belvedere M, Di Bella G, Dominguez L (2011) Altered ionized magnesium levels in mild-to-moderate Alzheimer's disease. *Magnesium Research* 24:S115-S121. PMID: 21951617

71. Andrasi E, Igaz S, Molnar Z, Mako S (2000) Disturbances of magnesium concentration in various brain areas in Alzheimer's disease. *Magnesium Research* 13:189-196. PMID: 11008926

72. Tzeng N, Chung C, Lin F et al. (2018) Magnesium oxide use and reduced risk of dementia: a retrospective, nationwide cohort study in Taiwan. *Current Medical Research and Opinion* 34:163-169. PMID: 28952385

73. Ozturk S, Cilliler A (2006) Magnesium supplementation in the treatment of dementia patients. *Medical Hypotheses* 67:1223-1225. PMID: 16790324

74. Yase Y, Yoshida S, Kihira T et al. (2001) Kii ALS dementia. *Neuropathology* 21:105-109. PMID: 11396674

75. Haraguchi T, Ishizu H, Takehisa Y et al. (2001) Lead content of brain tissue in diffuse neurofibrillary tangles with calcification (DNTC): the possibility of lead neurotoxicity. *Neuroreport* 12:3887-3890. PMID: 11742204

76. Singh A, Verma P, Balaji G et al. (2016) Nimodipine, an L-type calcium channel blocker attenuates mitochondrial dysfunctions to protect against 1-methyl-4-phenyl-1,2,3,6-tetrahydropyridine-induced Parkinsonism in mice. *Neurochemistry International* 99:221-232. PMID: 27395789

77. Surmeier D, Halliday G, Simuni T (2017) Calcium, mitochondrial dysfunction and slowing the progression of Parkinson's disease. *Experimental Neurology* 298:202-209. PMID: 28780195

78. Surmeier D, Schumacker P, Guzman J et al. (2017a) Calcium and Parkinson's disease. *Biochemical and Biophysical Research Communications* 483:1013-1019. PMID: 27590583

79. Glaser T, Arnaud Sampaio V, Lameu C, Ulrich H (2018) Calcium signalling: a common target in neurological disorders and neurogenesis. *Seminars in Cell & Developmental Biology* Dec 13. [Epub ahead of print]. PMID: 30529426

80. Liss B, Striessnig J (2019) The potential of L-type calcium channels as a drug target for neuroprotective therapy in Parkinson's disease. *Annual Review of Pharmacology and Toxicology* 59:263-289. PMID: 30625283

81. Nunez M, Hidalgo C (2019) Noxious iron-calcium connections in neurodegeneration. *Frontiers in Neuroscience* 13:48. PMID: 30809110

82. McLeary F, Rcom-H'cheo-Gauthier A, Goulding M et al. (2019) Switching on endogenous metal binding proteins in Parkinson's disease. *Cells* 8. PMID: 30791479

83. Bostanci M, Bagirici F (2013) Blocking of L-type calcium channels protects hippocampal and nigral neurons against iron neurotoxicity. The role of L-type calcium channels in iron-induced neurotoxicity. *The International Journal of Neuroscience* 123:876-882. PMID: 23768064

84. Schampel A, Kuerten S (2017) Danger: high voltage—the role of voltage-gated calcium channels in central nervous system pathology. *Cells* 6. PMID: 29140302

85. Tabata Y, Imaizumi Y, Sugawara M et al. (2018) T-type calcium channels determine the vulnerability of dopaminergic neurons to mitochondrial stress in familial Parkinson disease. *Stem Cell Reports* 11:1171-1184. PMID: 30344006

86. Gudala K, Kanukula R, Bansai D (2015) Reduced risk of parkinson's disease in users of calcium channel blockers: a meta-analysis. *International Journal of Chronic Diseases* 2015:697404. PMID: 26464872

87. Lang Y, Gong D, Fan Y (2015) Calcium channel blocker use and risk of Parkinson's disease: a meta-analysis. *Pharmacoepidemiology and Drug Safety* 24:559-566. PMID: 25845582

88. Lee Y, Lin C, Wu R et al. (2014) Antihypertensive agents and risk of Parkinson's disease: a nationwide cohort study. *PLoS One* 9:e98961. PMID: 24910980

89. Yamaguchi H, Shimada H, Yoshita K et al. (2019) Severe hypermagnesemia induced by magnesium oxide ingestion: a case series. *CEN Case Reports* 8:31-37. PMID: 30136128

90. Larsson S, Orsini N, Wolk A (2012) Dietary magnesium intake and risk of stroke: a meta-analysis of prospective studies. *The American Journal of Clinical Nutrition* 95:362-366. PMID: 22205313

91. Nie Z, Wang Z, Zhou B et al. (2013) Magnesium intake and incidence of stroke: meta-analysis of cohort studies. *Nutrition, Metabolism, and Cardiovascular Diseases* 23:169-176. PMID: 22789806

92. Adebamowo S, Jimenez M, Chiuve S et al. (2014) Plasma magnesium and risk of ischemic stroke among women. *Stroke* 45:2881-2886. PMID: 25116874

93. Bain L, Myint P, Jennings A et al. (2015) The relationship between dietary magnesium intake, stroke and its major risk factors, blood pressure and cholesterol, in the EPIC-Norfolk cohort. *International Journal of Cardiology* 196:108-114. PMID: 26082204

94. You S, Zhone C, Du H et al. (2017) Admission low magnesium level is associated with in-hospital mortality in acute ischemic stroke patients. *Cerebrovascular Disease* 44:35-42. PMID: 28419989

95. Tu X, Qiu H, Lin S et al. (2018) Low levels of serum magnesium are associated with poststroke cognitive impairment in ischemic stroke patients. *Neuropsychiatric Disease and Treatment* 14:2947-2954. PMID: 30464479

96. Singh H, Jalodia S, Gupta M et al. (2012) Role of magnesium sulfate in neuroprotection in acute ischemic stroke. *Annals of Indian Academy of Neurology* 15:177-180. PMID: 22919188

97. Wang L, Huang C, Wang H et al. (2012) Magnesium sulfate and nimesulide have synergistic effects on rescuing brain damage after transient focal ischemia. *Journal of Neurotrauma* 29:1518-1529. PMID: 22332641

98. Huang B, Khatibi N, Tong L et al. (2010) Magnesium sulfate treatment improves outcome in patients with subarachnoid hemorrhage: a meta-analysis study. *Translational Stroke Research* 1:108-112. PMID: 23002400

99. Hoane M (2007) Assessment of cognitive function following magnesium therapy in the traumatically injured brain. *Magnesium Research* 20:229-236. PMID: 18271492

100. Hoane M, Gilbert D, Barbre A, Harrison S (2008) Magnesium dietary manipulation and recovery of function following controlled cortical damage in the rat. *Magnesium Research* 21:29-37. PMID: 18557131

101. Zhang C, Zhao S, Zang Y et al. (2018) Magnesium sulfate in combination with nimodipine for the treatment of subarachnoid hemorrhage: a randomized controlled clinical study. *Neurological Research* 40:283-291. PMID: 29540123

102. Tan G, Yuan R, Wei C et al. (2018) Serum magnesium but not calcium was associated with hemorrhagic transformation in stroke overall and stroke subtypes: a case-control study in China. *Neurological Sciences* 39:1437-1443. PMID: 29804167

103. Goyal N. Tsivgoulis G, Malhotra K et al. (2018) Serum magnesium levels and outcomes in patients with acute spontaneous intracerebral hemorrhage. *Journal of the American Heart Association* 7(8). PMID: 29654197

Chapter 6

1. Britton J, Pavord I, Richards K et al. (1994) Dietary magnesium, lung function, wheezing, and airway hyperreactivity in a random adult population sample. *Lancet* 344:357-362. PMID: 7914305

2. Gilliland F, Berhane K, Li Y et al. (2002) Dietary magnesium, potassium, sodium, and children's lung function. *American Journal of Epidemiology* 155:125-131. PMID: 11790675

3. Daliparty V, Manu M, Mohapatra A (2018) Serum magnesium levels and its correlation with level of control in patients with asthma: a hospital-based, cross-sectional, prospective study. *Lung India* 35:407-410. PMID: 30168460

4. de Baaij J, Hoenderop J, Bindels R (2015) Magnesium in man: implications for health and disease. *Physiological Reviews* 95:1-46. PMID: 25540137

5. Kilic H, Kanbay A, Karalezi A et al. (2018) The relationship between hypomagnesemia and pulmonary function tests in patients with chronic asthma. *Medical Principles and Practice* 27:139-144. PMID: 29455196

6. Shaikh M, Malapati B, Gokani R et al. (2016) Serum magnesium and vitamin D levels as indicators of asthma severity. *Pulmonary Medicine* 2016:1643717. PMID: 27818797

7. Dominguez L, Barbagallo M, Di Lorenzo G et al. (1998) Bronchial reactivity and intracellular magnesium: a possible mechanism for the bronchodilating effects of magnesium in asthma. *Clinical Science* 95:137-142. PMID: 9680494

8. Albuali W (2014) The use of intravenous and inhaled magnesium sulphate in management of children with bronchial asthma. *The Journal of Maternal-Fetal & Neonatal Medicine* 27:1809-1815. PMID: 24345031

9. Kew K, Kirtchuk L, Michell C (2014) Intravenous magnesium sulfate for treating adults with acute asthma in the emergency department. *The Cochrane Database of Systematic Reviews* 5:CD0109090. PMID: 24865567

10. Alansari K, Ahmed W, Davidson B et al. (2015) Nebulized magnesium for moderate and severe pediatric asthma: a randomized trial. *Pediatric Pulmonology* 50:1191-1199. PMID: 25652104

11. Ling Z, Wu Y, Kong J et al. (2016) Lack of efficacy of nebulized magnesium sulfate in treating adult asthma: a meta-analysis of randomized controlled trials. *Pulmonary Pharmacology & Therapeutics* 41:40-47. PMID: 27651324

12. Su Z, Li R, Gai Z (2016) Intravenous and nebulized magnesium sulfate for treating acute asthma in children: a systematic review and meta-analysis. *Pediatric Emergency Care* Oct 4. [Epub ahead of print]. PMID: 27749796

13. Abuabat F, AlAlwan A, Masuadi E et al. (2019) The role of oral magnesium supplements for the management of stable bronchial asthma: a systematic review and meta-analysis. *NPJ Primary Care Respiratory Medicine* 29:4. PMID: 30778086

14. Shivanthan M, Rajapakse S (2014) Magnesium for acute exacerbation of chronic obstructive pulmonary disease: a systematic review of randomized trials. *Annals of Thoracic Medicine* 9:77-80. PMID: 24791169

15. Mukerji S, Shahpuri B, Clayton-Smith B et al. (2015) Intravenous magnesium sulphate as an adjuvant therapy in acute exacerbations of chronic obstructive pulmonary disease: a single centre, randomized, double-blinded, parallel group, placebo-controlled trial: a pilot study. *The New Zealand Medical Journal* 128:34-42. PMID: 26905985

16. Solooki M, Miri M, Mokhtari M et al. (2014) Magnesium sulfate in exacerbations of COPD in patients admitted to internal medicine ward. *Iranian Journal of Pharmaceutical Research* 13:1235-1239. PMID: 25587312

17. Comert S, Kiyan E, Okumus G et al. (2016) [Efficiency of nebulized magnesium sulphate in infective exacerbations of chronic obstructive pulmonary disease]. Article in Turkish. 64:17-26. PMID: 27266281

18. Hashim Ali Hussein S, Nielsen L, Konow Bogebjerg Dolberg M, Dahl R (2015) Serum magnesium and not vitamin D is associated with better QoL in COPD: a cross-sectional study. *Respiratory Medicine* 109:727-733. PMID: 25892292

Chapter 7

1. Fawcett W, Haxby E, Male D (1999) Magnesium: physiology and pharmacology. *British Journal of Anaesthesia* 83:302-320. PMID: 10618948

2. Long S, Romani A (2014) Role of cellular magnesium in human diseases. *Austin Journal of Nutrition and Food Sciences* 2(10). PMID: 25839058

3. He L, Zhang X, Liu B et al. (2016) Effect of magnesium ion on human osteoblast activity. *Brazilian Journal of Medical and Biological Research* 49. PMID: 27383121

4. Belluci M, Schoenmaker T, Rossa-Junior C et al. (2013) Magnesium deficiency results in an increased formation of osteoclasts. *The Journal of Nutritional Biochemistry* 24:1488-1498. PMID: 23517915

5. Mammoli F, Castiglioni S, Parenti S et al. (2019) Magnesium is a key regulator of the balance between osteoclast and osteoblast differentiation in the presence of vitamin D_3. *International Journal of Molecular Sciences* 20. PMID: 30658432

6. Galli S, Stocchero M, Andersson M et al. (2017) The effect of magnesium on early osseointegration in osteoporotic bone: a histological and gene expression investigation. *Osteoporosis International* 28:2195-2205. PMID: 28349251

7. Kunutsor S, Whitehouse M, Blom A, Laukkanen J (2017) Low serum magnesium levels are associated with increased risk of fractures: a long-term prospective cohort study. *European Journal of Epidemiology* 32:593-603. PMID: 28405867

8. Veronese N, Stubbs B, Solmi M et al. (2017) Dietary magnesium intake and fracture risk: data from a large prospective study. *The British Journal of Nutrition* 117:1570-1576. PMID: 28631583

9. Sojka J, Weaver C (1995) Magnesium supplementation and osteoporosis. *Nutrition Reviews* 53:71-74. PMID: 7770187

10. Welch A, Skinner J, Hickson M (2017) Dietary magnesium may be protective for aging of bone and skeletal muscle in middle and younger older age men and women: cross-sectional findings from the UK Biobank Cohort. *Nutrients* 9(11). PMID: 29084183

11. Boomsma D (2008) The magic of magnesium. *International Journal of Pharmaceutical Compounding* 12:306-309. PMID: 23969766

12. Uwitonze A, Razzaque M (2018) Role of magnesium in vitamin D activation and function. *The Journal of the American Osteopathic Association* 118:181-189. PMID: 29480918

13. Rude R, Singer F, Gruber H (2009) Skeletal and hormonal effects of magnesium deficiency. *Journal of the American College of Nutrition* 28:131-141. PMID: 19828898

14. Deng X, Song Y, Manson J et al. (2013) Magnesium, vitamin D status and mortality: results from US National Health and Nutrition Examination Survey (NHANES) 2001 to 2006 and NHANES III. *BMC Medicine* 11:187. PMID: 23981518

15. Mederle O, Balas M, Ioanoviciu S et al. (2018) Correlations between bone turnover markers, serum magnesium and bone mass density in postmenopausal osteoporosis. *Clinical Interventions in Aging* 13:1383-1389. PMID: 30122910

16. Li Y, Yue J, Yang C (2016) Unraveling the role of Mg(++) in osteoarthritis. *Life Sciences* 147:24-29. PMID: 26800786

17. Shmagel A, Onizuka N, Langsetmo L et al. (2018) Low magnesium intake is associated with increased knee pain in subjects with radiographic knee osteoarthritis: date from the Osteoarthritis Initiative. *Osteoarthritis and Cartilage* 26:651-658. PMID: 29454594

18. Zeng C, Wei J, Terkeltaub R et al. (2017) Dose-response relationship between lower serum magnesium level and higher prevalence of knee chondrocalcinosis. *Arthritis Research & Therapy* 19:236. PMID: 29065924

19. Zeng C, Wei J, Li H et al. (2015a) Relationship between serum magnesium concentration and radiographic knee osteoarthritis. *The Journal of Rheumatology* 42:1231-1236. PMID: 26034158

20. Chen R, Zhou X, Yin S et al. (2018) [Study on the protective mechanism of autophagy on cartilage by magnesium sulfate]. Article in Chinese. *Chinese Journal of Reparative and Reconstructive Surgery* 32:1340-1345. PMID: 30600669

21. Musik I, Kurzepa J, Luchowska-Kocot D et al. (2019) Correlations among plasma silicon, magnesium and calcium in patients with knee osteoarthritis—analysis in consideration of gender. *Annals of Agricultural and Environmental Medicine* 26:97-102. PMID: 30922037

22. Li H, Zeng C, Wei J et al. (2017) Associations of dietary and serum magnesium with serum high-sensitivity C-reactive protein in early radiographic knee osteoarthritis patients. *Modern Rheumatology* 27:669-674. PMID: 27588353

23. Zeng C, Wei J, Terkeltaub R et al. (2017) Dose-response relationship between lower serum magnesium level and higher prevalence of knee chondrocalcinosis. *Arthritis Research & Therapy* 19:236. PMID: 29065924

24. Li S, Ma F, Pang X et al. (2019) Synthesis of chondroitin sulfate magnesium for osteoarthritis treatment. *Carbohydrate Polymers* 212:387-394. PMID: 30832871

25. Rock E, Astier C, Lab C et al. (1995) Dietary magnesium deficiency in rats enhances free radical production in skeletal muscle. *The Journal of Nutrition* 125:1205-1210. PMID: 7738680

26. Beaudart C, Lacquet M, Touvier M et al. (2019) Association between dietary nutrient intake and sarcopenia in the SarcoPhAge study. *Aging Clinical and Experimental Research* Apr 6 [Epub ahead of print]. PMID: 30955158

27. Heffernan S, Horner K, De Vito G, Conway G (2019) The role of mineral and trace element supplementation in exercise and athletic performance: a systemic review. *Nutrients* 11(3). PMID: 30909645

Chapter 8

1. Wu J, Xun P, Tang Q et al. (2017) Circulating magnesium levels and incidence of coronary heart diseases, hypertension, and type 2 diabetes mellitus: a meta-analysis of prospective cohort studies. *Nutrition Journal* 16:60. PMID: 28927411

2. Xu Q, Wang J, Chen F et al. (2016) Protective role of magnesium isoglycyrrhizinate in non-alcoholic fatty liver disease and the associated molecular mechanisms. *International Journal of Molecular Medicine* 38:275-282. PMID: 27220460

3. El-Tanbouly D, Abdelsalam R, Attia A, Abdel-Aziz M (2015) Pretreatment with magnesium ameliorates lipopolysaccharide-induced liver injury in mice. *Pharmacological Reports* 67:914-920. PMID: 26398385

4. Eshraghi T, Eidi A, Mortazavi P et al. (2015) Magnesium protects against bile duct ligation-induced liver injury in male Wistar rats. *Magnesium Research* 28:32-45. PMID: 25967882

5. Eidi A, Mortazavi P, Moradi F et al. (2013) Magnesium attenuates carbon tetrachloride-induced hepatic injury in rats. *Magnesium Research* 26:1656-175. PMID: 24508950

6. Zou X, Wang Y, Peng C et al. (2018) Magnesium isoglycyrrhizinate has hepatoprotective effects in an oxaliplatin-induced model of liver injury. *International Journal of Molecular Medicine* 42:2020-2030. PMID: 30066834

7. Cohen-Hagai K, Feldman D, Turani-Feldman T et al. (2018) Magnesium deficiency and minimal hepatic encephalopathy among patients with compensated liver cirrhosis. *The Israel Medical Association Journal* 20:533-538. PMID: 30221864

8. Li Y, Ji C, Mei L et al. (2017) Oral administration of trace element magnesium significantly improving the cognition and locomotion in hepatic encephalopathy. *Scientific Reports* 7:1817. PMID: 28500320

9. Mei F, Yu J, Li M et al. (2019) Magnesium isoglycyrrhizinate alleviates liver injury in obese rats with acute necrotizing pancreatitis. *Pathology, Research and Practice* 215:106-114. PMID: 30396756

10. Schick V, Scheiber J, Mooren F et al. (2014) Effect of magnesium supplementation and depletion on the onset and course of acute experimental pancreatitis. *Gut* 63:1469-1480. PMID: 24277728

11. Guerrero-Romero F, Rodriguez-Moran M (2011) Magnesium improves the beta-cell function to compensate variation of insulin sensitivity: double-blind, randomized clinical trial. *European Journal of Clinical Investigation* 41:405-410. PMID: 21241290

12. Soltani N, Keshavarz M, Minaii B et al. (2005) Effects of administration of oral magnesium on plasma glucose and pathological changes in the aorta and pancreas of diabetic rats. *Clinical and Experimental Pharmacology & Physiology* 32:604-610. PMID: 16120185

13. Hanley M, Sayres L, Reiff E et al. (2019) Tocolysis: a review of the literature. *Obstetrical & Gynecological Survey* 74:50-55. PMID: 30648727

14. Jung E, Byun J, Kim Y et al. (2018) Antenatal magnesium sulfate for both tocolysis and fetal neuroprotection in premature rupture of the membranes before 32 weeks' gestation. *The Journal of Maternal-Fetal & Neonatal Medicine* 31:1431-1441. PMID: 28391733

15. Magee L, De Silva D, Sawchuck D et al. (2019) No. 376—magnesium sulphate for fetal neuroprotection. *Journal of Obstetrics and Gynaecology Canada* 41:505-522. PMID: 30879485

16. Enaruna N, Ande A, Okpere E (2013) Clinical significance of low serum magnesium in pregnant women attending the University of Benin Teaching Hospital. *Nigerian Journal of Clinical Practice* 16:448-453. PMID: 23974737

17. Durlach J, Pages N, Bac P et al. (2002) Magnesium deficit and sudden infant death syndrome (SIDS): SIDS due to magnesium deficiency and SIDS due to various forms of magnesium depletion: possible importance of the chronopathological form. *Magnesium Research* 15:269-278. PMID: 12635883

18. Rokhtabnak F, Djalali Motlagh S, Ghodraty M et al. (2017) Controlled hypotension during rhinoplasty: a comparison of dexmedetomidine with magnesium sulfate. *Anesthesiology and Pain Medicine* 7:e64032. PMID: 29696129

19. Bakhet W, Wahba H, El Fiky L, Debis H (2019) Magnesium sulphate optimises surgical field without attenuation of the stapaedius reflex in paediatric cochlear implant surgery. *Indian Journal of Anaesthesia* 63:304-309. PMID: 31000896

20. Christensen M, Petersen K, Bogevig S et al. (2018) Outcomes following calcium channel blocker exposures reported to a poison information center. *BMC Pharmacology & Toxicology* 19:78. PMID: 30482251

21. Nikbakht R, Taheri Moghadam M, Ghane'ee H (2014) Nifedipine compared to magnesium sulfate for treating preterm labor: a randomized clinical trial. *Iran Journal of Reproductive Medicine* 12:145-150. PMID: 24799873

22. Elliott J, Morrison J, Bofill J (2016) Risks and benefits of magnesium sulfate tocolysis in preterm labor (PTL). *AIMS Public Health* 3:348-356. PMID: 29546168

23. Ferre S, Li X, Adams-Huet B et al. (2019) Low serum magnesium is associated with faster decline in kidney function: the Dallas Heart Study experience. *Journal of Investigative Medicine* Mar 2. [Epub ahead of print]. PMID: 30826804

24. Xiong J, He T, Wang M et al. (2019) Serum magnesium, mortality, and cardiovascular disease in chronic kidney disease and end-stage renal disease patients: a systematic review and meta-analysis. *Journal of Nephrology* Mar 19 [Epub ahead of print]. PMID: 30888644

25. M de Francisco A, Rodriguez M (2013) Magnesium—its role in CKD. *Nefrologia* 33:389-399. PMID: 23640095

26. Cevette M, Vormann J, Franz K (2003) Magnesium and hearing. *Journal of the American Academy of Audiology* 14:202-212. PMID: 12940704

27. Attias J, Weisz G, Almog S et al. (1994) Oral magnesium intake reduces permanent hearing loss induced by noise exposure. *American Journal of Otolaryngology* 15:26-32. PMID: 8135325

28. Nageris B, Ulanovski D, Attias J (2004) Magnesium treatment for sudden hearing loss. *The Annals of Otology, Rhinology, and Laryngology* 113:672-675. PMID: 15330150

29. Choi Y, Miller J, Tucker K et al. (2014) Antioxidant vitamins and magnesium and the risk of hearing loss in the US general population. *The American Journal of Clinical Nutrition* 99:148-155. PMID: 24196403

30. Le Prell C, Ojano-Dirain C, Rudnick E et al. (2014) Assessment of nutrient supplement to reduce gentamicin-induced ototoxicity. *Journal of the Association for Research in Otolaryngology* 15:375-393. PMID: 24590390

31. Xiong M, Wang J, Yang C, Lai H (2013) The cochlea magnesium content is negatively correlated with hearing loss induced by impulse noise. *American Journal of Otolaryngology* 34:209-215. PMID: 23332299

32. Abaamrane L, Raffin F, Gal M et al. (2009) Long-term administration of magnesium after acoustic trauma caused by gunshot noise in guinea pigs. *Hearing Research* 247:137-145. PMID: 19084059

33. Cevette M, Barrs D, Patel A et al. (2011) Phase 2 study examining magnesium-dependent tinnitus. *The International Tinnitus Journal* 16:168-173. PMID: 22249877

34. Abouzari M, Abiri A, Djalilian H (2019) Successful treatment of a child with definite Meniere's disease with the migraine regimen. *American Journal of Otolaryngology* Feb 18. [Epub ahead of print]. PMID: 30803806

Chapter 9

1. Silberstein S, Loder E, Diamond S et al. (2007) Probably migraine in the United States: results of the American Migraine Prevalence and Prevention (AMPP) study. *Cephalalgia* 27:220-229. PMID: 17263769

2. Brennan K, Charles A (2010) An update on the blood vessel in migraine. *Current Opinion in Neurology* 23:266-274. PMID: 20216215

3. Pourshoghi A, Danesh A, Tabby D et al. (2015) Cerebral reactivity in migraine patients measured with functional near-infrared spectroscopy. *European Journal of Medical Research* 20:96. PMID: 26644117

4. Manju L, Nair R (2006) Magnesium deficiency augments myocardial response to reactive oxygen species. *Canadian Journal of Physiology and Pharmacology* 84:617-624. PMID: 16900246

5. Kim J, Jeon J, No H et al. (2011) The effects of magnesium pretreatment on reperfusion injury during living donor liver transplantation. *Korean Journal of Anesthesiology* 60:408-415. PMID: 21738843

6. Solaroglu A, Suat Dede F, Gelisen O et al. (2011) Neuroprotective effect of magnesium sulfate treatment on fetal brain in experimental intrauterine ischemia reperfusion injury. *The Journal of Maternal-Fetal & Neonatal Medicine* 24:1259-1261. PMID: 21504338

7. Akan M, Ozbilgin S, Boztas N et al. (2016) Effect of magnesium sulfate on renal ischemia-reperfusion injury in streptozotocin-induced diabetic rats. *European Review for Medical and Pharmacological Sciences* 20:1642-1655. PMID: 27160141

8. Amoni M, Kelly-Laubscher R, Petersen M, Gwanyanya A (2017) Cardioprotective and anti-arrhythmic effects of magnesium pretreatment against ischaemia/reperfusion injury in isoprenaline-induced hypertrophic rat heart. *Cardiovascular Toxicology* 17:49-57. PMID: 26696240

9. Celik Kavak E, Gulcu Bulmus F, Bulmus O et al. (2018) Magnesium: does it reduce ischemia/reperfusion injury in an adnexal torsion rat model? *Drug Design, Development and Therapy* 12:409-415. PMID: 29535502

10. Hamilton K, Robbins M (2019) Migraine treatment in pregnant women presenting to acute care: a retrospective observational study. *Headache* 59:173-179. PMID: 30403400

11. Veronese N, Demurtas J, Pesolillo G (2019) Magnesium and health outcomes: an umbrella review of systematic reviews and meta-analyses of observational and intervention studies. *European Journal of Nutrition* Jan 25. [Epub ahead of print]. PMID: 30684032

12. Grober U, Schmidt J, Kisters K (2015) Magnesium in prevention and therapy. *Nutrients* 7:8199-8226. PMID: 26404370

13. Assarzadegan F, Asgarzadeh S, Hatamabadi H et al. (2016) Serum concentration of magnesium as an independent risk factor in migraine attacks: a matched case-control study and review of the literature. *International Clinical Psychopharmacology* 31:287-292. PMID: 27140442

14. Silberstein S (2015) Preventive migraine treatment. *Continuum* 21:973-989. PMID: 26252585

15. Nattagh-Eshtivani E, Sani M, Dahri M et al. (2018) The role of nutrients in the pathogenesis and treatment of migraine headaches: review. *Biomedicine & Pharmacotherapy* 102:317-325. PMID: 29571016

16. Wells R, Beuthin J, Granetzke L (2019) Complementary and integrative medicine for episodic migraine: an update of evidence from the last 3 years. *Current Pain and Headache Reports* 23:10. PMID: 307901380

17. Xu F, Arakelyan A, Spitzberg A et al. (2019) Experiences of an outpatient infusion center with intravenous magnesium therapy for status migrainosus. *Clinical Neurology and Neurosurgery* 178:31-35. PMID: 30685601

18. Chiu H, Yeh T, Huang Y, Chen P (2016) Effects of intravenous and oral magnesium on reducing migraine: a meta-analysis of randomized controlled trials. *Pain Physician* 19:E97-E112. PMID: 26752497

19. Delavar Kasmaei H, Amiri M, Negida A et al. (2017) Ketorolac versus magnesium sulfate in migraine headache pain management; a preliminary study. *Emergency* 5:e2. PMID: 28286809

20. Baratloo A, Mirbaha S, Delavar Kasmaei H et al. (2017) Intravenous caffeine citrate vs. magnesium sulfate for reducing pain in patients with acute migraine headache; a prospective quasi-experimental study. *The Korean Journal of Pain* 30:176-182. PMID: 28757917

21. Abouzari M, Abiri A, Djalilian H (2019) Successful treatment of a child with definite Meniere's disease with the migraine regimen. *American Journal of Otolaryngology* Feb 18. [Epub ahead of print]. PMID: 30803806

22. Kovacevic G, Stevanovic D, Bogicevic D et al. (2017) A 6-month follow-up of disability, quality of life, and depressive and anxiety symptoms in pediatric migraine with magnesium prophylaxis. *Magnesium Research* 30:133-141. PMID: 29637898

23. von Luckner A, Riederer F (2018) Magnesium in migraine prophylaxis—is there an evidence-based rationale? A systematic review. *Headache* 58:199-209. PMID: 29131326

24. Karimi N, Razian A, Heidari M (2019) The efficacy of magnesium oxide and sodium valproate in prevention of migraine headache: a randomized, controlled, double-blind, crossover study. *Acta Neurologica Belgica* Feb 23. [Epub ahead of print]. PMID: 30798472

25. Mauskop A, Varughese J (2012) Why all migraine patients should be treated with magnesium. *Journal of Neural Transmission* 119:575-579. PMID: 22426836

26. Dzugan S, Dzugan K (2015) Is migraine a consequence of a loss of neurohormonal and metabolic integrity? A new hypothesis. *Neuro Endocrinology Letters* 36:421-429. PMID: 26707041

Chapter 10

1. Joy J, Coulter C, Duffull S, Isbister G (2011) Prediction of torsade de pointes from the QT interval: analysis of a case series of amisulpride overdoses. *Clinical Pharmacology and Therapeutics* 90:243-245. PMID: 21716272

2. Schade Hansen C, Pottegard A, Ekelund U et al. (2018) Association between QTc prolongation and mortality in patients with suspected poisoning in the emergency department: a transnational propensity score matched cohort study. *BMJ Open* 8:e020036. PMID: 29982199

3. Huffaker R, Lamp S, Weiss J, Kogan B (2004) Intracellular calcium cycling, early afterdepolarizations, and reentry in simulated long QT syndrome. *Heart Rhythm* 1:441-448. PMID: 15851197

4. Iseri L, French J (1984) Magnesium: nature's physiologic calcium blocker. *American Heart Journal* 108:188-193. PMID: 6375330\

5. Eisner D, Trafford A, Diaz M et al. (1998) The control of Ca release from the cardiac sarcoplasmic reticulum: regulation versus auto-regulation. *Cardiovascular Research* 38:589-604. PMID: 9747428

6. Wang M, Tashiro M, Berlin J (2004) Regulation of L-type calcium current by intracellular magnesium in rat cardiac myocytes. *The Journal of Physiology* 555:383-396. PMID: 14617671

7. Spencer C, Baba S, Nakamura K et al. (2014) Calcium transients closely reflect prolonged action potentials in iPSC models of inherited cardiac arrhythmia. *Stem Cell Reports* 3:269-281. PMID: 25254341

8. Manini A, Nelson L, Skolnick A et al. (2010) Electrocardiographic predictors of adverse cardiovascular events in suspected poisoning. *Journal of Medical Toxicology* 6:106-115. PMID: 20361362

9. Pollak P, Verjee Z, Lyon A (2011) Risperidone-induced QT prolongation following overdose correlates with serum drug concentration and resolves rapidly with no evidence of altered pharmacokinetics. *Journal of Clinical Pharmacology* 51:1112-1115. PMID: 20663990

10. Borak M, Sarc L, Mugerli D et al. (2019) Occupational inhalation poisoning with the veterinary antibiotic tiamulin. *Clinical Toxicology* Jun 21. [Epub ahead of print]. PMID: 31226893

11. Rosa M, Pappacoda S, D'Anna C et al. (2017) Ventricular tachycardia induced by propafenone intoxication in a pediatric patient. *Pediatric Emergency Care* Oct 31. [Epub ahead of print]. PMID: 29095281

12. Karturi S, Gudmundsson H, Akhtar M et al. (2016) Spectrum of cardiac manifestations from aconitine poisoning. *HeartRhythm Case Reports* 2:415-420. PMID: 28491724

13. Erenler A, Dogan T, Kocak C, Ece Y (2016) Investigation of toxic effects of mushroom poisoning on the cardiovascular system. *Basic & Clinical Pharmacology & Toxicology* 119:317-321. PMID: 26879235

14. Bui Q, Simpson S, Nordstrom K (2015) Psychiatric and medical management of marijuana intoxication in the emergency department. *The Western Journal of Emergency Medicine* 16:414-417. PMID: 25897916

15. Alinejad S, Kazemi T, Zamani N et al. (2015) A systematic review of the cardiotoxicity of methadone. *EXCLI Journal* 14:577-600. PMID: 26869865

16. Hassanian-Moghaddam H, Hakiminejhad M, Farnaghi F et al. (2017) Eleven years of children methadone poisoning in a referral center: a review of 453 cases. *Journal of Opioid Management* 13:27-36. PMID: 28345744

17. O'Connell C, Gerona R, Friesen M, Ly B (2015) Internet-purchased ibogaine toxicity confirmed with serum, urine, and product content levels. *The American Journal of Emergency Medicine* 33. PMID: 25687617

18. Paksu S, Duran L, Altuntas M et al. (2014) Amitriptyline overdose in emergency department of university hospital: evaluation of 250 patients. *Human & Experimental Toxicology* 33:980-990. PMID: 24505046

19. Kim Y, Lee J, Hong C et al. (2014) Heart rate-corrected QT interval predicts mortality in glyphosphate-surfactant herbicide-poisoned patients. *The American Journal of Emergency Medicine* 32:203-207. PMID: 24360317

20. Lin C, Liao S, Shih C, Hsu K (2014) QTc prolongation as a useful prognostic factor in acute paraquat poisoning. *The Journal of Emergency Medicine* 47:401-407. PMID: 25060011

21. Arora N, Berk W, Aaron C, Williams K (2013) Usefulness of intravenous lipid emulsion for cardiac toxicity from cocaine overdose. *The American Journal of Cardiology* 111:445-447. PMID: 23186600

22. Aslan S, Cakir Z, Emet M et al. (2013) Wildflower (*Hyoscyamus reticulatus*) causes QT prolongation. *Bratislavske Lekarske Listy* 114:333-336. PMID: 23731045

23. Berling I, Whyte I, Isbister G (2013) Oxycodone overdose causes naloxone responsive coma and QT prolongation. *QJM* 106:35-41. PMID: 23023890

24. Li S, Korkmaz S, Loganathan S et al. (2012) Acute ethanol exposure increases the susceptibility of the donor hearts to ischemia/reperfusion injury after transplantation in rats. *PLoS One* 7:e49237. PMID: 23155471

25. Nisse P, Soubrier S, Saulnier F, Mathieu-Nolf M (2009) Torsade de pointes: a severe and unknown adverse effect in indoramin self-poisoning. *International Journal of Cardiology* 133:e73-e75. PMID: 18191476

26. Villa A, Hong H, Lee H et al. (2012) [Acute indoramin poisoning: a review of 55 cases reported to the Paris Poison Centre from 1986 to 2010]. Article in French. *Therapie* 67:523-527. PMID: 27392392

27. Menegueti M, Basile-Filho A, Martins-Filho O, Auxiliadora-Martins M (2012) Severe arrhythmia after lithium intoxication in a patient with bipolar disorder admitted to the intensive care unit. *Indian Journal of Critical Care Medicine* 16:109-111. PMID: 22988367

28. Liu S, Lin J, Weng C et al. (2012) Heart rate-corrected QT interval helps predict mortality after intentional organophosphate poisoning. *PLoS One* 7:e36576. PMID: 22574184

29. Boegevig S, Rothe A, Tfelt-Hansen J, Hoegberg L (2011) Successful reversal of life threatening cardiac effect following dosulepin overdose using intravenous lipid emulsion. *Clinical Toxicology* 49:337-339. PMID: 21563912

30. Karademir S, Akcam M, Kuybulu A et al. (2011) Effects of fluorosis on QT dispersion, heart rate variability and echocardiographic parameters in children. *The Anatolian Journal of Cardiology* 11:150-155. PMID: 21342861

31. Eum K, Nie L, Schwartz J et al. (2011) Prospective cohort study of lead exposure and electrocardiographic conduction disturbances in the Department of Veterans Affairs Normative Aging Study. *Environmental Health Perspectives* 119:940-944. PMID: 21414889

32. Kieltucki J, Dobrakowski M, Pawlas N et al. (2017) The analysis of QT interval and repolarization morphology of the heart in chronic exposure to lead. *Human & Experimental Toxicology* 36:1081-1086. PMID: 27903879

33. Paudel G, Syed M, Kalantre S, Sharma J (2011) Pyrilamine-induced prolonged QT interval in adolescent with drug overdose. *Pediatric Emergency Care* 27:945-947. PMID: 21975494

34. Sayin M, Dogan S, Aydin M, Karabag T (2011) Extreme QT interval prolongation caused by mad honey consumption. *The Canadian Journal of Cardiology* 27. PMID: 21944273

35. Pollak P, Verjee Z, Lyon A (2011) Risperidone-induced QT prolongation following overdose correlates with serum drug concentration and resolves rapidly with no evidence of altered pharmacokinetics. *Journal of Clinical Pharmacology* 51:1112-1115. PMID: 20663990

36. Mohammed R, Norton J, Geraci S et al. (2010) Prolonged QTc interval due to escitalopram overdose. *Journal of the Mississippi State Medical Association* 51:350-353. PMID: 21370605

37. Chan C, Chan M, Tse M et al. (2009) Life-threatening torsades de pointes resulting from "natural" cancer treatment. *Clinical Toxicology* 47:592-594. PMID: 19586358

38. Chang J, Weng T, Fang C (2009) Long QT syndrome and torsades de pointes induced by acute sulpiride poisoning. *The American Journal of Emergency Medicine* 27. PMID: 19857426

39. Schwartz M, Patel M, Kazzi Z, Morgan B (2008) Cardiotoxicity after massive amantadine overdose. *Journal of Medical Toxicology* 4:173-179. PMID: 18821491

40. Service J, Waring W (2008) QT prolongation and delayed atrio-ventricular conduction caused by acute ingestion of trazodone. *Clinical Toxicology* 46:71-73. PMID: 18167038

41. Tilelli J, Smith K, Pettignano R (2006) Life-threatening bradyar-rhythmia after massive azithromycin overdose. *Pharmacotherapy* 26:147-150. PMID: 16506357

42. Onvlee-Dekker I, De Vries A, Ten Harkel A (2007) Carbon monoxide poisoning mimicking long-QT induced syncope. *Archives of Disease in Childhood* 92:244-245. PMID: 17337682

43. Howell C, Wilson A, Waring W (2007) Cardiovascular toxicity due to venlafaxine poisoning in adults: a review of 235 consecutive cases. *British Journal of Clinical Pharmacology* 64:192-197. PMID: 17298480

44. Ortega Carnicer J, Ruiz Lorenzo F, Manas Garcia D, Ceres Alabau F (2006) [Early onset of torsades de pointes and elevated levels of serum troponin I due to acute arsenic poisoning]. Article in Spanish. *Medicina Intensiva* 30:77-80. PMID: 16706333

45. Chen C (2014) Health hazards and mitigation of chronic poisoning from arsenic in drinking water: Taiwan experiences. *Reviews on Environmental Health* 29:13-19. PMID: 24552958

46. Isbister G, Murray L, John S et al. (2006) Amisulpride deliberate self-poisoning causing severe cardiac toxicity including QT prolongation and torsade de pointes. *The Medical Journal of Australia* 184:354-356. PMID: 16584372

47. Friberg L, Isbister G, Duffull S (2006) Pharmacokinetic-pharmacodynamic modelling of QT interval prolongation following citalopram overdoses. *British Journal of Clinical Pharmacology* 61:177-190. PMID: 16433872

48. Downes M, Whyte I, Isbister G (2005) QTc abnormalities in deliberate self-poisoning with moclobemide. *Internal Medicine Journal* 35:388-391. PMID: 15958107

49. Thakur A, Aslam A, Aslam A et al. (2005) QT interval prolongation in diphenhydramine toxicity. *International Journal of Cardiology* 98:341-343. PMID: 15686790

50. Strachan E, Kelly C, Bateman D (2004) Electrocardiogram and cardiovascular changes in thioridazine and chlorpromazine poisoning. *European Journal of Clinical Pharmacology* 60:541-545. PMID: 15372128

51. Balit C, Isbister G, Hackett L, Whyte I (2003) Quetiapine poisoning: a case series. *Annals of Emergency Medicine* 42:751-758. PMID: 14634598

52. Isbister G, Balit C (2003) Bupropion overdose: QTc prolongation and its clinical significance. *The Annals of Pharmacotherapy* 37:999-1002. PMID: 12841807

53. Franco V (2015) Wide complex tachycardia after bupropion overdose. *The American Journal of Emergency Medicine* 33. PMID: 26311156

54. Isbister G, Hackett L (2003) Nefazodone poisoning: toxicokinetics and toxicodynamics using continuous data collection. *Journal of Toxicology. Clinical Toxicology* 41:167-173. PMID: 12733855

55. Assimes T, Malcolm I (1998) Torsade de pointes with sotalol overdose treated successfully with lidocaine. *The Canadian Journal of Cardiology* 14:753-756. PMID: 9627533

56. Legras A, Piquemal R, Furet Y et al. (1996) Buflomedil poisoning: five cases with cardiotoxicity. *Intensive Care Medicine* 22:57-61. PMID: 8857439

57. Krahenbuhl S, Sauter B, Kupferschmidt H et al. (1995) Case report: reversible QT prolongation with torsades de pointes in a patient with pimozide intoxication. *The American Journal of the Medical Sciences* 309:315-316. PMID: 7771501

58. Saviuc P, Danel V, Dixmerias F (1993) Prolonged QT interval and torsade de pointes following astemizole overdose. *Journal of Toxicology. Clinical Toxicology* 31:121-125. PMID: 8433408

59. Reingardene D (1989) [A case of acute poisoning by amiodarone]. Article in Russian. *Anesteziologiia i Reanimatologiia* 4:62-63. PMID: 2817505

60. Aunsholt N (1989) Prolonged Q-T interval and hypokalemia caused by haloperidol. *Acta Psychiatrica Scandinavica* 79:411-412. PMID: 2735214

61. Lopez-Valdes J (2017) [Haloperidol poisoning in pediatric patients]. Article in Spanish. *Gaceta Medica de Mexico* 153:125-128. PMID: 28128816

62. Giermaziak H (1989) [Organic changes in rabbits and rats in thiometon poisoning. II. Relation between ECG curve changes in rabbits and rats and cholinesterase inhibition and lysosomal hydrolase activation in acute thiometon poisoning]. Article in Polish. *Medycyna Pracy* 40:133-138. PMID: 2593812

63. Vill H (1959) [Extreme lengthening of the QT-interval in electrocardiography in acute pervitin poisoning]. Article in German. *Cardiologia* 34:190-196. PMID: 13638992

64. Tzivoni D, Keren A, Cohen A et al. (1984) Magnesium therapy for torsades de pointes. *The American Journal of Cardiology* 53:528-530. PMID: 6695782

65. Pajoumand A, Shadnia S, Rezaie A et al. (2004) Benefits of magnesium sulfate in the management of acute human poisoning by organophosphorus insecticides. *Human & Experimental Toxicology* 23:565-569. PMID: 15688984

66. Vijayakumar H, Kannan S, Tejasvi C et al. (2017) Study of effect of magnesium sulphate in management of acute organophosphorous pesticide poisoning. *Anesthesia, Essays and Researches* 11:192-196. PMID: 28298783

67. Jamshidi F, Yazdanbakhsh A, Jamalian M et al. (2018) Therapeutic effect of adding magnesium sulfate in treatment of organophosphorus poisoning. *Open Access Macedonian Journal of Medical Sciences* 6:2051-2056. PMID: 30559859

68. Basher A, Rahman S, Ghose A et al. (2013) Phase II study of magnesium sulfate in acute organophosphate pesticide poisoning. *Clinical Toxicology* 51:35-40. PMID: 23311540

69. Wang M, Tseng C, Bair S (1998) Q-T interval prolongation and pleomorphic ventricular tachyarrhythmia ('Torsade de pointes') in organophosphate poisoning: report of a case. *Human & Experimental Toxicology* 17:587-590. PMID: 9821023

70. Emamhadi M, Mostafazadeh B, Hassanijirdehi M (2012) Tricyclic antidepressant poisoning treated by magnesium sulfate: a randomized, clinical trial. *Drug and Chemical Toxicity* 35:300-303. PMID: 22309432

71. Othong R, Devlin J, Kazzi Z (2015) Medical toxicologists' practice patterns regarding drug-induced QT prolongation in overdose patients: a survey in the United States of America, Europe, and Asia Pacific region. *Clinical Toxicology* 53:204-209. PMID: 25706450

72. Brvar M, Chan M, Dawson A et al. (2018) Magnesium sulfate and calcium channel blocking drugs as antidotes for acute organophosphorus insecticide poisoning—a systematic review and meta-analysis. *Clinical Toxicology* 56:725-736. PMID: 29557685

73. Carafoli E, Stauffer T (1994) The plasma membrane calcium pump: functional domains, regulation of the activity, and tissue specificity of isoform expression. *Journal of Neurobiology* 25:312-324. PMID: 8195792

74. Barber D, Hunt J, Ehrich M (2001) Inhibition of calcium-stimulated ATPase in the hen brain P2 synaptosomal fraction by organophosphorus esters: relevance to delayed neuropathy. *Journal of Toxicology and Environmental Health. Plan A* 63:101-113. PMID: 11393797

75. Ajilore B, Alli A, Oluwadairo T (2018) Effects of magnesium chloride on *in vitro* cholinesterase and ATPase poisoning by organophosphate (chlorpyrifos). *Pharmacology Research & Perspectives* 6:e00401. PMID: 29736246

76. Ofoefule S, Okonta M (1999) Adsorption studies of ciprofloxacin: evaluation of magnesium trisilicate, kaolin and starch as alternatives for the management of ciprofloxacin poisoning. *Bollettino Chimico Farmaceutico* 138:239-242. PMID: 10464971

77. Romani A (2008) Magnesium homeostasis and alcohol consumption. *Magnesium Research* 21:197-204. PMID: 19271417

78. Poikolainen K, Alho H (2008) Magnesium treatment in alcoholics: a randomized clinical trial. *Substance Abuse Treatment, Prevention, and Policy* 3:1. PMID: 18218147

79. Vijayakumar H, Kannan S, Tejasvi C et al. (2017) Study of effect of magnesium sulphate in management of acute organophosphorous pesticide poisoning. *Anesthesia, Essays and Researches* 11:192-196. PMID: 28298783

80. Levy T (2011) *Primal Panacea.* Henderson, NV: MedFox Publishing

81. Chugh S, Malhotra S, Kumar P, Malhotra K (1991b) Reversion of ventricular and supraventricular tachycardia by magnesium sulphate therapy in aluminium phosphide poisoning. Report of two cases. *The Journal of the Association of Physicians of India* 39:642-643. PMID: 1814883

82. Chugh S, Kolley T, Kakkar R et al. (1997) A critical evaluation of anti-peroxidant effect of intravenous magnesium in acute aluminium phosphide poisoning. *Magnesium Research* 10:225-230. PMID: 9483483

83. Chugh S, Dushyant, Ram S et al. (1991a) Incidence & outcome of aluminium phosphate poisoning in a hospital study. *The Indian Journal of Medical Research* 94:232-235. PMID: 1937606

84. Hena Z, McCabe M, Perez M et al. (2018) Aluminum phosphide poisoning: successful recovery of multiorgan failure in a pediatric patient. *International Journal of Pediatrics & Adolescent Medicine* 5:155-158. PMID: 30805553

85. Sharma A, Dishant, Gupta V et al. (2014) Aluminum phosphide (celphos) poisoning in children: a 5-year experience in a tertiary care hospital from northern India. *Indian Journal of Critical Care Medicine* 18:33-36. PMID: 24550611

86. Agrawal V, Bansal A, Singh R et al. (2015) Aluminum phosphide poisoning: possible role of supportive measures in the absence of specific antidote. *Indian Journal of Critical Care Medicine* 19:109-112. PMID: 25722553

87. Chugh S, Chugh K, Ram S, Malhotra K (1991) Electrocardiographic abnormalities in aluminium phosphide poisoning with special reference to its incidence, pathogenesis, mortality and histopathology. *Journal of the Indian Medical Association* 89:32-35. PMID: 2056173

88. Karamani A, Mohammadpour A, Zirak M et al. (2018) Antidotes for aluminum phosphide poisoning—an update. *Toxicology Reports* 5:1053-1059. PMID: 30406022

89. Zheltova A, Kharitonova M, Iezhitsa I, Spasov A (2016) Magnesium deficiency and oxidative stress: an update. *BioMedicine* 6:20. PMID: 27854048

90. Yamaguchi T, Uozu S, Isogai S et al. (2017) Short hydration regimen with magnesium supplementation prevents cisplatin-induced nephrotoxicity in lung cancer: a retrospective analysis. *Supportive Care in Cancer* 25:1215-1220. PMID: 27966021

91. Kumar G, Solanki M, Xue X et al. (2017) Magnesium improves cisplatin-mediated tumor killing while protecting against cisplatin-induced nephrotoxicity. *American Journal of Physiology. Renal Physiology* 313:F339-F350. PMID: 28424213

92. Zou X, Wang Y, Peng C et al. (2018) Magnesium isoglycyrrhizinate has hepatoprotective effects in an oxaliplatin-induced model of liver injury. *International Journal of Molecular Medicine* 42:2020-2030. PMID: 30066834

93. Babaknejad N, Moshtaghie A, Nayeri H et al. (2016) Protective role of zinc and magnesium against cadmium nephrotoxicity in male Wistar rats. *Biological Trace Element Research* 174:112-120. PMID: 27038621

94. Babaknejad N, Bahrami S, Moshtaghie A et al. (2018) Cadmium testicular toxicity in male Wistar rats: protective roles of zinc and magnesium. *Biological Trace Element Research* 185:106-115. PMID: 29238917

95. Ghaffarian-Bahraman A, Shahroozian I, Jafari A, Ghazi-Khansari M (2014) Protective effect of magnesium and selenium on cadmium toxicity in the isolated perfused rat liver system. *Acta Medica Iranica* 52:872-878. PMID: 25530047

96. Buha A, Bulat Z, Dukic-Cosic D, Matovic V (2012) Effects of oral and intraperitoneal magnesium treatment against cadmium-induced oxidative stress in plasma of rats. *Arhiv Za Higijenu Rada I Toksikologiju* 63:247-254. PMID: 23152374

97. Salem M, Kasinski N, Munoz R, Chernow B (1995) Progressive magnesium deficiency increases mortality from endotoxin challenge: protective effects of acute magnesium replacement therapy. *Critical Care Medicine* 23:108-118. PMID: 8001362

98. El-Tanbouly D, Abdelsalam R, Attia A, Abdel-Aziz M (2015) Pretreatment with magnesium ameliorates lipopolysaccharide-induced liver injury in mice. *Pharmacological Reports* 67:914-920. PMID: 26398385

99. Williamson R, McCarthy C, Kenny L, O'Keeffe G (2016) Magnesium sulphate prevents lipopolysaccharide-induced cell death in an *in vitro* model of the human placenta. *Pregnancy Hypertension* 6:356-360. PMID: 27939482

100. Almousa L, Salter A, Langley-Evans S (2018) Magnesium deficiency heightens lipopolysaccharide-induced inflammation and enhances monocyte adhesion in human umbilical vein endothelial cells. *Magnesium Research* 31:39-48. PMID: 30398154

101. Almousa L, Salter A, Langley-Evane S (2018a) Varying magnesium concentration elicits changes in inflammatory response in human umbilical vein endothelial cells (HUVECs). *Magnesium Research* 31:99-109. PMID: 30530425

102. Kang J, Yoon S, Sung Y, Lee S (2012) Magnesium chenoursodeoxycholic acid ameliorates carbon tetrachloride-induced liver fibrosis in rats. *Experimental Biology and Medicine* 237:83-92. PMID: 22185916

103. Tan Q, Hu Q, Zhu S et al. (2018) Licorice root extract and magnesium isoglycyrrhizinate protect against triptolide-induced hepatotoxicity via up-regulation of the Nrf2 pathway. *Drug Delivery* 25:1213-1223. PMID: 29791258

104. Blinova E, Halzova M, Blinov D (2016) A protective role for magnesium 2-aminoethansulfonate in paracetamol and ethanol-induced liver injury in pregnant rats. Article in English and Russian. *Experimental & Clinical Gastroenterology* 10:50-53. PMID: 29889373

105. Tabrizian K, Khodayari H, Rezaee R et al. (2018) Magnesium sulfate protects the heart against carbon monoxide-induced cardiotoxicity in rats. *Research in Pharmaceutical Sciences* 13:65-72. PMID: 29387113

106. Bagheri G, Rezaee R, Tsarouhas K et al. (2019) Magnesium sulfate ameliorates carbon monoxide-induced cerebral injury in male rats. *Molecular Medicine Reports* 19:1032-1039. PMID: 30569139

107. Stanley M, Kelers K, Boller E, Boller M (2019) Acute barium poisoning in a dog after ingestion of handheld fireworks (party sparklers). *Journal of Veterinary Emergency and Critical Care* 29:201-207. PMID: 30861291

108. Kao W, Deng J, Chiang S et al. (2004) A simple, safe, and efficient way to treat severe fluoride poisoning—oral calcium or magnesium. *Journal of Toxicology. Clinical Toxicology* 42:33-40. PMID: 15083934

109. Hfaiedh N, Murat J, Elfeki A (2012) A combination of ascorbic acid and α-tocopherol or a combination of Mg and Zn are both able to reduce the adverse effects of lindane-poisoning on rat brain and liver. *Journal of Trace Elements in Medicine and Biology* 26:273-278. PMID: 22677539

110. Shen J, Song L, Muller K et al. (2016) Magnesium alleviates adverse effects of lead on growth, photosynthesis, and ultrastructural alterations of *Torreya grandis* seedlings. *Frontiers in Plant Science* 7:1819. PMID: 27965704

111. Matovic V, Plamenac Bulat Z, Djukic-Cosic D, Soldatovic D (2010) Antagonism between cadmium and magnesium: a possible role of magnesium in therapy of cadmium intoxication. *Magnesium Research* 23:19-26. PMID: 20228012

112. Tan Q, Hu Q, Zhu S et al. (2018) Licorice root extract and magnesium isoglycyrrhizinate protect against triptolide-induced hepatotoxicity via up-regulation of the Nrf2 pathway. *Drug Delivery* 25:1213-1223. PMID: 29791258

Chapter 11

1. Neveu A (1959) [*La Polio Guerie! Traitement Cytophylactique de la Poliomyelite par le Chlorure de Magnesium*]. Book in French. ("Polio healed. Cytophylactic treatment of polio with magnesium chloride"). Paris, France: La Vie Claire

2. Rodale J (with Taub H) (1968) *Magnesium, the Nutrient that could Change Your Life.* Pyramid Publications, Inc: New York, NY

3. Neveu A (1958) [*Le Chlorure de Magnesium: Traitement Cytophylactique des Maladies Infectieuses*]. Book in French. ("Cytophylactic treatment of infectious diseases by magnesium chloride"). Paris, France: Librairie Le Francois

4. Neveu A (1961) *Le Chlorure de Magnesium Dans L'Elevage: Traitment Cytophylactique des Maladies Infectieuses.* Librairie Le Francois: Paris, France

5. Dekopol B (2018) [*Le Chlorure de Magnesium Histoire et Manuel Pratique: Traitement des maladies infectieuses chez l'homme et les animaux*]. Book in French. ("Magnesium chloride history and practical manual: treatment of infectious diseases in humans and animals"). Le Jardin de l'Ataraxie. Amazon Kindle

6. Levy T (2011) *Primal Panacea.* Henderson, NV: MedFox Publishing

7. Klenner F (1948) Virus pneumonia and its treatment with vitamin C. *Southern Medicine and Surgery* 110:36-38. PMID: 18900646

8. Klenner F (1949) The treatment of poliomyelitis and other virus diseases with vitamin C. *Southern Medicine and Surgery* 111:209-214. PMID: 18147027

9. Klenner F (1951) Massive doses of vitamin C and the virus diseases. *Southern Medicine and Surgery* 113:101-107. PMID: 14855098

10. Klenner F (1952) The vitamin and massage treatment for acute poliomyelitis. *Southern Medicine and Surgery* 114:194-197. PMID: 12984224

11. Klenner F (1971) Observations on the dose and administration of ascorbic acid when employed beyond the range of a vitamin in human pathology. *Journal of Applied Nutrition* Winter, pp. 61-88.

12. Klenner F (1974) Significance of high daily intake of ascorbic acid in preventive medicine. *Journal of Preventive Medicine* 1:45-69.

13. Rapp F, Butel J, Wallis C (1965) Protection of measles virus by sulfate ions against thermal inactivation. *Journal of Bacteriology* 90:132-135. PMID: 16562007

14. Wallis C, Morales F, Powell J, Melnick J (1966) Plaque enhancement of enteroviruses by magnesium chloride, cysteine, and pancreatin. *Journal of Bacteriology* 91:1932-1935. PMID: 4287074

15. Delbet P (1944) [*Politique Preventive du Cancer*]. Book in French. ("Preventive Cancer Policy"). France: La Vie Claire

16. Rodale J (with Taub H) (1968) *Magnesium, the Nutrient that could Change Your Life.* Pyramid Publications, Inc: New York, NY

17. Vergini R (1994) [*Curarsi con il Magnesio*]. Book in Italian. ("To Cure Yourself with Magnesium"). Italy: Red Edizioni

18. di Fabio A (1992) The art of getting well: magnesium chloride hexahydrate therapy. *The Arthritis Trust of America,* reprinted in *Townsend Letter for Doctors,* November, 1992, p. 992.

19. Zeng J, Ren L, Yuan Y et al. (2013) Short-term effect of magnesium implantation on the osteomyelitis modeled animals induced by *Staphylococcus aureus. Journal of Materials Science. Materials in Medicine* 24:2405-2416. PMID: 23793564

20. Li F, Wu W, Xiang L et al. (2015) Sustained release of VH and rhBMP-2 from nanoporous magnesium-zinc-silicon xerogels for osteomyelitis treatment and bone repair. *International Journal of Nanomedicine* 10:4071-4080. PMID: 26124660

21. Li Y, Liu G, Zhai Z et al. (2014) Antibacterial properties of magnesium *in vitro* and in an *in vivo* model of implant-associated methicillin-resistant *Staphylococcus aureus* infection. *Antimicrobial Agents and Chemotherapy* 58:7586-7591. PMID: 25288077

22. Rahim M, Eifler R, Rais B, Mueller P (2015) Alkalization is responsible for antibacterial effects of corroding magnesium. *Journal of Biomedical Materials Research. Part A* 103:3526-3532. PMID: 25974048

23. Welch K, Latifzada M, Frykstrand S, Stromme M (2016) Investigation of the antibacterial effect of mesoporous magnesium carbonate. *ACS Omega* 1:907-914. PMID: 30023495

24. Bai N, Tan C, Li Q, Xi Z (2017) Study on the corrosion resistance and anti-infection of modified magnesium alloy. *Bio-Medical Materials and Engineering* 28:339-345. PMID: 28869427

25. Andres N, Sieben J, Baldini M et al. (2018) Electroactive Mg^{2+}-hydroxyapatite nanostructured networks against drug-resistant bone infection strains. *ACS Applied Materials & Interfaces* 10:19534-19544. PMID: 29799727

26. Van Laecke S, Vermeiren P, Nagler E et al. (2016) Magnesium and infection risk after kidney transplantation: an observational cohort study. *The Journal of Infection* 73:8-17. PMID: 27084308

27. Thongprayoon C, Cheungpasitporn W, Erickson S (2015) Admission hypomagnesemia linked to septic shock in patients with systemic inflammatory response syndrome. *Renal Failure* 37:1518-1521. PMID: 26335852

28. Hupp S, Ribes S, Seele J et al. (2017) Magnesium therapy improves outcome in *Streptococcus pneumoniae* meningitis by altering pneumolysin pore formation. *British Journal of Pharmacology* 174:4295-4307. PMID: 28888095

29. Chung Y, Hsieh F, Lin Y et al. (2015) Magnesium lithospermate B and rosmarinic acid, two compounds present in *Salvia miltiorrhiza*, have potent antiviral activity against enterovirus 71 infections. *European Journal of Pharmacology* 755:127-133. PMID: 25773498

30. Rafiei S, Rezatofighi S, Ardakani M, Madadgar O (2015) In vitro anti-foot-and-mouth disease virus activity of magnesium oxide nanoparticles. *IET Nanobiotechnology* 9:247-251. PMID: 26435276

31. Ravell J, Otim I, Nabalende H et al. (2018) Plasma magnesium is inversely associated with Epstein-Barr virus load in peripheral blood and Burkitt lymphoma in Uganda. *Cancer Epidemiology* 52:70-74. PMID: 29248801

32. Zhu L, Yin H, Sun H et al. (2019) The clinical value of aquaporin-4 in children with hand, food, and mouth disease and the effect of magnesium sulfate on its expression: a prospective randomized clinical trial. *European Journal of Clinical Microbiology & Infectious Diseases* 38:1343-1349. PMID: 31028503

33. Das B, Moumita S, Ghosh S et al. (2018) Biosynthesis of magnesium oxide (MgO) nanoflakes by using leaf extract of *Bauhinia purpurea* and evaluation of its antibacterial property against *Staphylococcus aureus*. *Materials Science & Engineering. C, Materials for Biological Applications* 91:436-444. PMID: 30033274

34. Hussein E, Ahmed S, Mokhtar A et al. (2018) Antiprotozoal activity of magnesium oxide (MgO) nanoparticles against *Cyclospora cayetanensis* oocysts. *Parasitology International* 67:666-674. PMID: 29933042

35. Nguyen N, Grelling N, Wetteland C et al. (2018) Antimicrobial activities and mechanisms of magnesium oxide nanoparticles (nMgO) against pathogenic bacteria, yeasts, and biofilms. *Scientific Reports* 8:16260. PMID: 30389984

Chapter 12

1. Halliwell B (2006) Reactive species and antioxidants. Redox biology is a fundamental theme of aerobic life. *Plant Physiology* 141:312-322. PMID: 16760481

2. Levy T (2002) *Curing the Incurable. Vitamin C, Infectious Diseases, and Toxins* Henderson, NV: MedFox Publishing

3. Long C, Maull K, Krishnan R et al. (2003) Ascorbic acid dynamics in the seriously ill and injured. *The Journal of Surgical Research* 109:144-148. PMID: 12643856

4. Berger M, Oudemans-van Straaten H (2015) Vitamin C supplementation in the critically ill patient. *Current Opinion in Clinical Nutrition and Metabolic Care* 18:193-201. PMID: 25635594

5. Haraszthy V, Zambon J, Trevisan M et al. (2000) Identification of periodontal pathogens in atheromatous plaques. *Journal of Periodontology* 71:1554-1560. PMID: 11063387

6. Mattila K, Pussinen P, Paju S (2005) Dental infections and cardiovascular diseases: a review. *Journal of Periodontology* 76(11 Suppl):2085-2088. PMID: 16277580

7. Mahendra J, Mahendra L, Kurian V et al. (2010) 16S rRNA-based detection of oral pathogens in coronary atherosclerotic plaque. *Indian Journal of Dental Research* 21:248-252. PMID: 20657096

8. Mahendra J, Mahendra L, Nagarajan A, Mathew K (2015) Prevalence of eight putative periodontal pathogens in atherosclerotic plaque of coronary artery disease patients and comparing them with noncardiac subjects: a case-control study. *Indian Journal of Dental Research* 26:189-195. PMID: 26096116

9. Ott S, El Mokhtari N, Musfeldt M et al. (2006) Detection of diverse bacterial signatures in atherosclerotic lesions of patients with coronary artery disease. *Circulation* 113:929-937. PMID: 16490835

10. Willis G, Fishman S (1955) Ascorbic acid content of human arterial tissue. *Canadian Medical Association Journal* 72:500-503. PMID: 14364385

Chapter 13

1. Levy T (2013) *Death by Calcium: Proof of the toxic effects of dairy and calcium supplements,* Henderson, NV: MedFox Publishing

Chapter 14

1. Levy T (2013) *Death by Calcium: Proof of the toxic effects of dairy and calcium supplements,* Henderson, NV: MedFox Publishing

2. Whittaker P, Tufaro P, Rader J (2001) Iron and folate in fortified cereals. *Journal of the American College of Nutrition* 20:247-254. PMID: 11444421

3. Reifen R, Matas Z, Zeidel L et al. (2000) Iron supplementation may aggravate inflammatory status of colitis in a rat model. *Digestive Diseases and Sciences* 45:394-397. PMID: 10711457

4. Carrier J, Aghdassi E, Platt I et al. (2001) Effect of oral iron supplementation on oxidative stress and colonic inflammation in rats with induced colitis. *Alimentary Pharmacology & Therapeutics* 15:1989-1999. PMID: 11736731

5. Yu S, Feng Y, Shen Z, Li M (2011) Diet supplementation with iron augments brain oxidative stress status in a rat model of psychological stress. *Nutrition* 27:1048-1052. PMID: 21454054

6. Gao W, Li X, Gao Z, Li H (2014) Iron increases diabetes-induced kidney injury and oxidative stress in rats. *Biological Trace Element Research* 160:368-375. PMID: 24996958

7. Volani C, Paglia G, Smarason S et al. (2018) Metabolic signature of dietary iron overload in a mouse model. *Cells* Dec 11 7. PMID: 30544931

8. Korkmaz V, Ozkaya E, Seven B et al. (2014) Comparison of oxidative stress in pregnancies with and without first trimester iron supplement: a randomized double-blind controlled trial. *The Journal of Maternal-Fetal & Neonatal Medicine* 27:1535-1538. PMID: 24199687

9. Lymperaki E, Tsikopoulos A, Makedou K et al. (2015) Impact of iron and folic acid supplementation on oxidative stress during pregnancy. *Journal of Obstetrics and Gynaecology* 35:803-806. PMID: 25692315

10. Scholl T (2005) Iron status during pregnancy: setting the stage for mother and infant. *The American Journal of Clinical Nutrition* 81:1218S-1222S. PMID: 15883455

11. Tiwari A, Mahdi A, Chandyan S et al. (2011) Oral iron supplementation leads to oxidative imbalance in anemic women: a prospective study. *Clinical Nutrition* 30:188-193. PMID: 20888091

12. Deugnier Y, Bardou-Jacquet E, Laine F (2017) Dysmetabolic iron overload syndrome (DIOS). *Presse Medicale* 46:e306-e311. PMID: 29169710

13. Fibach E, Rachmilewitz E (2017) Iron overload in hematological disorders. *Presse Medicale* 46:e296-e305. PMID: 29174474

14. Kolnagou A, Kontoghiorghe C, Kontoghiorghes G (2018) New targeted therapies and diagnostic methods for iron overload diseases. *Frontiers in Bioscience* 10:1-20. PMID: 28930516

15. Weinberg E (2009) Is addition of iron to processed foods safe for iron replete consumers? *Medical Hypotheses* 73:948-949. PMID: 19628337

16. Weinberg E (2000) Iron-enriched rice: the case for labeling. *Journal of Medicinal Food* 3:189-191. PMID: 19236176

17. Paul S, Gayen D, Datta S, Datta K (2016) Analysis of high iron rice lines reveals new miRNAs that target iron transporters in roots. *Journal of Experimental Botany* 67:5811-5824. PMID: 27729476

18. Yalcintepe L, Halis E (2016) Modulation of iron metabolism by iron chelation regulates intracellular calcium and increases sensitivity to doxorubicin. *Bosnian Journal of Basic Medical Sciences* 16:14-20. PMID: 26773173

19. Hildalgo C, Nunez M (2007) Calcium, iron and neuronal function. *IUBMB Life* 59:280-285. PMID: 17505966

20. Lee D, Park J, Lee H et al. (2016) Iron overload-induced calcium signals modulate mitochondrial fragmentation in HT-22 hippocampal neuron cells. *Toxicology* 365:17-24. PMID: 27481217

21. Nunez M, Hidalgo C (2019) Noxious iron-calcium connections in neurodegeneration. *Frontiers in Neuroscience* 13:48. PMID: 30809110

22. Peterson E, Shapiro H, Li Y et al. (2016) Arsenic from community water fluoridation: quantifying the effect. *Journal of Water and Health* 14:236-242. PMID: 27105409

23. Tankeu A, Ndip Agbor V, Noubiap J (2017) Calcium supplementation and cardiovascular risk: a rising concern. *Journal of Clinical Hypertension* 19:640-646. PMID: 28466573

24. Levy T (2013) *Death by Calcium: Proof of the toxic effects of dairy and calcium supplements,* Henderson, NV: MedFox Publishing

25. Bolland M, Grey A, Avenell A et al. (2011) Calcium supplements with or without vitamin D and risk of cardiovascular events: reanalysis of the Women's Health Initiative limited access dataset and meta-analysis. *BMJ* 342:d2040. PMID: 21505219

26. Bolland M, Avenell A, Baron J et al. (2010) Effect of calcium supplements on risk of myocardial infarction and cardiovascular events: meta-analysis. *BMJ* 341:c3691. PMID: 20671013

27. Michaelsson K, Melhus H, Warensjo Lemming E et al. (2013) Long term calcium intake and rates of all cause and cardiovascular mortality: commonly based prospective longitudinal cohort study. *BMJ* 346:f228. PMID: 23403980

28. Trump B, Berezesky I (1996) The role of altered [Ca2+]i regulation in apoptosis, oncosis, and necrosis. *Biochimica et Biophysica Acta* 1313:173-178. PMID: 8898851

29. Touyz R, Schiffrin E (1993) The effect of angiotensin II on platelet intracellular free magnesium and calcium ionic concentrations in essential hypertension. *Journal of Hypertension* 11:551-558. PMID: 8390527

30. Li M, Inoue K, Si H, Xiong Z (2011) Calcium-permeable ion channels involved in glutamate receptor-independent ischemic brain injury. *Acta Pharmacologica Sinica* 32:734-740. PMID: 21552295

31. Rakkar K, Bayraktutan U (2016) Increases in intracellular calcium perturb blood-brain barrier via protein kinase C-alpha and apoptosis. *Biochimica et Biophysica Acta* 1862:56-71. PMID: 26527181

32. Kass G, Wright J, Nicotera P, Orrenius S (1988) The mechanism of 1-methyl-4-phenyl-1,2,3,6-tetrahydropyridine toxicity: role of intracellular calcium. *Archives of Biochemistry and Biophysics* 260:789-797. PMID: 2963592

33. Pothoulakis C, Sullivan R, Melnick D et al. (1988) *Clostridium difficile* toxin A stimulates intracellular calcium release and chemotactic response in human granulocytes. *The Journal of Clinical Investigation* 81:1741-1745. PMID: 2838520

34. Liu L, Chang X, Zhang Y et al. (2018) Fluorochloridone induces primary cultured Sertoli cells apoptosis: involvement of ROS and intracellular calcium ions-mediated ERK1/2 activation. *Toxicoloty In Vitro* 47:228-237. PMID: 29248592

35. Shin S, Hur G, Kim Y et al. (2000) Intracellular calcium antagonist protects cultured peritoneal macrophages against anthrax lethal toxin-induced cytotoxicity. *Cell Biology and Toxicology* 16:137-144. PMID: 10917569

36. Wang X, Chen J, Wang H et al. (2017) Memantine can reduce ethanol-induced caspase-3 activity and apoptosis in H4 cells by decreasing intracellular calcium. *Journal of Molecular Neuroscience* 62:402-411. PMID: 28730337

37. Vezir O, Comelekoglu U, Sucu N et al. (2017) N-acetylcysteine-induced vasodilatation is modified by K_{ATP} channels, Na^+/K^+-ATPase activity and intracellular calcium concentration: an *in vitro* study. *Pharmacological Reports* 69:738-745. PMID: 28577450

38. Kawamata H, Manfredi G (2010) Mitochondrial dysfunction and intracellular calcium dysregulation in ALS. *Mechanisms of Ageing and Development* 131:517-526. PMID: 20493207

39. Bravo-Sagua R, Parra V, Lopez-Crisosto C et al. (2017) Calcium transport and signaling in mitochondria. *Comprehensive Physiology* 7:623-634. PMID: 28333383

40. Tian P, Hu Y, Schilling W et al. (1994) The nonstructural glycoprotein of rotavirus affects intracellular calcium levels. *Journal of Virology* 68:251-257. PMID: 8254736

41. Orrenius S, Burkitt M, Kass G et al. (1992) Calcium ions and oxidative cell injury. *Annals of Neurology* 32 Suppl:S33-S42. PMID: 1510379

42. Prasad A, Bloom M, Carpenter D (2010) Role of calcium and ROS in cell death induced by polyunsaturated fatty acids in murine thymocytes. *Journal of Cellular Physiology* 225:829-836. PMID: 20589836

43. Surmeier D, Guzman J, Sanchez-Padilla J, Schumacker P (2011) The role calcium and mitochondrial oxidant stress in the loss of substantia nigra pars compacta dopaminergic neurons in Parkinson's disease. *Neuroscience* 198:221-231. PMID: 21884755

44. Billings F (1930) Focal infection as the cause of general disease. *Bulletin of the New York Academy of Medicine* 6:759-773. PMID: 19311755

45. Auld J (1927) An address on focal infection in relation to systemic disease. *The Canadian Medical Association Journal* 17:294-297. PMID: 20316215

46. Daland J (1922) Diagnosis of focal infection. *Transactions of the American Climatological and Clinical Association* 38:66-71. PMID: 21408811

47. Nakamura T (1924) A study on focal infection and elective localization in ulcer of the stomach and in arthritis. *Annals of Surgery* 79:29-43. PMID: 17864965

48. Cecil R (1934) Focal infection—some modern aspects. *California and Western Medicine* 40:397-402. PMID: 18742882

49. Henry C (1920) Focal infection. *The Canadian Medical Association Journal* 10:593-604. PMID: 20312306

50. Kulacz R, Levy T (2014) *The Toxic Tooth: How a root canal could be making you sick,* Henderson, NV: MedFox Publishing

51. Levy T (2017) *Hidden Epidemic: Silent oral infections cause most heart attacks and breast cancers,* Henderson, NV: MedFox Publishing

52. Levy T (2017) *Hidden Epidemic: Silent oral infections cause most heart attacks and breast cancers,* Henderson, NV: MedFox Publishing

53. Kulacz R, Levy T (2002) *The Roots of Disease: Connecting Dentistry & Medicine,* Bloomington, IN: Xlibris Publishing

54. Kulacz R, Levy T (2014) *The Toxic Tooth: How a root canal could be making you sick,* Henderson, NV: MedFox Publishing

55. Levy T (2017) *Hidden Epidemic: Silent oral infections cause most heart attacks and breast cancers,* Henderson, NV: MedFox Publishing

56. Levy T (2001) *Optimal Nutrition for Optimal Health,* New York, NY: Keats Publishing

57. Levy T (2013) *Death by Calcium: Proof of the toxic effects of dairy and calcium supplements,* Henderson, NV: MedFox Publishing

Chapter 15

1. Barrasa G, Gonzalez Canete N, Boasi L (2018) Age of postmenopause women: effect of soy isoflavone in lipoprotein and inflammation markers. *Journal of Menopausal Medicine* 24:176-182. PMID: 30671410

2. Barrow J, Turan N, Wangmo P et al. (2018) The role of inflammation and potential use of sex steroids in intracranial aneurysms and subarachnoid hemorrhage. *Surgical Neurology International* 9:150. PMID: 30105144

3. Son H, Kim N, Song C et al. (2018) 17β-Estradiol reduces inflammation and modulates antioxidant enzymes in colonic epithelial cells. *The Korean Journal of Internal Medicine* Oct 22 [Epub ahead of print]. PMID: 30336658

4. Vermillion M, Ursin R, Attreed S, Klein S (2018) Estriol reduces pulmonary immune cell recruitment and inflammation to protect female mice from severe influenza. *Endocrinology* 159:3306-3320. PMID: 30032246

5. Cheng C, Wu H, Wang M et al. (2019) Estrogen ameliorates allergic airway inflammation by regulating activation of NLRP3 in mice. *Bioscience Reports* Jan 8 39. PMID: 30373775

6. Liu T, Ma Y, Zhang R et al. (2019) Resveratrol ameliorates estrogen deficiency-induced depression- and anxiety-like behaviors and hippocampal inflammation in mice. *Psychopharmacology* Jan 4 [Epub ahead of print]. PMID: 30607478

7. Peng X, Qiao Z, Wang Y et al. (2019) Estrogen reverses nicotine-induced inflammation in chondrocytes via reducing the degradation of ECM. *International Journal of Rheumatic Diseases* Feb 11 [Epub ahead of print]. PMID: 30746895

8. Collins P, Rosano G, Jiang C et al. (1993) Cardiovascular protection by oestrogen—a calcium antagonist effect? *Lancet* 341:1264-1265. PMID: 8098404

9. Muck A, Seeger H, Bartsch C, Lippert T (1996) Does melatonin affect calcium influx in human aortic smooth muscle cells and estradiol-mediated calcium antagonism? *Journal of Pineal Research* 20:145-147. PMID: 8797181

10. Sugishita K, Li F, Su Z, Barry W (2003) Anti-oxidant effects of estrogen reduce [Ca2+]i during metabolic inhibition. *Journal of Molecular and Cellular Cardiology* 35:331-336. PMID: 12676548

11. Sribnick E, Del Re A, Ray S et al. (2009) Estrogen attenuates glutamate-induced cell death by inhibiting Ca2+ influx through L-type voltage-gated Ca2+ channels. *Brain Research* 1276:159-170. PMID: 19389388

12. Dobrydneva Y, Williams R, Morris G, Blackmore P (2002) Dietary phytoestrogens and their synthetic structural analogues as calcium channel blockers in human platelets. *Journal of Cardiovascular Pharmacology* 40:399-410. PMID: 12198326

13. Facchinetti F, Borella P, Valentini M et al. (1988) Premenstrual increase of intracellular magnesium levels in women with ovulatory, asymptomatic menstrual cycles. *Gynecological Endocrinology* 2:249-256. PMID: 3227989

14. Chaban V, Mayer E, Ennes H, Micevych P (2003) Estradiol inhibits ATP-induced intracellular calcium concentration increase in dorsal root ganglia neurons. *Neuroscience* 118:941-948. PMID: 12732239

15. Wang X, Guo H, Wang Y, Yi X (2007) [Effects of 17beta-estradiol on the intracellular calcium of masticatory muscles myoblast *in vitro*]. [Article in Chinese] *West China Journal of Stomatology* 25:611-613. PMID: 18306639

16. Xi Q, Hoenderop J, Bindels R (2009) Regulation of magnesium reabsorption in DCT. *Pflugers Archiv: European Journal of Physiology* 458:89-98. PMID: 18949482

17. Cameron I, Pool T, Smith N (1980) Intracellular concentration of potassium and other elements in vaginal epithelial cells stimulated by estradiol administration. *Journal of Cellular Physiology* 104:121-125. PMID: 7440641

18. de Padua Mansur A, Silva T, Takada J et al. (2012) Long-term prospective study of the influence of estrone levels on events in postmenopausal women with or at high risk for coronary artery disease. *ScientificWorldJournal* 2012:363595. PMID: 22701354

19. Schairer C, Adami H, Hoover R, Persson I (1997) Cause-specific mortality in women receiving hormone replacement therapy. *Epidemiology* 8:59-65. PMID: 9116097

20. Mikkola T, Tuomikoski P, Lyytinen H et al., (2015) Estradiol-based postmenopausal hormone therapy and risk of cardiovascular and all-cause mortality. *Menopause* 22:976-983. PMID: 25803671

21. Alexandersen P, Tanko L, Bagger Y et al. (2006) The long-term impact of 2-3 of hormone replacement therapy on cardiovascular mortality and atherosclerosis in healthy women. *Climacteric* 9:108-118. PMID: 16698657

22. Li S, Rosenberg L, Wise L et al. (2013) Age at natural menopause in relation to all-cause and cause-specific mortality in a follow-up study of US black women. *Maturitas* 75:246-252. PMID: 23642541

23. La S, Lee J, Kim D et al. (2016) Low magnesium levels in adults with metabolic syndrome: a meta-analysis. *Biological Trace Element Research* 170:33-42. PMID: 26208810

24. Guerrero-Romano F, Jaquez-Chairez F, Rodriguez-Moran M (2016) Magnesium in metabolic syndrome: a review based on randomized, double-blind clinical trials. *Magnesium Research* 29:146-153. PMID: 27834189

25. Sarrafzadegan N, Khosravi-Boroujeni H, Lotfizadeh M et al. (2016) Magnesium status and the metabolic syndrome: a systematic review and meta-analysis. *Nutrition* 32:409-417. PMID: 26919891

26. Finan B, Yang B, Ottaway N et al. (2012) Targeted estrogen delivery reverses the metabolic syndrome. *Nature Medicine* 18:1847-1856. PMID: 23142820

27. Xu J, Xiang Q, Lin G et al. (2012) Estrogen improved metabolic syndrome through down-regulation of VEGF and HIF-1α to inhibit hypoxia of periaortic and intra-abdominal fat in ovariectomized female rats. *Molecular Biology Reports* 39:8177-8185. PMID: 22570111

28. Korljan B, Bagatin J, Kokic S et al. (2010) The impact of hormone replacement therapy on metabolic syndrome components in perimenopausal women. *Medical Hypotheses* 74:162-163. PMID: 19665311

29. Alemany M (2012) Do the interactions between glucocorticoids and sex hormones regulate the development of the metabolic syndrome? *Frontiers in Endocrinology* 3:27. PMID: 22649414

30. Mauvais-Jarvis F, Clegg D, Hevener A (2013) The role of estrogens in control of energy balance and glucose homeostasis. *Endocrine Reviews* 34:309-338. PMID: 23460719

31. Xue W, Deng Y, Wang Y, Sun A (2016) Effect of half-dose and standard-dose conjugated equine estrogens combined with natural progesterone on dydrogesterone on components of metabolic syndrome in healthy postmenopausal women: a randomized controlled trial. *Chinese Medical Journal* 129:2773-2779. PMID: 27900987

32. Levy T (2013) *Death by Calcium: Proof of the toxic effects of dairy and calcium supplements,* Henderson, NV: MedFox Publishing

33. Bianchi V (2018) The anti-inflammatory effects of testosterone. *Journal of the Endocrine Society* 3:91-107. PMID: 30582096

34. Hall J, Jones R, Jones T et al. (2006) Selective inhibition of L-type Ca2+ channels in A7r5 cells by physiological levels of testosterone. *Endocrinology* 147:2675-2680. PMID: 16527846

35. Scragg J, Dallas M, Peers C (2007) Molecular requirements for L-type Ca2+ channel blockade by testosterone. *Cell Calcium* 42:11-15. PMID: 17173968

36. Oloyo A, Sofola O, Nair R et al. (2011) Testosterone relaxes abdominal aorta in male Sprague-Dawley rats by opening potassium (K(+)) channel and blockade of calcium (Ca(2+)) channel. *Pathophysiology* 18:247-253. PMID: 21439799

37. Jones T, Kelly D (2018) Randomized controlled trials—mechanistic studies of testosterone and the cardiovascular system. *Asian Journal of Andrology* 20:120-130. PMID: 29442075

38. Marin D, Bolin A, dos Santos Rde C et al. (2010) Testosterone suppresses oxidative stress in human neutrophils. *Cell Biochemistry and Function* 28:394-402. PMID: 20589735

39. Campelo A, Cutini P, Massheimer V (2012) Testosterone modulates platelet aggregation and endothelial cell growth through nitric oxide pathway. *The Journal of Endocrinology* 213:77-87. PMID: 22281525

40. Kelly D, Jones T (2013) Testosterone: a metabolic hormone in health and disease. *Journal of Endocrinology* 217:R25-R45. PMID: 23378050

41. Rovira-Llopis S, Banuls C, de Maranon A et al. (2017) Low testosterone levels are related to oxidative stress, mitochondrial dysfunction and altered subclinical atherosclerotic markers in type 2 diabetic male patients. *Free Radical Biology & Medicine* 108:155-162. PMID: 28359952

42. Hackett G, Heald A, Sinclair A et al. (2016) Serum testosterone, testosterone replacement therapy and all-cause mortality in men with type 2 diabetes: retrospective consideration of the impact of PDE5 inhibitors and statins. *International Journal of Clinical Practice* 70:244-253. PMID: 26916621

43. Bentmar Holgersson M, Landgren F, Rylander L, Lundberg Giwercman Y (2017) Mortality is linked to low serum testosterone levels in younger and middle-aged men. *European Urology* 71:991-992. PMID: 27993426

44. Nakashima A, Ohkido I, Yokoyama K et al. (2017) Associations between low serum testosterone and all-cause mortality and infection-related hospitalization in male hemodialysis patients: a prospective cohort study. *Kidney International Reports* 2:1160-1168. PMID: 29270524

45. Bianchi V (2018) Testosterone, myocardial function, and mortality. *Heart Failure Reviews* 23:773-788. PMID: 29978359

46. Meyer E, Wittert G (2018) Endogenous testosterone and mortality risk. *Asian Journal of Andrology* 20:115-119. PMID: 29384142

47. Holmboe S, Skakkebaek N, Juul A et al. (2017) Individual testosterone decline and future mortality risk in men. *European Journal of Endocrinology* 178:123-130. PMID: 29066571

48. Sharma R, Oni O, Gupta K et al. (2015) Normalization of testosterone level is associated with reduced incidence of myocardial infarction and mortality in men. *European Heart Journal* 36:2706-2715. PMID: 26248567

49. Hackett G, Cole N, Mulay A et al. (2019) Long-term testosterone therapy in type 2 diabetes is associated with reduced mortality without improvement in conventional cardiovascular risk factors. *BJU International* 123:519-529. PMID: 30216622

50. Nakashima A, Ohkido I, Yokoyama K et al. (2017) Associations between low serum testosterone and all-cause mortality and infection-related hospitalization in male hemodialysis patients: a prospective cohort study. *Kidney International Reports* 2:1160-1168. PMID: 29270524

51. Bianchi V, Locatelli V (2018) Testosterone a key factor in gender related metabolic syndrome. *Obesity Reviews* 19:557-575. PMID: 29356299

52. Skogastierna C, Hotzen M, Rane A, Ekstrom L (2014) A supraphysiological dose of testosterone induces nitric oxide production and oxidative stress. *European Journal of Preventive Cardiology* 21:1049-1054. PMID: 23471592

53. Cinar V, Polat Y, Baltaci A, Mogulkoc R (2011) Effects of magnesium supplementation on testosterone levels of athletes and sedentary subjects at rest and after exhaustion. *Biological Trace Element Research* 140:18-23. PMID: 20352370

54. Maggio M, De Vita F, Lauretani F et al. (2014) The interplay between magnesium and testosterone in modulating physical function in men. *International Journal of Endocrinology* 2014:525249. PMID: 24723948

55. Rotter I, Kosik-Bogacka D, Dolegowska B et al. (2015) Relationship between serum magnesium concentration and metabolic and hormonal disorders in middle-aged and older men. *Magnesium Research* 28:99-107. PMID: 26507751

56. Antinozzi C, Marampon F, Corinaldesi C et al. (2017) Testosterone insulin-like effects: an *in vitro* study on the short-term metabolic effects of testosterone in human skeletal muscle cells. *Journal of Endocrinological Investigation* 40:1133-1143. PMID: 28508346

57. Deutscher S, Bates M, Caines M et al. (1989) Relationships between serum testosterone, fasting insulin and lipoprotein levels among elderly men. *Atherosclerosis* 75:13-22. PMID: 2649112

58. Graham E, Selgrade J (2017) A model of ovulatory regulation examining the effects of insulin-mediated testosterone production on ovulatory function. *Journal of Theoretical Biology* 416:149-160. PMID: 28069449

59. Knight E, Christian C, Morales P et al. (2017) Exogenous testosterone enhances cortisol and affective responses to social-evaluative stress in dominant men. *Psychoneuroendocrinology* 85:151-157. PMID: 28865351

60. Norman A (2012) The history of the discovery of vitamin D and its daughter steroid hormone. *Annals of Nutrition & Metabolism* 61:199-206. PMID: 23183289

61. Barbonetti A, Vassallo M, Felzani G et al. (2016) Association between 25(OH)-vitamin D and testosterone levels: evidence from men with chronic spinal cord injury. *The Journal of Spinal Cord Medicine* 39:246-252. PMID: 26312544

62. No author (1932) Insulin and the healing of fractures. *Edinburgh Medical Journal* 39:268. PMID: 29640619

63. Gurd F (1937) Postoperative use of insulin in the nondiabetic: with special reference to wound healing. *Annals of Surgery* 106:761-769. PMID: 17857076

64. Rosenthal S (1968) Acceleration of primary wound healing by insulin. *Archives of Surgery* 96:53-55. PMID: 5635406

65. Vatankhah N, Jahangiri Y, Landry G et al. (2017) Effect of systemic insulin treatment on diabetic wound healing. *Wound Repair and Regeneration* 25:288-291. PMID: 28120507

66. Apikoglu-Rabus S, Izzettin F, Turan P, Ercan F (2010) Effect of topical insulin on cutaneous wound healing of rats with or without acute diabetes. *Clinical and Experimental Dermatology* 35:180-185. PMID: 19594766

67. Lima M, Caricilli A, de Abreu L et al. (2012) Topical insulin accelerates wound healing in diabetes by enhancing the AKT and ERK pathways: a double-blind placebo-controlled clinical trial. *PLoS One* 7:e36974. PMID: 22662132

68. Oryan A, Alemzadeh E (2017) Effects of insulin on wound healing: a review of animal and human evidences. *Life Sciences* 174:59-67. PMID: 28263805

69. Greenway S, Filler L, Greenway F (1999) Topical insulin in wound healing: a randomized, double-blind, placebo-controlled trial. *Journal of Wound Care* 8:526-528. PMID: 10827659

70. Zhang X, Chinkes D, Sadagopa Ramanujam V, Wolfe R (2007) Local injection of insulin-zinc stimulates DNA synthesis in skin donor site wound. *Wound Repair and Regeneration* 15:258-265. PMID: 17352759

71. Araujo M, Murashima A, Alves V et al. (2016) The topical use of insulin accelerates the healing of traumatic tympanic membrane perforations. *The Laryngoscope* 126:156-162. PMID: 2589194

72. Fai S, Ahem A, Mustapha M et al. (2017) Randomized controlled trial of topical insulin for healing corneal epithelial defects induced during vitreoretinal surgery in diabetics. *Asia-Pacific Journal of Ophthalmology* 6:418-424. PMID: 28828764

73. Wang A, Weinlander E, Metcalf B et al. (2017) Use of topical insulin to treat refractory neurotrophic corneal ulcers. *Cornea* 36:1426-1428. PMID: 28742619

74. Stephen S, Agnihotri M, Kaur S (2016) A randomized, controlled trial to assess the effect of topical insulin versus normal saline in pressure ulcer healing. *Ostomy/Wound Management* 62:16-23. PMID: 27356143

75. Martinez-Jimenez M, Aguilar-Garcia J, Valdes-Rodriguez R et al. (2013) Local use of insulin in wounds of diabetic patients: higher temperature, fibrosis, and angiogenesis. *Plastic and Reconstructive Surgery* 132:1015e-1019e. PMID: 24281606

76. Martinez-Jimenez M, Valadez-Castillo F, Aguilar-Garcia J et al. (2018) Effects of local use of insulin on wound healing in non-diabetic patients. *Plastic Surgery* 26:75-79. PMID: 29845043

77. Yu T, Gao M, Yang P et al. (2019) Insulin promotes macrophage phenotype transition through PI3K/Akt and PPAR-γ signaling during diabetic wound healing. *Journal of Cellular Physiology* 234:4217-4231. PMID: 30132863

78. Dai L, Ritchie G, Bapty B et al. (1999) Insulin stimulates Mg2+ uptake in mouse distal convoluted tubule cells. *The American Journal of Physiology* 277:F907-F913. PMID: 10600938

79. Cunningham J (1998) The glucose/insulin system and vitamin C: implications in insulin-dependent diabetes mellitus. *Journal of the American College of Nutrition* 17:105-108. PMID: 9550452

80. Chen M, Hutchinson M, Pecoraro R et al. (1983) Hyperglycemia-induced intracellular depletion of ascorbic acid in human mononuclear leukocytes. *Diabetes* 32:1078-1081. PMID: 6357907

81. Qutob S, Dixon S, Wilson J (1998) Insulin stimulates vitamin C recycling and ascorbate accumulation in osteoblastic cells. *Endocrinology* 139:51-56. PMID: 9421397

82. Paolisso G, Ravussin E (1995) Intracellular magnesium and insulin resistance: results in Pima Indians and Caucasians. *The Journal of Clinical Endocrinology and Metabolism* 80:1382-1385. PMID: 7714114

83. Hwang D, Yen C, Nadler J (1993) Insulin increases intracellular magnesium transport in human platelets. *The Journal of Clinical Endocrinology and Metabolism* 76:549-553. PMID: 8445010

84. Takaya J, Higashino H, Miyazaki R, Kobayashi Y (1998) Effects of insulin and insulin-like growth factor-1 on intracellular magnesium of platelets. *Experimental and Molecular Pathology* 65:104-109. PMID: 9828151

85. Takaya J, Higashino H, Kotera F, Kobayashi Y (2003) Intracellular magnesium of platelets in children with diabetes and obesity. *Metabolism* 52:468-471. PMID: 12701060

86. Delva P, Degan M, Trettene M, Lechi A (2006) Insulin and glucose mediate opposite intracellular ionized magnesium variations in human lymphocytes. *The Journal of Endocrinology* 190:711-718. PMID: 17003272

87. Takaya J, Yamato F, Kuroyanagi Y et al. (2010) Intracellular magnesium of obese and type 2 diabetes mellitus children. *Diabetes Therapy* 1:25-31. PMID: 22127671

88. Paolisso G, Barbagallo M (1997) Hypertension, diabetes mellitus, and insulin resistance: the role of intracellular magnesium. *American Journal of Hypertension* 10:346-355. PMID: 9056694

89. Takaya J, Higashino H, Kobayashi Y (2004) Intracellular magnesium and insulin resistance. *Magnesium Research* 17:126-136. PMID: 15319146

90. Morakinyo A, Samuel T, Adekunbi D (2018) Magnesium upregulates insulin receptor and glucose transporter-4 in streptozotocin-nicotinamide-induced type-2 diabetic rats. *Endocrine Regulations* 52:6-16. PMID: 29453923

91. Benni J, Patil P (2016) Non-diabetic clinical applications of insulin. *Journal of Basic and Clinical Physiology and Pharmacology* 27:445-456. PMID: 27235672

92. van den Berghe G, Wouters P, Weekers F et al. (2001) Intensive insulin therapy in critically ill patients. *The New England Journal of Medicine* 345:1359-1367. PMID: 11794168

93. Das U (2003) Insulin in sepsis and septic shock. *The Journal of the Association of Physicians of India* 51:695-700. PMID: 14621041

94. Capes S, Hunt D, Malmberg K, Gerstein H (2000) Stress hyperglycaemia and increased risk of death after myocardial infarction in patients with and without diabetes: a systematic overview. *Lancet* 355:773-778. PMID: 10711923

95. Maimaiti S, Frazier H, Anderson K et al. (2017) Novel calcium-related targets of insulin in hippocampal neurons. *Neuroscience* 364:130-142. PMID: 28939258

96. Long C, Maull K, Krishnan R et al. (2003) Ascorbic acid dynamics in the seriously ill and injured. *The Journal of Surgical Research* 109:144-148. PMID: 126438

97. Wilson J (2013) Evaluation of vitamin C for adjuvant sepsis therapy. *Antioxidants & Redox Signaling* 19:2129-2140. PMID: 23682970

98. Berger M, Oudemans-van Straaten H (2015) Vitamin C supplementation in the critically ill patient. *Current Opinion in Clinical Nutrition and Metabolic Care* 18:193-201. PMID: 25635594

99. Carr A, Rosengrave P, Bayer S et al. (2017) Hypovitaminosis C and vitamin C deficiency in critically ill patients despite recommended enteral and parenteral intakes. *Critical Care* 21:300. PMID: 29228951

100. Castelli A, Martorana G, Meucci E, Bonetti G (1982) Vitamin C in normal human mononuclear and polymorphonuclear leukocytes. *Acta Vitaminologica et Enzymologica* 4:189-196. PMID: 7148605

101. Evans R, Currie L, Campbell A (1982) The distribution of ascorbic acid between various cellular components of blood, in normal individuals, and its relation to the plasma concentration. *The British Journal of Nutrition* 47:473-482. PMID: 7082619

102. Ikeda T (1984) Comparison of ascorbic acid concentrations in granulocytes and lymphocytes. *The Tohoku Journal of Experimental Medicine* 142:117-118. PMID: 6719440

103. Yang X, Hosseini J, Ruddel M, Elin R (1989) Comparison of magnesium in human lymphocytes and mononuclear blood cells. *Magnesium* 8:100-105. PMID: 2755211

104. Hosseini J, Johnson E, Elin R (1983) Comparison of two separation techniques for the determination of blood mononuclear cell magnesium content. *Journal of the American College of Nutrition* 2:361-368. PMID: 6655160

105. O'Driscoll K, O'Gorman D, Taylor S, Boyle L (2013) The influence of a magnesium-rich marine extract on behavior, salivary cortisol levels and skin lesions in growing pigs. *Animal* 7:1017-1027. PMID: 23253104

106. Golf S, Happel O, Graef V, Seim K (1984) Plasma aldosterone, cortisol and electrolyte concentrations in physical exercise after magnesium supplementation. *Journal of Clinical Chemistry and Clinical Biochemistry* 22:717-721. PMID: 6527092

107. Golf S, Bender S, Gruttner J (1998) On the significance of magnesium in extreme physical stress. *Cardiovascular Drugs and Therapy* 12 Suppl 2:197-202. PMID: 97940

108. Dmitrasinovic G, Pesic V, Stanic D et al. (2016) ACTH, cortisol and IL-6 levels in athletes following magnesium supplementation. *Journal of Medical Biochemistry* 35:375-384. PMID: 28670189

109. Abbasi B, Kimiagar M, Sadeghniiat K et al. (2012) The effect of magnesium supplementation on primary insomnia in elderly: a double-blind placebo-controlled clinical trial. *Journal of Research in Medical Sciences* 17:1161-1169. PMID: 23853635

110. Brody S, Preut R, Schommer K, Schurmeyer T (2002) A randomized controlled trial of high dose ascorbic acid for reduction of blood pressure, cortisol, and subjective responses to psychological stress. *Psychopharmacology* 159:319-324. PMID: 11862365

111. Zor U, Her E, Talmon J et al. (1987) Hydrocortisone inhibits antigen-induced rise in intracellular free calcium concentration and abolishes leukotriene C4 production in leukemic basophils. *Prostaglandins* 34:29-40. PMID: 3685396

112. Sergeev P, Dukhanin A, Bulaev N (1992) [A combined effect of cortisol and concanavalin A on calcium ion contents in thymic lymphocytes]. [Article in Russion] *Biull Eksp Biol Med* 113:612-614. PMID: 1446030

113. Astashkin E, Khodorova A, Tumanova O et al. (1993) [The effect of arachidonic acid and hydrocortisone on the intracellular Ca2+ concentration in murine plasmacytoma JW cells]. [Article in Russian] *Biull Eksp Biol Med* 116:400-402. PMID: 8117964

114. ffrench-Mullen J (1995) Cortisol inhibition of calcium currents in guinea pig hippocampal CA1 neurons via G-protein-coupled activation of protein kinase C. *The Journal of Neuroscience* 15:903-911. PMID: 7823188

115. Hyde G, Seale A, Grau E, Borski R (2004) Cortisol rapidly suppresses intracellular calcium and voltage-gated calcium channel activity in prolactin cells of the tilapia (*Oreochromis mossambicus*). *American Journal of Physiology. Endocrinology and Metabolism* 286:E626-E633. PMID: 14656715

116. Han J, Lin W, Chen Y (2005) Inhibition of ATP-induced calcium influx in HT4 cells by glucocorticoids: involvement of protein kinase A. *Acta Pharmacologica Sinica* 26:199-204. PMID: 15663899

117. Gardner J, Zhang L (1999) Glucocorticoid modulation of Ca2+ homeostasis in human B lymphoblasts. *The Journal of Physiology* 514:385-396. PMID: 9852321

118. Yoshida T, Mio M, Tasaka K (1993) Ca(2+)-induced cortisol secretion from permeabilized bovine adrenocortical cells: the roles of calmodulin, protein kinase C and cyclic AMP. *Pharmacology* 46:181-192. PMID: 8387215

119. Siemieniuk R, Guyatt G (2015) Corticosteroids in the treatment of community-acquired pneumonia: an evidence summary. *Pol Arch Med Wewn* 125:570-575. PMID: 26020683

120. Florio S, Ciarcia R, Crispino L et al. (2003) Hydrocortisone has a protective effect on cyclosporin A-induced cardiotoxicity. *Journal of Cellular Physiology* 195:21-26. PMID: 12599205

121. Ciarcia R, Damiano S, Fiorito F et al. (2012) Hydrocortisone attenuates cyclosporin A-induced nephrotoxicity in rats. *Journal of Cellular Biochemistry* 113:997-1004. PMID: 22034142

122. Kraikitpanitch S, Haygood C, Baxter D et al. (1976) Effects of acetylsalicylic acid, dipyridamole, and hydrocortisone on epinephrine-induced myocardial injury in dogs. *American Heart Journal* 92:615-622. PMID: 983936

123. Levy T (2002) *Curing the Incurable: Vitamin C, infectious diseases, and toxins,* Henderson, NV: MedFox Publishing

124. Fujita I, Hirano J, Itoh N et al. (2001) Dexamethasone induces sodium-dependant vitamin C transporter in a mouse osteoblastic cell line MC3T3-E1. *The British Journal of Nutrition* 86:145-149. PMID: 11502226

125. Mikirova N, Levy T, Hunninghake R (2019) The levels of ascorbic acid in blood and mononuclear blood cells after oral liposome-encapsulated and oral non-encapsulated vitamin C supplementation, taken without and with IV hydrocortisone. *Journal of Orthomolecular Medicine* 34:1-8.

126. Mancini A, Di Segni C, Raimondo S et al. (2016) Thyroid hormones, oxidative stress, and inflammation. *Mediators of Inflammation* 2016:6757154. PMID: 27051079

127. Soto-Rivera C, Fichorova R, Allred E et al. (2015) The relationship between TSH and systemic inflammation in extremely preterm newborns. *Endocrine* 48:595-602. PMID: 24996532

128. Sahin E, Bektur E, Baycu C et al. (2019) Hypothyroidism increases expression of sterile inflammation proteins in rat heart tissue. *Acta Endocrinologica* 5:39-45. PMID: 31149058

129. Kvetny J, Heldgaard P, Bladbjerg E, Gram J (2004) Subclinical hypothyroidism is associated with a low-grade inflammation, increased triglyceride levels and predicts cardiovascular disease in males below 50 years. *Clinical Endocrinology* 61:232-238. PMID: 15272919

130. Anagnostis P, Efstathiadou Z, Slavakis A et al. (2014) The effect of L-thyroxine substitution on lipid profile, glucose homeostasis, inflammation and coagulation in patients with subclinical hypothyroidism. *International Journal of Clinical Practice* 68:857-863. PMID: 24548294

131. Vaya A, Gimenez C, Sarnago A et al. (2014) Subclinical hypothyroidism and cardiovascular risk. *Clinical Hemorheology and Microcirculation* 58:1-7. PMID: 25339098

132. Barnes B, Galton L (1976) *Hypothyroidism: The Unsuspected Illness.* New York, NY: Harper & Row

133. Kulacz R, Levy T (2014) *The Toxic Tooth: How a root canal could be making you sick.* Henderson, NV: MedFox Publishing

134. Levy T (2017) *Hidden Epidemic: Silent oral infections cause most heart attacks and breast cancers.* Henderson, NV: Medfox Publishing

135. Caplan D, Pankow J, Cai J et al. (2009) The relationship between self-reported history of endodontic therapy and coronary heart disease in the Atherosclerosis Risk in Communities Study. *Journal of the American Dental Association* 140:1004-1012. PMID: 19654253

136. Ott S, El Mokhtari N, Musfeldt M et al. (2006) Detection of diverse bacterial signatures in atherosclerotic lesions of patients with coronary heart disease. *Circulation* 113:929-937. PMID: 16490835

137. Ott S, El Mokhtari N, Rehman A et al. (2007) Fungal rDNA signatures in coronary atherosclerotic plaques. *Environmental Microbiology* 9:3035-3045. PMID: 17991032

138. Haraszthy V, Zambon J, Trevisan M et al. (2000) Identification of periodontal pathogens in atheromatous plaques. *Journal of Periodontology* 71:1554-1560. PMID: 11063387

139. Mattila K, Pussinen P, Paju S (2005) Dental infections and cardiovascular diseases: a review. *Journal of Periodontology* 76:2085-2088. PMID: 16277580

140. Mahendra J, Mahendra L, Kurian V et al. (2010) 16S rRNA-based detection of oral pathogens in coronary atherosclerotic plaque. *Indian Journal of Dental Research* 21:248-252. PMID: 20657096

141. Pessi T, Karhunen V, Karjalainen P et al. (2013) Bacterial signatures in thrombus aspirates of patients with myocardial infarction. *Circulation* 127:1219-1228. PMID: 23418311

142. Kabadi U (1986) Serum T3 and reverse T3 concentrations: indices of metabolic control in diabetes mellitus. *Diabetes Research* 3:417-421. PMID: 3816044

143. Lin H, Tang H, Leinung M et al. (2019) Action of reverse T3 on cancer cells. *Endocrine Research* Apr 3 [Epub ahead of print]. PMID: 30943372

144. Starr M (2009) *Hypothyroidism Type 2: The Epidemic.* Columbia, MO: Mark Starr Trust

145. Cicatiello A, Di Girolamo D, Dentice M (2018) Metabolic effects of the intracellular regulation of thyroid hormone: old players, new concepts. *Frontiers in Endocrinology* 9:474. PMID: 30254607

146. Schimmel M, Utiger R (1977) Thyroidal and peripheral production of thyroid hormones. Review of recent findings and their clinical implications. *Annals of Internal Medicine* 87:760-768. PMID: 412452

147. Bianco A, Kim B (2006) Deiodinases: implications of the local control of thyroid hormone action. *The Journal of Clinical Investigation* 116:2571-2579. PMID: 1701655o

148. Bianco A, da Conceicao R (2018) The deiodinase trio and thyroid hormone signaling. *Methods in Molecular Biology* 1801:67-83. PMID: 29892818

149. Cinar V (2007) The effects of magnesium supplementation on thyroid hormones of sedentars and Tae-Kwan-Do sportsperson at resting and exhaustion. *Neuro Endocrinology Letters* 28:708-712. PMID: 17984925

150. Ballard B, Torres L, Romani A (2008) Effect of thyroid hormone on Mg(2+) homeostasis and extrusion in cardiac cells. *Molecular and Cellular Biochemistry* 318:117-127. PMID: 18604605

151. Chincholikar S, Ambiger S (2018) Association of hypomagnesemia with hypocalcemia after thyroidectomy. *Indian Journal of Endocrinology and Metabolism* 22:656-660. PMID: 30294577

152. Ige A, Chidi R, Egbeluya E et al. (2019) Amelioration of thyroid dysfunction by magnesium in experimental diabetes may also prevent diabetes-induced renal impairment. *Heliyon* 5:e01660. PMID: 31193031

153. Wang K, Wei H, Zhang W et al., (2018) Severely low serum magnesium is associated with increased risks of positive anti-thyroglobulin antibody and hypothyroidism: a cross-sectional study. *Scientific Reports* 8:9904. PMID: 29967483

154. Zinman T, Shneyvays V, Tribulova N et al. (2006) Acute, nongenomic effect of thyroid hormones in preventing calcium overload in newborn rat cardiocytes. *Journal of Cellular Physiology* 207:220-231. PMID: 16331687

155. Gammage M, Franklyn J, Logan S (1987) Effects of amiodarone and thyroid dysfuction on myocardial calcium, serum calcium and thyroid hormones in the rat. *British Journal of Pharmacology* 92:363-370. PMID: 3676598

Chapter 16

1. Levy T. (2002) *Curing the Incurable. Vitamin C, Infectious Diseases, and Toxins.* Henderson, NV: MedFox Publishing

2. Klenner F (1971) Observations of the dose and administration of ascorbic acid when employed beyond the range of a vitamin in human pathology. *Journal of Applied Nutrition* 23:61-88.

3. Ayre S, Perez D, Perez, Jr. D (1986) Insulin potentiation therapy: a new concept in the management of chronic degenerative disease. *Medical Hypotheses* 20:199-210. PMID: 3526099

4. Damyanov C, Radoslavova M, Gavrilov V, Stoeva D (2009) Low dose chemotherapy in combination with insulin for the treatment of advanced metastatic tumors. Preliminary experience. *Journal of B.U.ON.* 14:711-715. PMID: 20148468

5. Qutob S, Dixon S, Wilson J (1998) Insulin stimulates vitamin C recycling and ascorbate accumulation in osteoblastic cells. *Endocrinology* 139:51-56. PMID: 9421397

6. Rumsey S, Daruwala R, Al-Hasani H et al. (2000) Dehydroascorbic acid transport by GLUT4 in Xenopus oocytes and isolated rat adipocytes. *The Journal of Biological Chemistry* 275:28246-28253. PMID: 10862609

7. Musselmann K, Kane B, Alexandrou B, Hassell J (2006) Stimulation of collagen synthesis by insulin and proteoglycan accumulation by ascorbate in bovine keratocytes *in vitro. Investigative Ophthalmology & Visual Science* 47:5260-5266. PMID: 17122111

8. Klenner F (1971) Observations of the dose and administration of ascorbic acid when employed beyond the range of a vitamin in human pathology. *Journal of Applied Nutrition* 23:61-88.

9. Marik P, Khangoora V, Rivera R et al. (2017) Hydrocortisone, vitamin C, and thiamine for the treatment of severe sepsis and septic shock: a retrospective before-after study. *Chest* 151:1229-1238. PMID: 27940189

10. Zabet M, Mohammadi M, Ramezani M, Khalili H (2016) Effect of high-dose ascorbic acid on vasopressor's requirement in septic shock. *Journal of Research in Pharmacy Practice* 5:94-100. PMID: 27162802

11. Cathcart R (1981) Vitamin C, titrating to bowel tolerance, anascorbemia, and acute induced scurvy. *Medical Hypotheses* 7:1359-1376. PMID: 7321921

12. Cathcart R (1985) Vitamin C: the nontoxic, nonrate-limited, antioxidant free radical scavenger. *Medical Hypotheses* 18:61-77. PMID: 4069036

13. Kurtz T, Morris, Jr. R (1983) Dietary chloride as a determinant of "sodium-dependent" hypertension. *Science* 222:1139-1141. PMID: 6648527

14. Kurtz T, Al-Bander H, Morris, Jr. R (1987) "Salt-sensitive" essential hypertension in men. Is the sodium ion alone important? *The New England Journal of Medicine* 317:1043-1048. PMID: 3309653

15. Pokorski M, Marczak M, Dymecka A, Suchocki P (2003) Ascorbyl palmitate as a carrier of ascorbate into neural tissues. *Journal of Biomedical Science* 10:193-198. PMID: 12595755

16. Pokorski M, Gonet B (2004) Capacity of ascorbyl palmitate to produce the ascorbyl radical *in vitro*: an electron spin resonance investigation. *Physiological Research* 53:311-316. PMID: 15209539

17. Pokorski M, Ramadan A, Marczak M (2004) Ascorbyl palmitate augments hypoxic respiratory response in the cat. *Journal of Biomedical Science* 11:465-471. PMID: 15153781

18. Ross D, Mendiratta S, Qu Z et al. (1999) Ascorbate 6-palmitate protects human erythrocytes from oxidative damage. *Free Radical Biology & Medicine* 26:81-89. PMID: 9890643

19. Loyd D, Lynch S (2011) Lipid-soluble vitamin C palmitate and protection of human high-density lipoprotein from hypochlorite-mediated oxidation. *International Journal of Cardiology* 152:256-257. PMID: 21872949

20. Gosenca M, Bester-Rogac M, Gasperlin M (2013) Lecithin based lamellar liquid crystals as a physiologically acceptable dermal delivery system for ascorbyl palmitate. *European Journal of Pharmaceutical Sciences* May 3. [Epub ahead of print]. PMID: 23643736

21. Sawant R, Vaze O, Wang T et al. (2012) Palmitoyl ascorbate liposomes and free ascorbic acid: comparison of anticancer therapeutic effects upon parenteral administration. *Pharmaceutical Research* 29:375-383. PMID: 21845505

22. Levy T. (2002) *Curing the Incurable. Vitamin C, Infectious Diseases, and Toxins.* Henderson, NV: MedFox Publishing

23. Simone II C, Simone N, Simone V, Simone C (2007) Antioxidants and other nutrients do not interfere with chemotherapy or radiation therapy and can increase kill and increase survival, part 1. *Alternative Therapies in Health and Medicine* 13:22-28. PMID: 17283738

24. Simone II C, Simone N, Simone V, Simone C (2007a) Antioxidants and other nutrients do not interfere with chemotherapy or radiation therapy and can increase kill and increase survival, part 2. *Alternative Therapies in Health and Medicine* 13:40-47. PMID: 17405678

25. Levy T. (2011) *Primal Panacea.* Henderson, NV: MedFox Publishing

26. Padayatty S, Sun A, Chen Q et al. (2010) Vitamin C: intravenous use by complementary and alternative medicine practitioners and adverse effects. *PLoS One* 5:e11414. PMID: 20628650

27. Curhan G, Willett W, Speizer F, Stampfer M (1999) Intake of vitamins B6 and C and the risk of kidney stones in women. *Journal of the American Society of Nephrology* 10:840-845. PMID: 10203369

28. Simon J, Hudes E (1999) Relation of serum ascorbic acid to serum vitamin B_{12}, serum ferritin, and kidney stones in US adults. *Archives of Internal Medicine* 159:619-624. PMID: 10090119

29. Curhan G, Willett W, Speizer F et al. (1997) Comparison of dietary calcium with supplemental calcium and other nutrients as factors affecting the risk for kidney stones in women. *Annals of Internal Medicine* 126:497-504. PMID: 9092314

30. Rawat A, Vaidya B, Khatri K et al. (2007) Targeted intracellular delivery of therapeutics: an overview. *Die Pharmazie* 62:643-658. PMID: 17944316

31. Yamada Y, Harashima H (2008) Mitochondrial drug delivery systems for macromolecule and their therapeutic application to mitochondrial diseases. *Advanced Drug Delivery Reviews* 60:1439-1462. PMID: 18655816

32. Goldenberg H, Schweinzer E (1994) Transport of vitamin C in animal and human cells. *Journal of Bioenergetics and Biomembranes* 26:359-367. PMID: 7844110

33. Liang W, Johnson D, Jarvis S (2001) Vitamin C transport systems of mammalian cells. *Molecular Membrane Biology* 18:87-95. PMID: 11396616

34. Welch R, Wang Y, Crossman, Jr. A (1995) Accumulation of vitamin C (ascorbate) and its oxidized metabolite dehydroascorbic acid occurs by separate mechanisms. *The Journal of Biological Chemistry* 270:12584-12592. PMID: 7759506

35. Ling S, Magosso E, Khan N et al. (2006) Enhanced oral bioavailability and intestinal lymphatic transport of a hydrophilic drug using liposomes. *Drug Development and Industrial Pharmacy* 32:335-345. PMID: 16556538

36. Lubin B, Shohet S, Nathan D (1972) Changes in fatty acid metabolism after erythrocyte peroxidation: stimulation of a membrane repair process. *The Journal of Clinical Investigation* 51:338-344. PMID: 5009118

37. Mastellone I, Polichetti E, Gres S et al., (2000) Dietary soybean phosphatidylcholines lower lipidemia: mechanisms at the levels of intestine, endothelial cell, and hepato-biliary axis. *The Journal of Nutritional Biochemistry* 11:461-466. PMID: 11091102

38. Buang Y, Wang Y, Cha J et al. (2005) Dietary phosphatidylcholine alleviates fatty liver induced by orotic acid. *Nutrition* 21:867-873. PMID: 15975496

39. Demirbile, S, Karaman A, Baykarabulut A et al. (2006) Polyenylphosphatidylcholine pretreatment ameliorates ischemic acute renal injury in rats. *International Journal of Urology* 13:747-753. PMID: 16834655

40. Levy T. (2002) *Curing the Incurable. Vitamin C, Infectious Diseases, and Toxins.* Henderson, NV: MedFox Publishing

41. Klenner F (1971) Observations of the dose and administration of ascorbic acid when employed beyond the range of a vitamin in human pathology. *Journal of Applied Nutrition* 23:61-88.

42. Lopez-Huertas E, Fonolla J (2017) Hydroxytyrosol supplementation increases vitamin C levels *in vivo*. A human volunteer trial. *Redox Biology* 11:384-389. PMID: 28063380

43. Grollman A, Lehninger A (1957) Enzymic synthesis of L-ascorbic acid in different animal species. *Archives of Biochemistry and Biophysics* 69:458-467. PMID: 13445217

44. Chatterjee I, Majumder A, Nandi B, Subramanian N (1975) Synthesis and some major functions of vitamin C in animals. *Annals of the New York Academy of Sciences* 258:24-47. PMID: 1106297

45. Nishikimi M, Koshizaka T, Ozawa T, Yagi K (1988) Occurrence in humans and guinea pigs of the gene related to their missing enzyme L-gulono-gamma-lactone oxidase. *Archives of Biochemistry and Biophysics* 267:842-846. PMID: 3214183

46. Adlard B, De Souza S, Moon S (1974) Ascorbic acid in fetal human brain. *Archives of Disease in Childhood* 49:278-282. PMID: 4830116

47. Salmenpera L (1984) Vitamin C nutrition during prolonged lactation: optimal in infants while marginal in some mothers. *The American Journal of Clinical Nutrition* 40:1050-1056. PMID: 6496385

48. Andersson M, Walker A, Falcke H (1956) An investigation of the rarity of infantile scurvy among the South African Bantu. *The British Journal of Nutrition* 10:101-105. PMID: 13315928

49. Kline A, Eheart M (1944) Variation in the ascorbic acid requirements for saturation of nine normal young women. *The Journal of Nutrition* 28:413-419.

50. Pijoan M, Lozner E (1944) Vitamin C economy in the human subject. *Bulletin of the Johns Hopkins Hospital* 75:303-314.

51. Williams R, Deason G (1967) Individuality in vitamin C needs. *Proceedings of the National Academy of Sciences of the United States of America* 57:1638-1641. PMID: 5231398

52. Odumosu A, Wilson C (1971) Metabolic availability of ascorbic acid in female guinea-pigs. *British Pharmacological Society* 42:637P-638P. PMID: 5116040

53. Odumosu A, Wilson C (1973) Metabolic availability of vitamin C in the guinea-pig. *Nature* 242:519-521. PMID: 4550033

54. Cummings M (1981) Can some people synthesize ascorbic acid? *The American Journal of Clinical Nutrition* 34:297-298. PMID: 7211730

55. Odumosu A, Wilson C (1970) The relationship between ascorbic acid concentrations and cortisol production during the development of scurvy in the guinea-pig. *British Journal of Pharmacology* 40:548P-549P. PMID: 5497811

56. Ginter E (1976) Ascorbic acid synthesis in certain guinea pigs. *International Journal for Vitamin and Nutrition Research* 46:173-179. PMID: 1032629

57. Benhabiles H, Gonzalez-Hilarion S, Amand S et al. (2017) Optimized approach for the identification of highly efficient correctors of nonsense mutations in human diseases. *PLoS One* 12:e0187930. PMID: 29131862

58. Linde L, Kerem B (2008) Introducing sense into nonsense in treatments of human genetic diseases. *Trends in Genetics* 24:552-563. PMID: 18937996

59. Perez B, Rodriguez-Pombo P, Ugarte M, Desviat L (2012) Readthrough strategies for therapeutic suppression of nonsense mutations in inherited metabolic disease. *Molecular Syndromology* 3:230-236. PMID: 23293581

60. Karijolich J, Yu Y (2014) Therapeutic suppression of premature termination codons: mechanisms and clinical considerations (review). *International Journal of Molecular Medicine* 34:355-362. PMID: 24939317

61. Keeling K, Xue X, Gunn G, Bedwell D (2014) Therapeutics based on stop codon readthrough. *Annual Review of Genomics and Human Genetics* 15:371-394. PMID: 24773318

62. Lee H, Dougherty J (2012) Pharmaceutical therapies to recode nonsense mutations in inherited diseases. *Pharmacology & Therapeutics* 136:227-266. PMID: 22820013

63. Baradaran-Heravi A, Balgi A, Zimmerman C et al. (2016) Novel small molecules potentiate premature termination codon read-through by aminoglycosides. *Nucleic Acids Research* 44:6583-6598. PMID: 27407112

64. Bidou L, Allamand V, Rousset J, Namy O (2012) Sense from nonsense: therapies for premature stop codon diseases. *Trends in Molecular Medicine* 18:679-688. PMID: 23083810

65. Fibach E, Prus E, Bianchi N et al. (2012) Resveratrol: antioxidant activity and induction of fetal hemoglobin in erythroid cells from normal donors and β-thalassemia patients. *International Journal of Molecular Medicine* 29:974-982. PMID: 22378234

66. Chowdhury et al. (2017) *International Journal of Advanced Research* 5:1816-1821.

67. Bianchi N, Zuccato C, Lampronti I et al. (2009) Fetal hemoglobin inducers from the natural world: a novel approach for identification of drugs for the treatment of {beta}-thalassemia and sickle-cell anemia. *Evidence-based Complementary and Alternative Medicine* 6:141-151. PMID: 18955291

Chapter 17

1. Wilson T, Datta S, Murrell J, Andrews C (1973) Relation of vitamin C levels to mortality in a geriatric hospital: a study of the effect of vitamin C administration. *Age and Ageing* 2:163-171. PMID: 4591257

2. Sahyoun N, Jacques P, Russell R (1996) Carotenoids, vitamins C and E, and mortality in an elderly population. *American Journal of Epidemiology* 144:501-511. PMID: 8781466

3. Khaw K, Bingham S, Welch A et al. (2001) Relation between plasma ascorbic acid and mortality in men and women in EPIC-Norfolk prospective study: a prospective population study. European Prospective Investigation into Cancer and Nutrition. *Lancet* 357:657-663. PMID: 11247548

4. Sotomayor C, Eisenga M, Gomes Neto A et al. (2017) Vitamin D depletion and all-cause mortality in renal transplant recipients. *Nutrients* 9. PMID: 28574431

5. Aune D, Keum N, Giovannucci E et al. (2018) Dietary intake and blood concentrations of antioxidants and the risk of cardiovascular disease, total cancer, and all-cause mortality: a systematic review and dose-response meta-analysis of prospective studies. *The American Journal of Clinical Nutrition* 108:1069-1091. PMID: 30475962

6. Huang Y, Wahlqvist M, Kao M et al. (2015) Optimal dietary and plasma magnesium statuses depend on dietary quality for a reduction in the risk of all-cause mortality in older adults. *Nutrients* 7:5664-5683. PMID: 26184299

7. Melamed M, Michos E, Post W, Astor B (2008) 25-hydroxyvitamin D levels and the risk of mortality in the general population. *Archives of Internal Medicine* 168:1629-1637. PMID: 18695076

8. Ginde A, Scragg R, Schwartz R, Camargo Jr. C (2009) Prospective study of serum 25-hydroxyvitamin D level, cardiovascular disease mortality, and all-cause mortality in older U.S. adults. *Journal of the American Geriatrics Society* 57:1595-1603. PMID: 19549021

9. Hutchinson M, Grimnes G, Joakimsen R et al. (2010) Low serum 25-hydroxyvitamin D levels are associated with increased all-cause mortality risk in a general population: the Tromso study. *European Journal of Endocrinology* 162:935-942. PMID: 20185562

10. Semba R, Houston D, Bandinelli S et al. (2010) Relationship of 25-hydroxyvitamin D with all-cause and cardiovascular disease mortality in older community-dwelling adults. *European Journal of Clinical Nutrition* 64:203-209. PMID: 19953106

11. Saliba W, Barnett O, Rennert H, Rennert G (2012) The risk of all-cause mortality is inversely related to serum 25(OH)D levels. *The Journal of Clinical Endocrinology and Metabolism* 97:2792-2798. PMID: 22648653

12. Schierbeck L, Rejnmark L, Tofteng C et al. (2012) Vitamin D deficiency in postmenopausal, healthy women predicts increased cardiovascular events: a 16-year follow-up study. *European Journal of Endocrinology* 167:553-560. PMID: 22875588

13. Thomas G, o Hartaigh B, Bosch J et al. (2012) Vitamin D levels predict all-cause and cardiovascular disease mortality in subjects with the metabolic syndrome: the Ludwigshafen Risk and Cardiovascular Health (LURIC) Study. *Diabetes Care* 35:1158-1164. PMID: 22399697

14. Schottker B, Haug U, Schomburg L et al. (2013) Strong associations of 25-hydroxyvitamin D concentrations with all-cause, cardiovascular, cancer, and respiratory disease mortality in a large cohort study. *The American Journal of Clinical Nutrition* 97:782-793. PMID: 23446902

15. Heath A, Kim I, Hodge A et al. (2019) Vitamin D status and mortality: a systemic review of observational studies. *International Journal of Environmental Research and Public Health* Jan 29; 16. PMID: 30700025

16. Burgi A, Gorham E, Garland C et al. (2011) High serum 25-hydroxyvitamin D is associated with a low incidence of stress fractures. *Journal of Bone and Mineral Research* 26:2371-2377. PMID: 21698667

17. Geleijnse J, Vermeer C, Grobbee D et al. (2004) Dietary intake of menaquinone is associated with a reduced risk of coronary heart disease: the Rotterdam Study. *The Journal of Nutrition* 134:3100-3105. PMID: 15514282

18. Juanola-Falgarona M, Salas-Salvado J, Martinez-Gonzalez M et al. (2014) Dietary intake of vitamin K is inversely associated with mortality risk. *The Journal of Nutrition* 144:743-750. PMID: 24647393

19. Einvik G, Klemsdal T, Sandvik L, Hjerkinn E (2010) A randomized clinical trial on n-3 polyunsaturated fatty acids supplementation and all-cause mortality in elderly men at high cardiovascular risk. *European Journal of Cardiovascular Prevention and Rehabilitation* 17:588-592. PMID: 20389249

20. Poole C, Halcox J, Jenkins-Jones S et al. (2013) Omega-3 fatty acids and mortality outcome in patients with and without type 2 diabetes after myocardial infarction: a retrospective, matched-cohort study. *Clinical Therapeutics* 35:40-51. PMID: 23246017

21. Lelli D, Antonelli Incalzi R, Ferrucci L et al. (2019) Association between PUFA intake and serum concentration and mortality in older adults: a cohort study. *Clinical Nutrition* Feb 23 [Epub ahead of print]. PMID: 30850268

22. Sen C, Khanna S, Roy S (2006) Tocotrienols: vitamin E beyond tocopherols. *Life Sciences* 78:2088-2098. PMID: 16458936

23. Lee G, Han S (2018) The role of vitamin E in immunity. *Nutrients* 10. PMID: 30388871

24. Pauling L (1991) Case report: lysine/ascorbate-related amelioration of angina pectoris. *Journal of Orthomolecular Medicine* 6:144-146.

25. Pauling L (1993) Third case report on lysine-ascorbate amelioration of angina pectoris. *Journal of Orthomolecular Medicine* 8:137-138.

26. Ivanov V, Roomi M, Kalinovsky et al. (2007) Anti-atherogenic effects of a mixture of ascorbic acid, lysine, proline, arginine, cysteine, and green tea phenolics in human aortic smooth muscle cells. *Journal of Cardiovascular Pharmacology* 49:140-145. PMID: 17414225

27. Rauf A, Imran M, Suleria H et al. (2017) A comprehensive review of the health perspectives of resveratrol. *Food & Function* 8:4284-4305. PMID: 29044265

28. Lopez-Huertas E, Fonolla J (2017) Hydroxytyrosol supplementation increases vitamin C levels *in vivo*. A human volunteer trial. *Redox Biology* 11:384-389. PMID: 28063380

29. Moeller S, Voland R, Tinker L et al. (2008) Associations between age-related nuclear cataract and lutein and zeaxanthin in the diet and serum in the Carotenoids in the Age-Related Eye Disease Study, an ancillary study of the Women's Health Initiative. *Archives of Ophthalmology* 126:354-364. PMID: 18332316

30. Christen W, Liu S, Glynn R et al. (2008) Dietary carotenoids, vitamins C and E, and risk of cataract in women: a prospective study. *Archives of Ophthalmology* 126:102-109. PMID: 18195226

Chapter 18

1. Kiberd B, Tennankore K, Daley C (2015) Increases in intravenous magnesium use among hospitalized patients: an institution cross-sectional experience. *Canadian Journal of Kidney Health and Disease* 2:24. PMID: 26106483

2. Cisaro F, Andrealli A, Calvo P et al. (2018) Bowel preparation for gastrointestinal endoscopic procedures with sodium picosulphate-magnesium citrate is an effective, safe, and well-tolerated option in pediatric patients: a single-center experience. *Gastroenterology Nursing* 41:312-315. PMID: 30063687

3. Tsuji S, Horiuchi A, Tamaki M et al. (2018) Effectiveness and safety of a new regimen of polyethylene glycol plus ascorbic acid for same-day bowel cleansing in constipated patients. *Acta Gastro-Enterologica Belgica* 81:485-489. PMID: 30645916

4. Abdoli A, Rahimi-Bashar F, Torabian S et al. (2019) Efficacy of simultaneous administration of nimodipine, progesterone, and magnesium sulfate in patients with severe traumatic brain injury: a randomized controlled trial. *Bulletin of Emergency and Trauma* 7:124-129. PMID: 31198800

5. Du L, Wenning L, Carvalho B et al. (2019) Alternative magnesium sulfate dosing regimens for women with preeclampsia: a population pharmacokinetic exposure-response modeling and simulation study. *Journal of Clinical Pharmacology* Jun 3. [Epub ahead of print]. PMID: 31157410

6. Soliman R, Abukhudair W (2019) The perioperative effect of magnesium sulfate in patients with concentric left ventricular hypertrophy undergoing cardiac surgery: a double-blinded randomized study. *Annals of Cardiac Anaesthesia* 22:246-253. PMID: 31274484

7. Uysal N, Kizildag S, Yuce Z et al. (2019) Timeline (bioavailability) of magnesium compounds in hours: which magnesium compound works best? *Biological Trace Element Research* 187:128-136. PMID: 29679349

8. Coudray C, Rambeau M, Feillet-Coudray et al. (2005) Study of magnesium bioavailability from ten organic and inorganic Mg salts in Mg-depleted rats using a stable isotope approach. *Magnesium Research* 18:215-223. PMID: 16548135

9. Neveu A (1961) *Le Chlorure de Magnesium Dans L'Elevage: Traitment Cytophylactique des Maladies Infectieuses.* Librairie Le Francois: Paris, France

10. Rodale J (with Taub H) (1968) *Magnesium, the Nutrient that could Change Your Life.* Pyramid Publications, Inc: New York, NY

11. Rapp F, Butel J, Wallis C (1965) Protection of measles virus by sulfate ions against thermal inactivation. *Journal of Bacteriology* 90:132-135. PMID: 16562007

12. Vink R (2016) Magnesium in the CNS: recent advances and developments. *Magnesium Research* 29:95-101. PMID: 27829572

13. Levy T (2004) *Curing the Incurable. Vitamin C, Infectious Diseases, and Toxins.* Henderson, NV: MedFox Publishing

14. Beyerbach K (1990) Transport of magnesium across biological membranes. *Magnesium and Trace Elements* 9:233-254. PMID: 2130822

15. Deason-Towne F, Perraud A, Schmitz C (2011) The Mg2+ transporter MagT1 partially rescues cell growth and Mg2+ uptake in cells lacking the channel-kinase TRPM7. *FEBS Letters* 585:2275-2278. PMID: 21627970

16. de Baaij J, Hoenderop J, Bindels R (2012) Regulation of magnesium balance: lessons learned from human genetic disease. *Clinical Kidney Journal* 5:i15-i24. PMID: 26069817

17. Mittermeier L, Demirkhanyan L, Stadlbauer B et al. (2019) TRPM7 is the central gatekeeper of intestinal mineral absorption essential for postnatal survival. *Proceedings of the National Academy of Sciences of the United States of America* Feb 15 [Epub ahead of print]. PMID: 30770447

18. Biesenbach P, Martensson J, Osawa E et al. (2018) Magnesium supplementation: pharmacokinetics in cardiac surgery patients with normal renal function. *Journal of Critical Care* 44:419-423. PMID: 29353118

19. McKeown A, Seppi V, Hodgson R (2017) Intravenous magnesium sulphate for analgesia after caesarean section: a systematic review. *Anesthesiology Research and Practice* 2017:9186374. PMID: 29333156

20. Shah T, Rubenstein A, Kosik E et al. (2018) Parturient on magnesium infusion and its effectiveness as an adjuvant analgesic after cesarean delivery: a retrospective analysis. *TheScientificWorldJournal* 2018:3978760. PMID: 30581373

21. Chiu H, Yeh T, Huang Y, Chen P (2016) Effects of intravenous and oral magnesium on reducing migraine: a meta-analysis of randomized controlled trials. *Pain Physician* 19:E97-E112. PMID: 26752497

22. Griffiths B, Kew K (2016) Intravenous magnesium sulfate for treating children with acute asthma in the emergency department. *The Cochrane Database of Systematic Reviews* 4:CD011050. PMID: 27126744

23. Jarahzadeh M, Harati S, Babaeizadeh H et al. (2016) The effect of magnesium sulfate infusion on reduction of pain after abdominal hysterectomy under general anesthesia: a double-blind, randomized clinical trial. *Electronic Physician* 8:2602-2606. PMID: 27648185

24. Mijalski C, Dakay K, Miller-Patterson C et al. (2016) Magnesium for treatment of reversible cerebral vasoconstriction syndrome: case series. *The Neurohospitalist* 6:111-113. PMID: 27366294

25. Brousseau D, Scott J, Badaki-Makun O et al. (2015) A multicenter randomized controlled trial of intravenous magnesium for sickle cell pain crisis in children. *Blood* 126:1651-1657. PMID: 26232172

26. Firouzi A, Maadani M, Kiani R et al. (2015) Intravenous magnesium sulfate: new method in prevention of contrast-induced nephropathy in primary percutaneous coronary intervention. *International Urology and Nephrology* 47:521-525. PMID: 25475196

27. Jacquemyn Y, Zecic A, Van Laere D, Roelens K (2015) The use of intravenous magnesium in non-preeclamptic pregnant women: fetal/neonatal neuroprotection. *Archives of Gynecology and Obstetrics* 291:969-975. PMID: 25501980

28. Solooki M, Miri M, Mokhtari M et al. (2014) Magnesium sulfate in exacerbations of COPD in patients admitted to internal medicine ward. *Iran Journal of Pharmaceutical Research* 13:1235-1239. PMID: 25587312

29. Mukerji S, Shahpuri B, Clayton-Smith B et al. (2015) Intravenous magnesium sulphate as an adjuvant therapy in acute exacerbations of chronic obstructive pulmonary disease: a single centre, randomized, double-blinded, parallel group, placebo-controlled trial: a pilot study. *The New Zealand Medical Journal* 128:34-42. PMID: 26905985

30. Gertsch E, Loharuka S, Wolter-Warmerdam K et al. (2014) Intravenous magnesium as acute treatment for headaches: a pediatric case series. *The Journal of Emergency Medicine* 46:308-312. PMID: 24182946

31. Marzban S, Haddadi S, Naghipour M et al. (2014) The effect of intravenous magnesium sulfate on laryngospasm after elective adenotonsillectomy surgery in children. *Anesthesiology and Pain Medicine* 4:e15960. PMID: 24660159

32. Albrecht E, Kirkham K, Liu S, Brull R (2013) Peri-operative intravenous administration of magnesium sulphate and postoperative pain: a meta-analysis. *Anaesthesia* 68:79-90. PMID: 23121612

33. Murphy J, Paskaradevan J, Eisler L et al. (2013) Analgesic efficacy of continuous intravenous magnesium infusion as an adjuvant to morphine for postoperative analgesia: a systematic review and meta-analysis. *Middle East Journal of Anaesthesiology* 22:11-20. PMID: 23833845

34. Yarad E, Hammond N (2013) Intravenous magnesium therapy in adult patients with an aneurysmal subarachnoid haemorrhage: a systematic review and meta-analysis.

35. Chowdhury J, Chaudhuri S, Bhattacharyya N et al. (2009) Comparison of intramuscular magnesium sulfate with low dose intravenous magnesium sulfate regimen for treatment of eclampsia. *The Journal of Gynaecological Research* 35:119-125. PMID: 19215558

36. Bhattacharjee N, Saha S, Ganguly R et al. (2011) A randomized comparative study between low-dose intravenous magnesium sulphate and standard intramuscular regimen for treatment of eclampsia. *Journal of Obstetrics and Gynaecology* 31:298-303. PMID: 21534749

37. Kidwell C, Lees K, Muir K et al. (2009) Results of the MRI substudy of the intravenous magnesium efficacy in stroke trial. *Stroke* 40:1704-1709. PMID: 19299636

38. Puliyel M, Pillai R, Korula S (2009) Intravenous magnesium sulphate infusion in the management of very severe tetanus in a child: a descriptive case report. *Journal of Tropical Pediatrics* 55:58-59. PMID: 18701521

39. Simpson J, Maxwell D, Rosenthal E, Gill H (2009) Fetal ventricular tachycardia secondary to long QT syndrome treated with maternal intravenous magnesium: case report and review of the literature. *Ultrasound in Obstetrics & Gynecology* 34:475-480. PMID: 19731233

40. Brill S, Sedgwick P, Hamann W, Di Vadi P (2002) Efficacy of intravenous magnesium in neuropathic pain. *British Journal of Anaesthesia* 89:711-714. PMID: 12393768

41. Heiden A, Frey R, Presslich O et al. (1999) Treatment of severe mania with intravenous magnesium sulphate as a supplementary therapy. *Psychiatry Research* 89:239-246. PMID: 10708270

42. Maggioni A, Orzalesi M, Mimouni F (1998) Intravenous correction of neonatal hypomagnesemia: effect on ionized magnesium. *The Journal of Pediatrics* 132:652-655. PMID: 9580765

43. Raimondi F, Migliaro F, Capasso L et al. (2008) Intravenous magnesium sulphate vs. inhaled nitric oxide for moderate, persistent pulmonary hypertension of the newborn. A multicenter, retrospective study. *Journal of Tropical Pediatrics* 54:196-199. PMID: 18048460

44. Huycke M, Naguib M, Stroemmel M et al. (2000) A double-blind placebo-controlled crossover trial of intravenous magnesium sulfate for foscarnet-induced ionized hypocalcemia and hypomagnesemia in patients with AIDS and cytomegalovirus infection. *Antimicrobial Agents and Chemotherapy* 44:2143-2148. PMID: 10898688

45. Schanler R, Smith Jr L, Burns P (1997) Effects of long-term maternal intravenous magnesium sulfate therapy on neonatal calcium metabolism and bone mineral content. *Gynecologic and Obstetric Investigation* 43:236-241. PMID: 9194621

46. Mauskop A, Altura BT, Cracco R, Altura BM (1995) Intravenous magnesium sulfate relieves cluster headaches in patients with low serum ionized magnesium levels. *Headache* 35:597-600. PMID: 8550360

47. Cox R, Osgood K (1994) Evaluation of intravenous magnesium sulfate for the treatment of hydrofluoric acid burns. *Journal of Toxicology. Clinical Toxicology* 32:123-136. PMID: 8145352

48. Kagawa T, Goto R, Iijima K et al. (1994) Intravenous magnesium sulfate as a preanesthetic medication: a double-blind study on its effects on hemodynamic stabilization at the time of tracheal intubation. *Journal of Anesthesia* 8:17-20. PMID: 28921191

49. Woods K, Fletcher S (1994) Long-term outcome after intravenous magnesium sulphate in suspected acute myocardial infarction: the second Leicester Intravenous Magnesium Intervention Trial (LIMIT-2). *Lancet* 343:816-819. PMID: 7908076

50. Gullestad L, Birkeland K, Molstad P et al. (1993) The effect of magnesium versus verapamil on supraventricular arrhythmias. *Clinical Cardiology* 16:429-434. PMID: 8504578

51. Kraus F (1993) Reversal of diastolic dysfunction by intravenous magnesium chloride. *The Canadian Journal of Cardiology* 9:618-620. PMID: 8221360

52. McNamara R, Spivey W, Skobeloff E, Jacubowitz S (1989) Intravenous magnesium sulfate in the management of acute respiratory failure complicating asthma. *Annals of Emergency Medicine* 18:197-199. PMID: 2916786

53. Rajala B, Abbasi R, Hutchinson H, Taylor T (1987) Acute pancreatitis and primary hyperparathyroidism in pregnancy: treatment of hypercalcemia with magnesium sulfate. *Obstetrics and Gynecology* 70:460-462. PMID: 3627603

54. Reisdorff E, Clark M, Walters B (1986) Acute digitalis poisoning: the role of intravenous magnesium sulfate. *The Journal of Emergency Medicine* 4:463-469. PMID: 3549866

55. Woods K, Fletcher S, Roffe C, Haider Y (1992) Intravenous magnesium sulphate in suspected acute myocardial infarction: results of the second Leicester Intravenous Magnesium Intervention Trial (LIMIT-2). *Lancet* 339:1553-1558. PMID: 1351547

56. Woods K, Fletcher S (1994) Long-term outcome after intravenous magnesium sulphate in suspected acute myocardial infarction: the second Leicester Intravenous Magnesium Intervention Trial (LIMIT-2). *Lancet* 343:816-819. PMID: 7908076

57. Shechter M, Hod H, Rabinowitz B et al. (2003) Long-term outcome of intravenous magnesium therapy in thrombolysis-ineligible acute myocardial infarction patients. *Cardiology* 99:205-210. PMID: 12845247

58. Saha P, Kaur J, Goel P et al. (2017) Safety and efficacy of low dose intramuscular magnesium sulphate (MgSO4) compared to intravenous regimen for treatment of eclampsia. *The Journal of Obstetrics and Gynaecology Research* 43:1543-1549. PMID: 28714170

59. Manarot M, Tongsong T, Khettglang T (1996) A comparison of serum magnesium sulfate levels in pregnant women with severe preeclampsia between intravenous and intramuscular magnesium sulfate regimens: a randomized controlled trial. *Journal of the Medical Association of Thailand* 79:76-82. PMID: 8868017

60. Pungavkar S (2014) Magnesium deposition in brain of pregnant patients administered intramuscular magnesium sulphate. *Magnetic Resonance Imaging* 32:241-244. PMID: 24418328

61. Al Hanbali O, Khan H, Sarfraz M et al. (2019) Transdermal patches: design and current approaches to painless drug delivery. *Acta Pharmaceutica* 69:197-215. PMID: 31259729

62. Benson H, Grice J, Mohammed Y et al. (2019) Topical and transdermal drug delivery: from simple potions to smart technologies. *Current Drug Delivery* 16:444-460. PMID: 30714524

63. Duscher D, Trotsyuk A, Maan Z et al. (2019) Optimization of transdermal deferoxiamine leads to enhanced efficacy in healing skin wounds. *Journal of Controlled Release* Jul 9. [Epub ahead of print]. PMID: 31299261

64. Heenatigala Palliyage G, Singh S, Ashby Jr C et al. (2019) Pharmaceutical topical delivery of poorly soluble polyphenols: potential role in prevention and treatment of melanoma. *AAPS PharmSciTech* 20:250. PMID: 31297635

65. Grober U, Werner T, Vormann J, Kisters K (2017) Myth or reality—transdermal magnesium? *Nutrients* 9:813. PMID: 28788060

66. Kass L, Rosanoff A, Tanner A et al. (2017) Effect of transdermal magnesium cream on serum and urinary magnesium levels in humans: a pilot study. *PLoS One* 12:e0174817. PMID: 28403154

67. Engen D, McAllister S, Whipple M et al. (2015) Effects of transdermal magnesium chloride on quality of life for patients with fibromyalgia: a feasibility study. *Journal of Integrative Medicine* 13:306-313. PMID: 26343101

68. Martin A, Finlay W (2015) Nebulizers for drug delivery to the lungs. *Expert Opinion on Drug Delivery* 12:889-900. PMID: 25534396

69. Stein S, Thiel C (2017) The history of therapeutic aerosols: a chronological review. *Journal of Aerosol Medicine and Pulmonary Drug Delivery* 30:20-41. PMID: 27748638

70. Blitz M, Blitz S, Hughes R et al. (2005) Aerosolized magnesium sulfate for acute asthma: a systematic review. *Chest* 128:337-344. PMID: 16002955

71. Modaresi M, Faghihinia J, Kelishadi R et al. (2015) Nebulized magnesium sulfate in acute bronchiolitis: a randomized controlled trial. *Indian Journal of Pediatrics* 82:794-798. PMID: 25731897

72. Comert S, Kiyan E, Okumus G et al. (2016) [Efficiency of nebulised magnesium sulphate in infective exacerbations of chronic obstructive pulmonary disease]. Article in Turkish. *Tuberkuloz ve Toraks* 64:17-26. PMID: 27266281

73. Yadav M, Chalumuru N, Gopinath R (2016) Effect of magnesium sulfate nebulization on the incidence of postoperative sore throat. *Journal of Anaesthesiology, Clinical Pharmacology* 32:168-171. PMID: 27275043

74. Mangat H, D'Souza G, Jacob M (1998) Nebulized magnesium sulphate versus nebulized salbutamol in acute bronchial asthma: a clinical trial. *The European Respiratory Journal* 12:341-344. PMID: 9727782

75. Sun Y, Gong C, Liu S et al. (2014) Effect of inhaled MgSO4 on FEV 1 and PEF in children with asthma induced by acetylcholine: a randomized controlled clinical trial of 330 cases. *Journal of Tropical Pediatrics* 60:141-147. PMID: 24343824

76. Ling Z, Wu Y, Kong J et al. (2016) Lack of efficacy of nebulized magnesium sulfate in treating adult asthma: a meta-analysis of randomized controlled trials. *Pulmonary Pharmacology & Therapeutics* 41:40-47. PMID: 27651324

77. Daengsuwan T, Watanatham S (2017) A comparative pilot study of the efficacy and safety of nebulized magnesium sulfate and intravenous magnesium sulfate in children with severe acute asthma. *Asian Pacific Journal of Allergy and Immunology* 35:108-112. PMID: 27996280

78. Shirk M, Donahue K, Shirvani J (2006) Unlabeled uses of nebulized medications. *American Journal of Health-System Pharmacy* 63:1704-1716. PMID: 16960254

79. Fleming D, Rumbaugh K (2018) The consequences of biofilm dispersal on the host. *Scientific Reports* 8:10738. PMID: 3001312

80. Olmedo G, Grillo-Puertas M, Cerioni L et al. (2015) Removal of pathogenic bacterial biofilms by combinations of oxidizing compounds. *Canadian Journal of Microbiology* 61:351-356. PMID: 25864510

81. Yahya M, Alias Z, Karsani S (2018) Antibiofilm activity and mode of action of DMSO alone and its combination with afatinib against Gram-negative pathogens. *Folia Microbiologica* 63:23-30. PMID: 28540585

82. Onishi S, Yoshino S (2006) Cathartic-induced fatal hypermagnesemia in the elderly. *Internal Medicine* 45:207-210. PMID: 16543690

83. Chen I, Huang H, Yang S et al. (2014) Prevalence and effectiveness of laxative use among elderly residents in a regional hospital affiliated nursing home in Hsinchu county. *Nursing and Midwifery Studies* 3:e13962. PMID: 25414891

84. Yamaguchi H, Shimada H, Yoshita K et al. (2019) Severe hypermagnesemia induced by magnesium oxide ingestion: a case series. *CEN Case Reports* 8:31-37. PMID: 30136128

85. Jones J, Heiselman D, Dougherty J, Eddy A (1986) Cathartic-induced magnesium toxicity during overdose management. *Annals of Emergency Medicine* 15:1214-1218. PMID: 3752654

86. Woodard J, Shannon M, Lacouture P, Woolf A (1990) Serum magnesium concentrations after repetitive magnesium cathartic administration. *The American Journal of Emergency Medicine* 8:297-300. PMID: 2194467

87. Kutsal E, Aydemir C, Eldes N et al. (2007) Severe hypermagnesemia as a result of excessive cathartic ingestion in a child without renal failure. *Pediatric Emergency Care* 23:570-572. PMID: 17726419

88. Collins E, Russell P (1949) Fatal magnesium poisoning following magnesium sulfate, glycerin, and water enema in primary megacolon. *Cleveland Clinic Quarterly* 16:162-166. PMID: 18132462

89. Vissers R, Purssell R (1996) Iatrogenic magnesium overdose: two case reports. *The Journal of Emergency Medicine* 14:187-191. PMID: 8740750

90. Digre K, Varner M, Schiffman J (1990) Neuroophthalmologic effects of intravenous magnesium sulfate. *American Journal of Obstetrics and Gynecology* 163:1848-1852. PMID: 2256494

91. Saris N, Mervaala E, Karppanen H et al. (2000) Magnesium. An update on physiological, clinical and analytical aspects. *Clinica Chimica Acta* 294:1-26. PMID: 10727669

92. Crozier T, Radke J, Weyland A et al. (1991) Haemodynamic and endocrine effects of deliberate hypotension with magnesium sulphate for cerebral-aneurysm surgery. *European Journal of Anaesthesiology* 8:115-121. PMID: 1874207

93. Jangra K, Malhotra S, Gupta A, Arora S (2016) Comparison of quality of the surgical field after controlled hypotension using esmolol and magnesium sulfate during endoscopic sinus surgery. *Journal of Anaesthesiology, Clinical Pharmacology* 32:325-328. PMID: 27625479

94. Modanlou Juibari H, Eftekharian H, Arabion H (2016) Intravenous magnesium sulfate to deliberate hypotension and bleeding after bimaxillary orthognathic surgery: a randomized double-blind controlled trial. *Journal of Dentistry* 17:276-282. PMID: 27840841

95. Hassan P, Saleh A (2017) Dexmedetomidine versus magnesium sulfate in anesthesia for cochlear implantation surgery in pediatric patients. *Anesthesia, Essays and Researches* 11:1064-1069. PMID: 29284876

96. Modir H, Modir A, Rezaei O, Mohammadbeigl A (2018) Comparing remifentanil, magnesium sulfate, and dexmedetomidine for intraoperative hypotension and bleeding and postoperative recovery in endoscopic sinus surgery and tympanomastoidectomy. *Medical Gas Research* 8:42-47. PMID: 30112164

97. Hamed M (2018) Comparative study between magnesium sulfate and lidocaine for controlled hypotension during functional endoscopic sinus surgery: a randomized controlled study. *Anesthesia, Essays and Researches* 12:715-718. PMID: 30283182

98. Bain E, Middleton P, Crowther C (2013) Maternal adverse effects of different antenatal magnesium sulphate regimens for improving maternal and infant outcomes: a systematic review. *BMC Pregnancy and Childbirth* 13:195. PMID: 24139447

99. Workinger J, Doyle R, Bortz J (2018) Challenges in the diagnosis of magnesium status. *Nutrients* 10:1202. PMID: 30200431

100. Nielsen F (2016) Guidance for the determination of status indicators and dietary requirements for magnesium. *Magnesium Research* 29:154-160. PMID: 28132953

101. Costello R, Elin R, Rosanoff A et al. (2016) Perspective: the case for an evidence-based reference interval for serum magnesium: the time has come. *Advances in Nutrition* 7:977-993. PMID: 28140318

102. Costello R, Nielsen F (2017) Interpreting magnesium status to enhance clinical care—key indicators. *Current Opinion in Clinical Nutrition and Metabolic Care* 20:504-511. PMID: 28806179

103. Sein H, Whye Lian C, Juan Loong K et al. (2014) Relationship between intracellular magnesium level, lung function, and level of asthma control in children with chronic bronchial asthma. *The Malaysian Journal of Medical Sciences* 21:30-36. PMID: 25977631

104. Elin R, Hosseini J (1985) Magnesium content of mononuclear blood cells. *Clinical Chemistry* 31:377-380. PMID: 3971556

105. Elin R (1987) Status of the mononuclear blood cell magnesium assay. *Journal of the American College of Nutrition* 6:105-107. PMID: 3584730

106. Reinhart R, Marx Jr J, Haas R, Desbiens N (1987) Intracellular magnesium of mononuclear cells from venous blood of clinically healthy subjects. *Clinica Chimica Acta* 167:187-195. PMID: 3665095

107. DiNicolantonio J, O'Keefe J, Wilson W (2018) Subclinical magnesium deficiency: a principal driver of cardiovascular disease and a public health crisis. *Open Heart* 5:e000668. PMID: 29387426

108. Lim P, Jacob E, Dong S, Khoo O (1969) Values for tissue magnesium as a guide in detecting magnesium deficiency. *Journal of Clinical Pathology* 22:417-421. PMID: 5798629

109. Frost L, Danielsen H, Dorup I et al. (1993) Skeletal muscle magnesium content during cyclosporin and azathioprine treatment in renal transplant recipients. *Nephrology, Dialysis, Transplantation* 8:79-83. PMID: 8381943

110. Haigney M, Silver B, Tanglao E et al. (1995) Noninvasive measurement of tissue magnesium and correlation with cardiac levels. *Circulation* 92:2190-2197. PMID: 7554201

111. Haigney M, Berger R, Schulman S et al. (1997) Tissue magnesium levels and the arrhythmic substrate in humans. *Journal of Cardiovascular Electrophysiology* 8:980-986. PMID: 9300294

112. Haigney M, Wei S, Kaab S et al. (1998) Loss of cardiac magnesium in experimental heart failure prolongs and destabilizes repolarization in dogs. *Journal of the American College of Cardiology* 31:701-706. PMID: 9502656

Index